PRAISE
TRANSFORMATIONAL HEALING

"Don Juan (Carlos Castaneda) teaches us that a new awareness can be as subtle as the wings of a moth. Jamie L. Saloff teaches us that awareness can be as joyous or heartbreaking as a 'Body Song.' After reading her story and experiencing Jamie's material, I will never again ignore the wellspring symphony within my body (symptoms, synchronicities, perceptions, associations). For whether my body honors me with a comedic, tragic, or joyous expression, I now know it is a linchpin of wisdom and it is singing to me, for me."

Sunday Larson, author of *The Spinning Game: A Sedona Story* and "To Free Your Fearless Voice / Write Like a Woman" workshops

"Most of the time we play 'Let's Make a Deal' with ourselves—hoping we'll pick the right door; this book doesn't just get you to the right door . . . it kicks it down!"

Chuck Behrens, author of *The Candle Maker*

TRANSFORMATIONAL *healing*

Five Surprisingly Simple Keys Designed to
Redirect Your Life Toward Wellness, Purpose, and Prosperity

Jamie L. Saloff

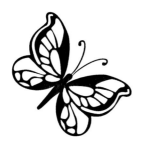

**SENT
BOOKS**

Requests for permissions should be addressed to:
Sent Books
P. O. Box 339
Edinboro, PA, 16412

Layout Designed by Sent Books
Cover Design by Mary Fisher Designs
Drawings by Mark G. Saloff
Jamie's Photo by E. J. Morris
Fonts: Century Schoolbook, Invitation, Capitals, President, Optima,
    Bickham Script, Renfield's Lunch, and Butterflies

Saloff, Jamie L.
    Transformational Healing: Five Surprisingly Simple Keys
    Designed to Redirect Your Life Toward Wellness, Purpose,
    and Posperity / Jamie L. Saloff
        p.   cm.
    ISBN 0-9707258-7-6 / 13 digit ISBN 978-0-9740642-0-8 : $24.95
    Includes: Index and bibliographic data.
    1. Healing (Self-help) 2. Intuition 3. Spirituality
    4. Altered states of consciousness (Psychology).
    5. Goal Setting. I. Title.
        2005

Library of Congress Control Number: 2001012345
Copyright information available upon request.

First Edition

Published in the United States of America on acid-free paper.

Although many offered a helping hand,
in the end, I had to create my own well-being.

in Memory of:

Thelma Kirsch and Patricia Boyles

TABLE OF CONTENTS

Dream it,
live it,
produce it,
pound it out,
let it rip,
get it going,
sweat a little,
love a lot,
bare it all,
be true to yourself.
Question, but do not doubt.

TABLE OF CONTENTS

CHAPTER SIX:
MISTAKEN PERCEPTIONS 43

SECTION II: COMMITMENT

CHAPTER SEVEN:
COMMITMENT, DEDICATION, AND DISCIPLINE 63

CHAPTER EIGHT:
OVERCOMING FEAR AND RECOGNIZING TRUTH 89

SECTION III: FINDING AND FULFILLING
THE DESIRES OF YOUR HEART

CHAPTER NINE:
MAPPING OUR DESIRES 97

SECTION IV: CONNECTION
COMMUNICATING WITH GOD AND OUR HIGHER SELF

CHAPTER TWENTY:
THE STILL, SMALL VOICE A GUIDE TO LEAD US 233

CHAPTER TWENTY-ONE:
TAKING YOUR CONNECTION TO THE NEXT LEVEL 257

Table of Contents

TABLE OF CONTENTS

INTRODUCTION:

"The Chinese word for transformation consists of two ideograms, both danger and opportunity."
Tom Kenyon,
Brain States

MY STORY

After having been diagnosed with cancer at only twenty-four years old, I knew my chances of living to old age weren't good. Both of my parents and all four of my grandparents had died of severe illnesses. I knew their fate would soon be mine unless I found a way to wholly heal my life and improve my odds.

For the next ten years, I read every book I could find on healing. But, for me, none of the methods seemed to work. I felt I needed a more personalized method that addressed the unique individual that I am—that we all are.

One night, determined to unlock the secret to wellness, I went upstairs and shut myself in the bedroom, vowing not to come out until I had found what I had sought for so long—the means to heal my life from illness, pain, and the overall chaos then controlling my day-to-day life.

Working with nothing more than a pack of mini sticky notes, some colored markers, and a piece of poster board, I wrote single words and short phrases on the notes and dropped them in related clusters onto the poster board.

Several hours later, I emerged with a smile. I had

"Now I knew from personal experience that disease can be healed, if we are willing to change the way we think and believe and act!"

Louise L. Hay,
You Can Heal Your Life

found the meaning of the disease that had once tried to destroy my life. In fact, I'd found the reason behind every ailment or injury that had ever plagued me. The experience also gave me a new realization—we never need suffer from any ailments at all.

Amazingly, the more I used the system, the more my life began to heal, not only physically, but everything else in my life began to improve as well. I no longer spent every day worrying about all those things I might never do because, now, I was doing them.

You see, when I learned how to find meaning in my ailments, I also learned how our ailments are a part of an elaborate, innate system designed to lead us to what we desire most. (Isn't that incredible?) Soon I was easily turning my onetime dreams into realities.

Not long after, I recognized I had an even bigger dream than anything I'd achieved so far. My deepest desire was to share what I'd learned with others so they could improve their lives as well. I figured that if everyone had the knowledge I did, the world would be a better place because everybody would be healthier and happier. Wouldn't that be great?

The best thing is how these methods are designed to be unique to the user. That means no matter who is using them, they will find the personal answers they need to heal their lives.

And that is the purpose of this book, to explain how I implemented these methods in my life so that you can use them as building blocks for healing whatever needs remedied in yours.

If you are ready to heal your life, physically, emotionally, and spiritually, then turn the page and take the simple assessment that begins on the next page.

"The word INCURABLE, which is so frightening to so many people, means to me that this particular condition cannot be cured by any outer means and that we must go within to find the cure!"
Louise L. Hay,
You Can Heal Your Life

CHAPTER ONE: HOW HEALTHY ARE YOU?

1

TAKE A SIMPLE TEST

Have you recently suffered from a sinus infection, a sore back, strained muscles, migraines, allergies, hemorrhoids, the flu, or any minor affliction? Have you received treatment for heart disease, high blood pressure, diabetes, arthritis, prostate, MS, or even cancer? At any given moment, most of us have some malady we're nursing, whether or not we have discussed it or been treated by our physician.

One of the most amazing things to me is how many different maladies each of us might have at any given moment—even if we consider ourselves "healthy." As you work though the simple test that follows, you may be surprised too.

Why are there so many *Body Songs* vying for your attention? What messages are trying to get through? Have you blocked your internal reception from receiving messages so that your higher mind now has no alternative other than to get your attention through something you *will* notice—such as pain?

While we are acutely aware of any major concerns: cancer, arthritis, migraines, and other diseases and disorders, most of

"Now primed to hear people speak woundology, I believe I was meant to challenge the assumptions that I and many others then held dear—especially the assumption that everyone who is wounded or ill wants the full recovery of their health."

Carolyn Myss,
Why People Don't Heal and How They Can

"You call this body matter, when awake, or when asleep in a dream. That matter can report pain, or that mind is IN matter, reporting sensations, is but a dream at all times. . . . When your belief in pain ceases, the pain stops; for matter has no intelligence of its own."
Mary Baker Eddy,
Miscellaneous Writings

us also seem to have a collection of sideline ailments we can call on at a moment's notice: migraines, tendinitis, backaches, carporal tunnel, toothaches, heartburn, sinus problems, constipation, allergies, sprained or strained muscles, cold sores, and more. The latter are more like parlor tricks we can utilize as excuses, crutches, and catalysts for simple conversation where it's almost as if we are in competition with one another to see who has had the worst experience.

For many of our minor ailments, we don't see a doctor and, often, we don't even medicate them. Why is that? Could it be they are not all that important? They seem to be important enough to notice, important enough to talk about, yet we seem to sense that in the scope of things, they're not something we need to be too concerned about. Why not?

What you need to ask yourself is this, if they are not important enough for treatment then why are they consuming your conversations and your thoughts? Could it be they have a message for you if you would only listen? Could it be that you are noticing the message but are just not sure what it might mean?

While you might think the best of situations would be to remain entirely malady free, that's not entirely true. Except for those few highly enlightened individuals who have fine-tuned their minds with God, your ailments are actually a part of your body's built-in messaging system designed to get your attention when all else fails. I'll discuss all of this later in the book; in the meantime, take the simple test that follows and see where you stand.

THE FULL BODY ASSESSMENT

Note: please see a doctor for treatment of any major ailment. I am not a physician and cannot offer you any medical advice. However, after you have attended to whatever necessary treatments your medical professional might advise, feel free to employ my methods as detailed throughout the book.

What I would like you to do is to simply assess where you are now healthwise. I want you to reveal the least of your maladies as well as your worst. Begin by making a copy of the diagram on the next page (or draw your own), then follow the instructions below:

1. Mark down every ache, pain, or symptom you currently are experiencing. Draw small images to describe your ailments when you can. As a rule of thumb, if an ailment has been recurrent and/or has shown itself within the last few days, or if the ailment is a long-term, chronic problem such as PMS, arthritis, back pain, migraines, etc., then include it.

2. Don't forget those minor inconveniences and annoyances such as blisters, cold sores, calluses, toe corns, warts, hemorrhoids, bruises, even paper cuts. Need further ideas? Just walk down the aisles of your local drugstore and you'll see the countless array of remedies available for these maladies.

3. Include a notation of any scars since they are a near-permanent mark on your body, calling for your recognition of them. If we have no more issues associated with them or are not to recall the particular incident any further, then why has our body not yet erased the evidence of it? Could it be this lifetime mark carries with it an ongoing message associated with our innate challenges or higher purpose? Do not discount these marks on subsequent reviews, either, as you may find the message that comes to you from them changes from time to time.

4. When you are done, list each item from the worst to least. You will need this information later on in the book.

6. Return to this exercise from time to time to do a quick assessment of your healthful condition.

7. If you need help interpreting any particular symptom, check my website for additional information as well as for online workshops and personal coaching.

HOW HEALTHY ARE YOU?

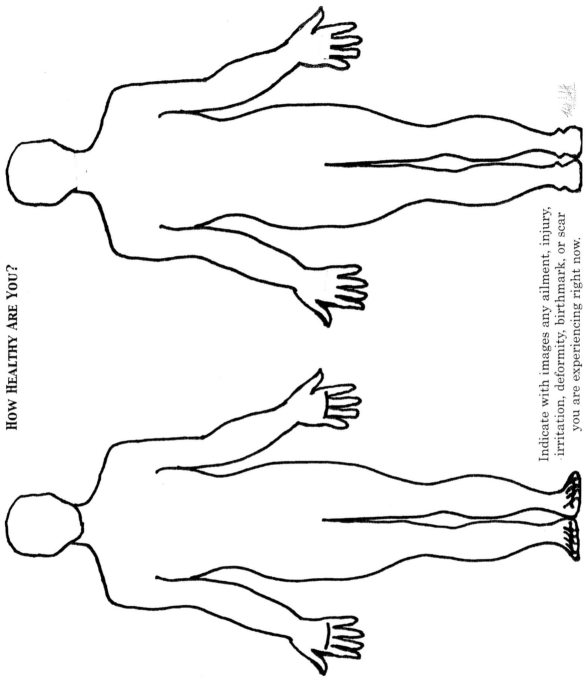

Indicate with images any ailment, injury, irritation, deformity, birthmark, or scar you are experiencing right now.

How Healthy Are You?

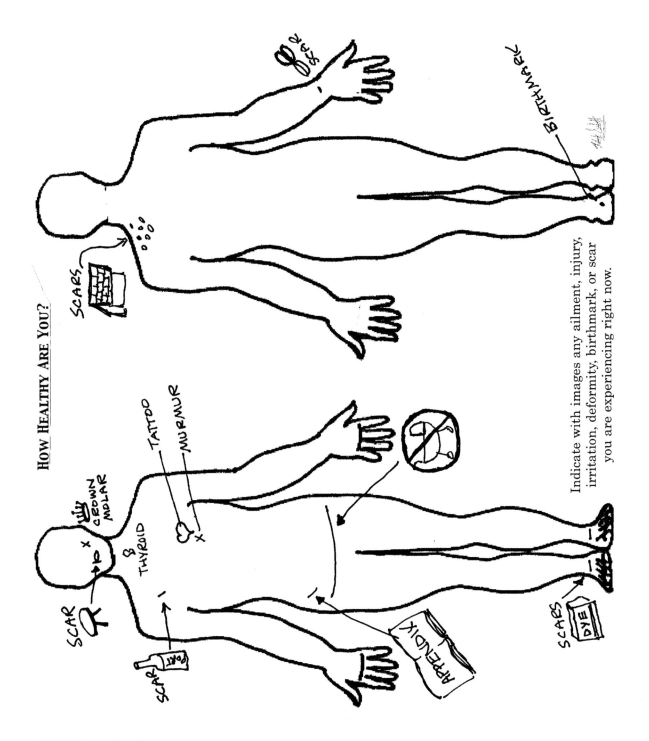

Indicate with images any ailment, injury, irritation, deformity, birthmark, or scar you are experiencing right now.

CHAPTER TWO: WHAT IS A BODY SONG?

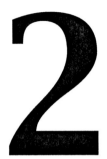

After a visit to my chiropractor, where I had been receiving treatment for injuries from an automobile accident, I picked up my journal and began to write. I'd recently learned how to tap into the deeper recesses of my mind and reap a wealth of valuable healing information by using archetypes, visual images, and word associations. Starting with the joint and bone aches my chiropractor had been treating, I drifted through my writing, hopping from one association to the next, waiting to see what incredible connection my mind would reveal this time.

In a way that only the mind can understand, I suddenly remembered the movie *The Goonies,* and my thoughts jumped to their strange pirate organ made from human bones. With this unique instrument, the Goonie kids were attempting to decipher its hidden musical messages. If they played the right chords, the pirates' secret passage began to open. If they played the wrong ones, the ground they stood on crumbled away.

Using my self-taught method, I found parallels between the Goonie's spooky organ and my visit to the chiropractor. My doctor and I had talked about the

"For us to become whole and healthy, we must balance the body, mind and spirit. We need to take good care of our bodies. We need to have a positive mental attitude about ourselves and about life. And we need to have a strong spiritual connection. When these three things are balanced, we rejoice in living. No doctor, no health practitioner can give us this unless we choose to take part in our healing process.

Louise L. Hay,
Heal Your Body

different ailments, aches, and pains that could be caused from a simple misalignment of the spine, some of which could be cured instantly with a basic adjustment. I'd proven this myself a time or two by going into his office with a sore throat and runny nose, and leaving less than fifteen minutes later without them. And this was but the simplest of ailments that an adjustment could quickly cure.

The idea that a slight misalignment of the spinal column could cause a physical ailment intrigued me. What caused the spinal column to change positions? Did the subconscious mind play a role?

How *does* the body create an ailment? Why is it that one morning we wake up fine and the next we find ourselves ill, in pain, or dysfunctional? Why do some people die of AIDS while others carry the HIV virus for years unaffected? Why do normal, healthy cells suddenly turn rogue and cancerous? Why are some people ill all the time while others go their entire lives without ever entering a hospital? Is there some deep, internal force controlling these symptoms from within us and, if so, for what purpose? Could the spine be a part of a more complicated, subconscious mechanism used for the purpose of creating symptoms reflective of our hidden emotional needs? Like the Goonies playing their unusual organ, is our body sending us clues we can use to heal and further benefit our lives?

With all these things in mind, I began referring to my physical symptoms as *Body Songs,* because I felt these ailments, no matter how severe or insignificant, were a message from within, designed to bring my body back into *harmony* with my higher purpose. Like poetic lyrics, these *Body Songs* played in riddles on my physical being so that I might discover their previously unrecognized emotional connection. It is in these connections that I found a powerful life-directional guide.

Thus, *Body Songs* are *any physical malady, disease, disorder, ailment, or injury—even if accidental—which offers us an opportunity to look deeper at our lives and its situations.* They are a message from within. Most often, an ailment is a symptom of a blocked dream or passion that is part of our higher purpose, a cry from deep within our soul to rekindle our passion and once again move us forward towards our dream.

"To me all disease stands in the same way and just as I have analyzed them, I find that they are the invention of man and they can be dissipated unless the impression is so strong that it is beyond the power of the operator to explain it."
Phineas Parkhust Quimby,
Health and Disease

"Illness is a way for people who have shut down their feelings to reopen their feeling centers and reconnect with their selves."
Author Unknown

BODY SONGS HAVE ONE OF FOUR PURPOSES WHICH ARE:

1. To *remove an emotional block* which is preventing us from fulfilling our highest purpose.

2. To encourage us to repair a hidden emotional pain or forgotten indiscretion that we have buried deep within and have failed to *release and/or forgive*.

3. To create a situation that will be instrumental in helping us *overcome an innate challenge*.

4. To *lead us to persons or situations* that can provide knowledge, experiences, or contacts we need to fulfill our purpose or goals.

A *Body Song* is *always* in direct proportion to the immediate need. The more urgent the need, the more severe the symptoms.

CORE DIRECTIVES

Deep within our being is the core of who we are and why we are. Above all else, this is what's most important to the body's underlying operating system. Even though our healthy body seems very important to us, to our core, health is secondary. Instead, our highest purpose is first and foremost. The body will do whatever is necessary to preserve and pursue that purpose even if it means sacrificing some physical function or bearing tremendous physical pain. While it seems ridiculous that our body would allow us to suffer pain for any reason—it's much easier to believe that our pain is due to some punishment, sin, or bad luck on our part—yet, the body does react in this way.

A *Body Song* is a catch valve. If we build emotional blocks that prevent us from reaching our predestined goal, our body devises a way to pull the blocks down. The more we pull in the wrong direction, the harder the safety catch pulls back.

When I was young, a friend took me to a large amusement park. We rode many different rides. Standing in line

"And if thy right eye offend thee, pluck it out, and cast it from thee, for it is profitable for thee that one of thy members should perish, and not that thy whole body should be cast into hell."
Matthew 5:29,
King James Version

13

at one of them, the sign depicted storybook character Mr. Toad[1] and his wild automobile ride. Toad had no regard for rules, regulations, roads, people, or even trees that might be in his way. I could not wait to get behind the wheel of that car so I could drive like Toad.

Of course, the park couldn't have patrons driving recklessly all over the place; thus, the cars were attached to the track by a safety bar. If the car turned too far right or too far left, the bar prevented the car from leaving the track. While this was not my idea of 'a wild ride,' it did prevent the park from facing countless lawsuits.

Our bodies have a safety bar too. During one of my more serious hospital stays, I nearly died. The doctors explained to my husband, as I lay unconscious in intensive care, that my body would shut down my vital organs, one at a time, in an attempt to *preserve my life*. But if my kidneys shut down, I would not survive. Fortunately, that didn't happen.

I later found an example in nature that helped me understand what happened to me. One of the plants I'd received while in the hospital began to drop its leaves. Whether too little sun, too much water, or some other problem, I did not know. I only knew that soon the plant had no leaves and became quite useless with nothing but an empty stalk.

The plant knew it could sacrifice its leaves as they weren't vital to its survival. Its *roots* were. By sacrificing its leaves, the plant prolonged the life of its core even though, to me, a plant without leaves had no use.

We often see our *physical* body as our most vital part. When we are hampered by ailments—whether temporary or permanent—we don't always realize how that lack or limited function has somehow furthered our higher purpose—something we may have given little or no credence to at all.

In the case of my plant, eventually, something destroyed the root, and I threw the dead stalk away. Had I been able to strengthen the root, the plant would have once again thrived. In our lives, our root is our highest purpose *even if it is unknown to us*—which brings up another point.

Do I need to know my purpose or the meaning of the ailment in order to gain the benefit? No. Many lives are changed every day without conscious knowledge of either

"If you understand or if you don't, if you believe or if you doubt. There's a universal justice; and the eyes of truth are always watching you."
Michael Cretu,
Cross of Changes

14

one. The body's internal system is designed to work regardless of whether or not we know.

But what if we did? What if we knew our purpose and actively pursued it, would we need ailments at all?

An ailment is a means for the underlying emotional body to gain our conscious attention. While it doesn't need our help to accomplish its goal, we can considerably enhance the situation if we do.

Think of it this way. If I climb to the top of a ski run and attempt to slide down without skis, the sheer slope and slipperiness—with the help of Mother Gravity—will bring me to the bottom of the hill. The result will not be pretty, but I will arrive at my desired destination.

If, however, I put on skis and guide myself down the slope with any manner of skill, I will arrive at the same destination not only quicker but also far better for it.

Therefore, if I interpret the underlying message of an ailment and begin to actively correct whatever emotional block caused it to manifest in the first place, I can shortcut its effects since the symptom will no longer be needed.

After my cancer diagnosis, I had no choice but to take the path directed by its circumstances—or die. Having cancer *forced* me to stand up for myself. The circumstances and situations surrounding my illness demanded it. I knew this and accepted it as the disease's personal message to me without ever knowing an ailment could be interpreted. Once I began to walk in the proper direction, the disease's message was no longer needed; thus, its symptoms were no longer needed, and they went away.

At the time I began to take my stand, I had not yet received any treatment for my cancer. I had only received countless tests over a two-month period. Nevertheless, my diagnoses went from nodular sclerosing Hodgkins Stage III (the worst) to Stage I (the earliest stage of the disease).

By taking action against the underlying emotional blocks, my outcome changed, my diagnosis changed, my treatment for cure changed, my outlook on life changed.

However, in those days, my actions were based purely on circumstances, not knowledge. I had blindly stumbled on my cure. Because I didn't understand the scope of what I had found, I subsequently spent years trying to understand what happened so I could duplicate it again in my own life, but also so I could share it with others.

"If I had the operation to remove the cancerous growth and also cleared the mental pattern that was causing the cancer, then it would not return. If cancer or any other illness returns, I do not believe it is because they did not 'get it all out,' but rather that the patient has made no mental changes. He or she just recreates the same illness, perhaps in a different part of the body."

Louise L. Hay,
You Can Heal Your Life

"There is Miss LeRoux whom we all know. She is stone blind in one eye, and has been for four years. . . .[But] God Almighty met the fellow's faith; the woman's eye opened right then, and she stood before that congregation and covering the good eye, read with the eye that had been blind, the entire chapter."

Gordon Lindsay,
The New John G. Lake Sermons

Today, I know that ailments have meaning. If we seek out those meanings and act on them, we can alter their course—sometimes instantly. (Think about that for a moment. . . . *Instantly*.)

In the same way my chiropractor's realignment of my spinal column can remove my cold symptoms, the realignment of my *mind* to its higher purpose can change my life's course.

But how many of us consciously know and pursue our purpose? How can we react effectively if we do not know what our body is reacting against?

Through the exercises that follow, you will learn how to interpret an ailment and learn its underlying message. You will also learn how to uncover your highest purpose.

In addition, you will. . .

1. Gain understanding about your ailments and how to react against them.

2. Learn how to remove the emotional blocks and fears preventing you from living life to its fullest.

3. Learn the meaning of your heritage and how the messages it brings can lend direction in your life.

4. Gain understanding about how being aware of your innate challenges will bring you the desires of your heart.

5. Learn how ailments actually empower your life and lead you toward fulfilling your highest purpose and most heartfelt dreams.

Chapter Three:
For the Journey
on Which You Are About
to Embark

3

Here are the fundamentals you need to know to make the best use of the exercises that follow.

The Main Purpose of These Exercises and Texts

1. These exercises are designed to delve deeply into your heart and mind to uncover the emotional connections between your physical condition and your life circumstances. By understanding how your reactions to certain situations relate to your physical condition, you can appropriately alter your reactions and, in turn, alter your physical symptoms.

2. This book is also about finding purpose, and in doing so, whole health—body, mind, and spirit. A person who has revealed their purpose to their conscious mind will pursue it with passion and vigor. They will have a renewed life. They will live with enthusiasm and have a happier, healthier outlook.

Yes, YOU have a purpose; we all do. By uncovering it, defining it, clarifying it, you'll gain clear direction and will

"So Brahma hid man's divinity within man himself; for it is there that man never thinks of looking but searches restlessly instead, all over the earth."
Lydia J. Schrader Gray,
Children of the New Age

be able to make confident decisions each step along the way. Your body will respond in kind by giving you the health you need to pursue your purpose and most heartfelt dreams.

You do not need extensive training in order to interpret a situation or to correlate the given signs and symbols. In fact, every child already knows how to do this. Each interpretation begins by simply relaxing the mind and allowing it to flow freely on word associations and images. *(You will find more details on this in Appendix A: How to Do Word Association Exercises.)*

Imagination is perhaps the most powerful gift ever given to us by God to use as we will. And yet we often box this power and store it away declaring it 'silly' or 'childish,' thus totally ignoring a powerful and creative tool readily and freely available to us all.

The wonderful thing about these intuitive interpretations is how they are decidedly unique and personal to our own experience and means of understanding. No one can tell us better than ourselves what lies beneath the surface of our skin. We are not monochrome clones with one-size-fits-all thinking. We are one-of-a-kind individuals seeking specialized answers.

3. Remember, this is intended to be a journey of healing, so don't become so absorbed and focused on your ailments that you make them worse. Discover the interpretation, then focus on a positive outcome and on goals designed to direct your life to its fullest potential.

4. Finally, the purpose of these exercises and texts is *not* to offer medical advice. *Please* seek a qualified professional for any medical condition.

Regardless of whether your search takes you through traditional, medical means or through alternative, holistic avenues, medical practitioners can play an important role in your search for total well-being, either by assisting with relief from symptoms or by providing a new contact, direction, or archetype in which to further your purposeful journey.

SECTION ONE: RELIEF

> "Pain is an indication that something is threatening the organism, while pleasure indicates that the situation is resolved and all is well, freeing our attention for other things."
>
> Lindsay C. Gibson,
> *Who You Were Meant to Be*

Chapter Four: Finding Relief

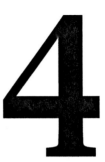

(Note: While I begin my discussion on the topic of Relief, in my own healing, no one key was more important than any other. Rather, each of the five keys harmoniously intertwine and balance each other.)

When I began to more fully understand healing on a holistic level, a process that transcended the physical body and brought well-being to all levels of my life—heart, mind, and soul—I discovered five essential keys. Those five keys are: *Relief, Goals and Desires, Connection, Commitment, and Synchronicity.*

In my own journey, *relief* became an important key to healing because I found that whenever I suffered pain, whether physical or emotional, I could not focus on forward movement, pursue my goals or purpose, or even function efficiently in my daily life. When in pain, pain became the focus of my life.

Pain blocked my connection to my higher self and to God. Without connection, I had no direction and lost enthusiasm for life. Thus relief, which gave me a time to reconnect, became just as vital as the connection itself.

"There are two motivating factors that drive us: Seeking pleasure and avoiding pain."
Sherry Maria Gideons,
Champion bodybuilder

Regardless of how short, those few moments of relief helped me through my toughest hours.

Once, while visiting my allergist, I had a terrible sinus infection. As I sat in the physician's office for several hours undergoing skin testing, I could barely breathe and had to constantly reach for tissues. I felt miserable. The allergist, who probably got tired of listening to my sniffles, handed me a prescription decongestant tablet saying:

> *"Sometimes you just need a space of relief so your body can get back to the task of healing."*

I took the pill and for the next couple of hours I could breathe easily.

Think of relief as the training wheels on a child's bicycle. Knowing those wheels are there gives the child confidence and time to learn balance—a necessary skill needed to ride a bike. Relief gives us a space of clear thinking to overcome the barrier put in our way. Relief gives us confidence to look for our next step and to plan a new course of action. Relief is recovering the peace of heart and mind left behind in the face of tragedy or devastation.

Whether relief comes from traditional medical means, holistic, alternative routes, or meditative emotional therapies does not matter. That it comes is all that matters.

I had no guide such as this book to help me. For the most part, I groped around in the dark trying this, trying that, experimenting with anything that might lead to wellness and a higher state of being. I had so many things from which I needed relief that I could only react to whatever was happening at the moment. My pains included physical ailments as well as emotional blocks and fears that caused me hours of anxiety. Financial worries caused a different kind of pain also in need of relief.

As, one by one, I conquered and removed my painful burdens, I uncovered the true me that had been buried beneath. I found periods of relief that allowed me the freedom to think beyond what pill I could take, to find purpose and meaning for my life

Finding relief is no easy task. Pain has a way of dragging a person down to sheer basic needs. Pain strips away the false masks that we wear and leaves us in the raw. It has the ability to make us forget common courtesies and to

"The Lord replied, 'The times when you have seen only one set of footprints is when I carried you.'"

Mary Stevenson,
Footprints in the Sand

create within our hearts a lasting bitterness. Pain is perhaps one of the most powerful vehicles of change the body has, for neither man or woman, president or king, soldier or child can resist its forceful hand.

I cannot tell you where to find relief because each situation and individual is unique. What I can tell you are some ways I found relief and offer the following advice: *Never give up!* Keep looking for the answer that is right for you. Keep searching for relief and total inner wellness. By the time you've finished reading this book, you will understand the five keys of healing and will learn strategies to further you along the way of total wellness.

"Never give up, never give up, never ever give up."
Jimmy Valvano,
Legendary NC State
basketball coach

MEDICAL RELIEF

For decades, I suffered from countless menstrual problems. Then one afternoon, while sitting in the doctor's office discussing yet another round of temporary, Band-Aid fixes, I asked for a hysterectomy. Why? Because he admitted I would eventually need one anyway, and because I was desperate for relief—*now*.

I had suffered with this situation for over twenty-three years. I wanted it to stop. While each fix worked temporarily, none were permanent. My troubles always recurred. On at least three occasions, I'd been hospitalized and received blood transfusions. I'd spent countless hours in gynecological offices and thousands of dollars on so-called cures. Some months I would not menstruate at all. Others, I'd menstruate for eight to fourteen days, and on more than one occasion, those days turned to weeks or just ran into the next month without a break in the cycle at all. I even menstruated during the eighth month of my first pregnancy.

I needed relief. At that point, I was willing to do *anything* to get it. Admittedly, I had yet to learn all I know now about ailments, and if faced with the same problem today, I might make a different decision. Back then, I could not begin to think about how to reach my deeper inner self or to even be curious about emotional healing. I was so beaten down from years and years of health problems, I could only think of and reach for relief, and that is what the hysterectomy brought me—relief.

"The greatest mistake physicians make is that they attempt to cure the body without attempting to cure the mind; yet the mind and body are one and should not be treated separately."
Plato

Afterwards, when my life and physical state of health returned to balance, I had the presence of mind to dig deeper, seeking out the emotional connection that lay hidden beneath the surface. Then, and only then, could I work on connecting and understanding what all that pain and suffering had been about. *(See: Appendix B for more.)*

Surgery is a radical, invasive approach. The same can be said of my cancer treatment where I received monitored doses of radiation therapy. There aren't many cures more caustic to the body than radiation. Today I might consider a more holistic approach before consenting to something so drastic. But at that time, I needed relief so desperately that I accepted any means within my reach.

I am sharing these things because I think sometimes we feel *guilty* if we cannot heal ourselves without a doctor's care. We forget that we have been raised and heavily programmed within a society deeply ingrained in the belief of doctors' pills, treatments, and surgeries. It is very difficult to escape something so much a part of our belief systems. Don't feel bad if this is the only route you see open to you. Just because you may have sought help from the traditional medical field doesn't mean this book cannot help you or that you have somehow failed in healing your life. You haven't. First and foremost in the search for healing is seeking and finding *relief*—by whatever means necessary. If you need a medical doctor that's fine. Put aside your guilt, seek out the needed and oh-so-necessary relief. Then come back to this book and learn the deeper, underlying meaning of all that has transpired. Finish the healing already begun by reaching within and understanding the ailment's purposeful message. Hear the true direction given by your inner *Body Songs*.

"All healing takes place from within. Our spirits heal our body. A doctor's sure hands may perform surgery, and medicine may provide ideal circumstances for health, but it is the spirit then that effects the healing."

Betty J. Eadie,
Embraced by the Light

ALTERNATIVE MEDICINES AND CARE

After my car accident, I suffered from terrible back and neck pain that prevented me from participating in family activities as well as doing simple jobs around the house, like vacuuming or raking. Even sitting at my computer caused me excruciating pain.

Had I worn a cast, a brace, even a bandage, my family would have gladly understood my refusal to ride in our

24

boat, join them for a game of golf, or in-line skate. But I had no visible injury. Even my physician could find no clear reason for my pain. As weeks turned into months, my family stopped asking to help, stopped offering concern, and in fact, were sometimes thoughtless in their remarks. They couldn't see anything visibly wrong with me so they reasoned I must not really be sick. Their lack of consideration left me feeling even worse. Why couldn't I get well?

My medical doctor gave me a prescription for muscle relaxants. These made me nauseous and sleepy, so I took them only when the pain became too much to bear. The rest of the time, I functioned in a mental fog.

As if that wasn't enough, my lawyer recommended I keep a daily log of how I felt. I wrote entries like:

> *"This morning I feel depressed and overwhelmed. I'm tired of fighting. Tired of waking up and feeling like an old lady before the day even begins."*

> *"The last few days have been hell. Right now I have a knot in my mid-upper back the size of a fist. It's been there a couple of days. People wonder why I'm withdrawing from activities, why I want to be alone. . . . I'm just trying to hide from the pain."*

> *"I took some time to look back at the past writings here. I find the words depressing. I try not to complain to my friends and family about all I have been through, but these written words are a constant reminder of all my suffering. In another few months it will be two years and here I am still in pain every day, still constantly reminded of the accident, still afraid to do many things."*

> *"Every day I find myself hesitating, should I do this? Will it hurt me? Even simple things like reaching for an item high on a shelf, or looking under the bed, or vacuuming, anything that requires a*

"When you ask for a healing, you never know what your body is going to tell you. It may tell you to stop or start eating something, express some feelings to a friend, quit your job, or go see a doctor. The key is to ask and then listen for a response."

Shakti Gawain,
Living in the Light

25

range of motion. I keep silent, but dearly wish I didn't have this constant fear looking over my shoulder, the continuing pain in my back and neck, the lingering memories of June 20, 1996."

"I feel sorry for anyone who has to read this. I keep writing the same thing over and over—living it too. I feel like that groundhog movie with Bill Murray where he lives the same awful day over and over and over."

This had to be the absolute worst way to start each day since these writings merely reinforced how miserable I felt and how I'd given up hope. Having reminded myself at the start of the day how much I'd suffered, what did I have to look forward to for the rest of my waking hours?

After a year of this, I took my son to see a chiropractor[1] never thinking he might be able to help *me*. When he learned of my situation, he said he believed he could assist me in finding some relief. I had given up all hope of ever being pain free again, so I agreed to try anything that could give me my life back.

From my x-rays, the chiropractor discovered that due to the car accident, I had suffered a reverse curvature of the spine (a cervical kyphosis). With dedicated, long-term treatment from him, I found the relief I'd sought for so long. I am deeply indebted to this man for not only lending his skills with his hands and spinal adjustments, but also his laughter and smile. With his help, I gradually regained relief from the pain that had held me for so long. Having at last found relief, I could then work through the emotional connections. Soon I returned to all the activities I'd once given up. I dusted off my golf clubs, brought out my in-line skates, and gladly picked up a rake.

Now, alternative medicines and treatments range from chiropractic to acupuncture, from naturopathic to ayurveda, and continuing down a long list of remedies that are natural, spiritual, wholistic. What works for one person, has no effect on another. What some call bogus may save another person's life. The important thing is that if whatever method you explore brings *you* relief, then go for it. No matter what it is, if your belief system accepts it as plausible and your intuition is driving you toward it, then allow yourself to try it. What you learn from the experience and from the people involved in managing it may be an important key not only in your finding whole health but also in finding your personal path and purpose. This is true whether or not your experience with them is positive or negative.

RELIEF FOR THE MIND

Relief doesn't have to mean taking a pill, having surgery, or receiving a treatment of some kind. If the mind can be distracted from its focus on the pain, either through work or other mental activity, a period of relief can be obtained just as effectively by those means.

As part of the testing during my cancer diagnosis, my doctors scheduled a procedure called a *lymphangiogram*. For this, a team of two doctors pumped dye into my lymph system—a tiny, vein-like system that circulates lymph fluid to the body's lymph nodes—through incisions cut in the tops of my feet. The dye allowed the lymph nodes to be x-rayed and viewed for symptoms of cancer.

Except—there were problems. The procedure didn't go as planned, and the process took longer than the doctors expected. In their rush to finish up and get to their next appointment, they neglected to prescribe the promised pain medication, so I didn't receive any.

I soon learned that what goes in, must come out. The chemical dye oozing over the raw incisions burned immensely and left me in terrible pain from which I could find no relief. To ease this now intense pain, they eventually offered me a single Tylenol.

I suffered for hours. The more I suffered, the worse I felt. The pain constantly turned on itself and grew as it sucked away my focus from everything else. The pain and my agony grew so great, my husband could no longer stay by my side. This was the only time through all my ordeals that he ever got up and left. He later said I'd undergone treatments worse than a laboratory animal.

Alone in my hospital bed and late into the night I moaned, I groaned, I cried. The hospital staff offered little in the way of compassion or care because, as one doctor

"The greatest discovery of any generation is that human beings can alter their lives by altering the attitudes of their minds."
Albert Schweitzer

"Eventually most people who have recurrent attacks will develop a chronic pattern. . . . 'The only chair I can sit on has to have a hard seat and a straight back, and on and on. And the pain becomes the primary focus of their lives. . . . They become obsessed with it."
John Sarno,
Healing Back Pain

> "If I can convince the conscious mind that [the pain] is not serious and not worthy of its attention, better yet that it is a phony, a charade, and that rather than fear it one should ridicule it, that most of the structural diagnoses are not valid and that the only things worthy of one's attention are repressed feelings, what has been accomplished? We will have made [the pain] useless."
>
> John Sarno,
> *Healing Back Pain*

> "The void gives us an opportunity to end some part of our development, and to prepare the ground for new growth. Whether or not we know it consciously, we are undergoing a psychic reorganization of our attracting field of purpose."
>
> Carol Adrienne,
> *The Purpose of Your Life*

put it, 'I have a hundred other patients far worse off than you.' I knew I had to find some way to distract my mind from the engulfing pain.

I switched on the TV. At two in the morning, the only programming available was a Spanish-speaking show. Not able to understand a word, I attempted to watch the pictures trying to figure out what the show could be about. Focused on the riddle of the program, I distracted my mind from the pain and found relief. I even experienced a kind of euphoric high[2] as my body relaxed and finally released all its pent-up tension.

Whenever I remember this situation, I am amazed by how the mind could multiply what should have been no worse than a minor abrasion into something of catastrophic proportions and then turn in a matter of minutes to a place of not only being pain free, but actually creating for itself a drug of sorts to give the mind peace. I have used this 'bait-and-switch' tactic many times, distracting myself from pain by entertaining my mind with something else.

There have been several times in my life where tragedy or calamity left me in a cloud of depression. These periods often lasted for several months. I can't explain how it feels when all enthusiasm for life has been lost. Only those who have been there will truly understand. Regardless of my many blessings, I had no desire to function and could see no escape from my situation. I truly wanted nothing more than to die. I'd tried medications; I'd tried sleeping through the pain. I'd tried praying. I'd spent hours reading. Anything to distract my mind. Nothing seemed to work. In these most severe of cases of depression, I found that by taking some kind of *action* I would, at last, find relief. As soon as I could focus my mind on a worthy project, *something that felt purposeful and important*, I no longer had time to dwell on the void, and it dissipated.

YOGA

There are some pains of the mind that are buried too deeply to find. For whatever reason, they are too painful for us to view. They remain in our body causing subsequent symptoms and *Body Songs*. One way to eradicate them is through yoga, deep tissue massage, or other disciplines of directed movement such as Tai Chi or Qigong.

While working with author Tom Bird through his Intensive Writer's program, he diligently prodded me to take up some form of yoga. *Yoga!?* I thought, imagining myself twisted in contorted knots, standing on my head, and bending in ways nature never intended. *No way!* That wasn't for me. I had no interest in yoga whatsoever and couldn't see how practicing it could in any way help me with the many physical problems I faced. And even if it could, where would I find the time? My life was utterly chaotic at the time. I barely had time to take a shower, let alone take up a new practice of bending and stretching.

What Tom already knew, but didn't specifically say, was that yoga, which held the body in such a way as to test it, but not hurt it, could reach down into the body's core past the reach of the subconscious mind where it could find and release my deeply embedded emotional pains.

Fortunately, Tom did not let up on me. He continually kept on me about it until I agreed to at least try it. I purchased Brian Kest's video *Energize!*

While this particular video may not have been the best starting point (the exercises were more advanced than my ability) in my case, it worked. The first time I played the video, I stood watching Brian with my mouth gaping open and my mind saying, *What? Are you crazy? You have to be out of your mind to try that!* But I did try it. The next day, I followed the video doing only about one-tenth (or less) of the moves. I did only what I could comfortably do. When I was done, something incredible happened. I actually felt *energized!*

The following morning, I knew I had to do it again. I wanted to feel that way all the time. Of course, on day two, I was a little sore from day one, so I could not even do all that I did on the first day, yet I knew I would be better off moving through the soreness, than allowing my body to recede back into its stiff immobility.

I continued doing yoga in my own haphazard way for almost a year, eventually being able to do most the moves in the video to some degree. Being able to do these moves brought me physical and emotional relief but also gave me a sense of satisfaction and self esteem. I had accomplished something beyond my wildest expectations and I felt great

"The original intention of exercise was to heal and to maintain health."

Brian Kest,
as told to Philip Self,
Yogi Bare

for having done so. In addition, that sense of accomplishment encouraged me to try other things I'd once thought out of my reach, many of which I also accomplished.

Here are some other reasons I found yoga beneficial and empowering to me:

- Yoga allowed me to *easily* become more limber and flexible (and believe me, I did not know how stiff I'd become until I attempted some of those positions).

- Yoga released pent up tension from my muscles that allowed me to be more relaxed and calm. This gave me a more centered and peaceful feeling even in times of chaos and stress.

- Releasing tension from my muscles allowed a clear pathway for internal energies to flow and unblocked energy centers allowing them to work properly.

- Yoga helped me to build good muscle tone and reduce fat.

- Yoga gave me increased confidence and self-esteem by being able to eventually master (or at least improve my ability on) different yoga positions.

- Yoga also helped me to get in touch with my body—*physically*. (And this is very important for making a connection and for getting in touch with the emotional side of the physical body.) Being able to feel my hamstrings, the stretch of my spine, the flow of my breath, the pull in my shoulders, the ache in my groin, the relaxations of my belly, allowed me to also feel my other senses throughout the day. This pulled me into the present where living takes place and took me away from the imagined future or exaggerated past.

Thus, yoga, or any intense practice similar to it, offers a good means of relief, particularly for releasing and healing from emotional distresses that cannot be dealt with on a conscious level. In addition, it offers a daily discipline that helps maintain a strong, ongoing connection. *(See: Section IV)*

"Practice with me to bring calm, well-being, and vitality to your day. In the beginning, the benefits of these exercises may seem small, but as you continue, I believe you will find the rewards are truly great."

Rodney Yee,
AM PM Yoga

30

FINANCIAL RELIEF

Although our financial standing is not a physical factor in our health, our money worries *are*, and I would be remiss if I didn't at least mention financial relief in this chapter.

As I write this, according to the latest figures available from the Federal Reserve, America's debt has reached nearly two trillion dollars, doubling over the past ten years. Obviously, many of us need relief from this overpowering burden.

If you are deeply in debt, finding the relief you need will not be easy. You will need a dedicated commitment to correct it. Much of our financial standing is entwined amid our beliefs about money. Because of this, many of the exercises in this book will help you rethink how you feel and react towards money. In the meantime, begin looking for ways you can ease your burden one small step at a time and, if necessary, seek professional help. Just as in pain management, accept even small victories of relief and build on them wherever you can.

I would like to share with you how I found my own, small piece of financial relief. My parents had both grown up during the Great Depression and had come from homes where money was always scarce. In turn, they lived frugal lives, rarely splurging on anything that wasn't useful or necessary. When I married, I carried their beliefs and practices with me just as they had. In our lean years, particularly as a stay-at-home mom, my clipping coupons and buying only out of necessity helped us get by. But as we grew more financially secure, my habits didn't change. I remained in an impoverished mindset.

Part of this mindset could also be attributed to my not ever having any money to call my own. In fact, I knew very little about how we spent our money or where. Fortunately, my husband decided to teach me these things. But learning about money did not give me the freedom to make any of our financial decisions, and, more importantly, I never felt I had any right to spend what I saw as *his* money (even though this was an inappropriate belief). Particularly at Christmastime, I would become depressed since I could not even purchase a Christmas gift for him without asking for the money or without feeling as if he'd technically bought his own gift.

"You should never acquire long-term debt for possessions with short-term value."
Suze Orman,
(Paraphrased)

"If we glance around society we are easily able to determine who has abundant thoughts and who does not. Because whoever believes life should be a struggle, struggles. and whoever believes that money always slips through the fingers, never has any."
Susanna Thorpe-Clark,
Changing the Thought

"Over and over again, people talk to me about not having enough money. But there's no place in them for money to live because they don't like it. Why would money come to you. . . if you don't really like it?"
Lynn V. Andrews,
Love and Power

"Many people still believe—not rationally, but in their Tribal 'gut'—that God rewards good behavior financially, and punishes negative behavior the same way."

Carolyn Myss,
Why People Don't Heal

"Don't ever allow a man to be thrifty with you, my dear, or he'll become frugal when it comes to ways of love."

Sybile from *The Spinning Game, A Sedona Story*,
Sunday Larson

"'I am going to start taking an hour or two first thing in the morning to do my writing,' I said to my husband. 'Fine,' he said. He had reached the point where he would agree with whatever to humor the neurotic wife; to him it was just another of my brain farts. But to me it was the most important sentence I ever spoke. With that statement I stopped being a housewife who sometimes stole time to write, and I started being a writer. Conform, go crazy—or become an artist. By becoming a writer—by becoming who I truly was—I became well."

Nancy Springer, author
scsffs.org[3]

Eventually, he gave me a small allowance, telling me, *"I want you to spend this only on yourself and on anything you'd like to have."* For a while, having that twenty dollars a week felt like a million. I bought myself books, CDs, makeup, and other things I'd felt guilty about buying in the past. However, I still faced the same old feelings if I wanted a big ticket item like a new computer. Twenty dollars a week couldn't buy those kinds of things.

I did not want to take a job outside the home, especially after I had started homeschooling my boys. And really, we'd come to a place financially where my working wasn't necessary. But one day, the opportunity came where I could work from home. Since I did computer piecework, it didn't pay very much, but the job brought more than the twenty dollars a week I'd been getting from my husband. This new cash flow permitted me the freedom to continue volunteer work and other activities I enjoyed, something a nine-to-five job wouldn't have allowed, while also giving me the financial freedom I'd often longed for.

Then I made one of the most important decisions I've ever made in my life. I decided the money I earned from this work was *mine*. I opened my own checking account and became the sole proprietor of its means and ends. I also decided to get my own credit card.

My husband and I have never agreed about this. He asked me a perfectly legitimate question more than once, "Why is my money, *our* money, but your money, *your* money?" I could only tell him, "This is how it has to be."

I don't know if he will ever understand the importance of my having my own money because he has no frame of reference to understand what it feels like not having a say in how we spend our money or why. *My money* had to be *my money* in order for me to heal myself both emotionally and financially.

From this small step forward, I still had much to learn in regard to my beliefs about money and in maintaining my rights to it. But, in time, my money has continued to grow. I can buy more than CDs and books. I have earned myself a little piece of freedom and, yes, very gratefully, *relief*.

Later, I will offer more strategies on beliefs and change. Many of them can be applied toward how you feel and respond in financial situations, even though they don't specifically say so. Keep in mind that your financial standing is a reflection of the inner you. In Section IV we will work with reflections and I'll explain how you can unravel their mystery. For now, simply begin in any way you can to find relief for the situation. If money is pulling your health down, then strive diligently for some type of relief and take whatever steps are necessary to find it.

When you find relief, know it will be fleeting until you not only address the physical symptoms but also the underlying emotional ones. The keys presented in this book will help you use your moments of relief to your greatest advantage and further you along a path of wellness.

Before we can talk about those kinds of things, however, we must first start with the basics, the ailment itself, the reason you may be reading this book in the first place. Above all, remember to hold fast to hope. There is an unseen power in such a belief that will keep you going in even the most difficult of times.

"Now faith is the substance of things hoped for, the evidence of things not seen."

Mark 9:24,
King James Version

33

CHAPTER FIVE: HOW TO INTERPRET AN AILMENT

5

EXERCISE 1—HOW TO INTERPRET AN AILMENT

Note: For best results, read through the entire exercise first, then begin. You may choose to record the exercise onto a cassette tape for convenient playback. In addition, please review *Appendix A: How to Do the Word Association Exercises*, before continuing.

Focus on one ailment and symptom at a time as multiple symptoms will produce multiple connections and understandings.

STEP ONE—GO WITHIN

Begin by visualizing the interior of your body and its normal function.

'See' your lungs filling with air, tickling the tiny hairs of your trachea, expanding your chest. 'See' your bones in movement with their corresponding muscles and ligaments. 'See' your heart beating, its chambers opening,

"We are not to deny the presence of the illness or problem, we are simply to deny its power over our divine right to remove it."

Betty J. Eadie,
Embraced by the Light

then closing, and passing blood and oxygen from one ventricle to the next. 'See' your blood flowing through your arteries and veins, exchanging nutrients, nourishing your body throughout.

STEP TWO—VISUALIZE YOUR AILMENT

Now change your focus to 'see' the area or areas where the ailment resides. Begin by comparing normal function to what you imagine is taking place. In this first stage, you are trying to determine what might actually be happening.

Whether a broken bone, body ache, or malignancy, view it with the mind's eye, attempting to understand its malfunction and condition.

STEP THREE—FIND KEY WORDS

Begin to put these thoughts into key words such as 'swollen,' 'burns,' 'throbs,' 'aches.' At first, your impressions will be vague. Keep working on them until they feel more defined.

At the same time, keep clarifying what is really happening. As you focus on what you are truly feeling, you may need to question or restate your initial impressions. You may need to physically touch yourself in the vicinity of the pain in order to verify its position. Don't be surprised if the pain seems to change location to a degree or if your initial impression changes. These are common occurrences and further signs you can learn from this ailment.

> *No, it doesn't seem to be muscular after all, rather it feels more like it's emanating from the bone. . .*
>
> *No, it isn't the full length of the leg as I first thought, rather, it's more in the area of the knee. . .*
>
> *I thought it to be in my ankle, but now I 'see' it is in my foot.*

Using *word association (See: Appendix A)*, begin writing these impressions in the form of key words on index

"They may come as memories or visual images or inner sensations of various kinds. Especially they may state themselves in the form of similes or metaphors in addition to expressing the literal facts of past experience. Let your attitude be receptive enough that the continuity of your life as a whole can present itself to your both in symbolic forms and in literal factual statements."

Ira Progoff,
At a Journal Workshop

36

cards or sticky notes. Let these thoughts take you wherever they will, continuing until the flow falters or an association 'rings true,' then move on to the next step.

Remember, the goal is not to be medically accurate, even though you might be looking with a physician's eye. Rather, the goal is to pick up clues as to the underlying message produced by this symptom or malady.

Feel free to include whatever impressions, feelings, images, or memories that pop into your mind at this time. Although they may not feel related, you may find an unexpected correlation as you move on.

As you go deeper into this interpretive exercise, you will move away from *actualities* and more into *symbolic* correlations and interpretations.

STEP FOUR—ASKING QUESTIONS

As you continue 'seeing' inside yourself and looking at the area of concern, ask yourself the following questions:

a. Can I compare this function to something that takes place in nature? Do plants or animals function in a similar way?

b. Can I find a comparison with a man-made device such as a computer, an automobile, or a manufactured machine?

c. Focus for a moment, trying to understand how this comparison parallels the ailment.

d. Why does nature or this man-made object function in this way?

Look for parallels between how nature functions or the machine works and how this area of focus in your body operates. Then form a symbolic definition of the malady utilizing the images just brought out.

> I see my cancer cells as rebels who have usurped control, going against their natural course and calling.

> My body aches remind me of mini streams of lava flowing over the muscle.

"If it reminds me of that, I wonder if it might function like that—in some way that helps the critter or plant survive?"
Kerry Ruef,
The Private Eye

Because these interpretations are based on at-that-moment impressions and on individual perceptions, two people with the same malady will have two very different symbolic descriptions and, more than likely, very different underlying emotional connections for their ailment.

For example, a friend and I once compared our associations of depression. Mine felt like a balance scale with all the weight placed on one side. In actuality, I'd been suffering from a hormone imbalance. Her impressions led her to symbolize a car stuck in the mud, something she later associated with her relationship towards her father and his holding her back.

Step Five—Going Deeper

Next, ask yourself:

a. What kinds of situations were taking place in my environment at the time this ailment began?

b. Could any of these situations be symbolically described in a similar way as the interpretation of the ailment?

For instance, in the case of my cancer cells 'usurping control,' I later paralleled that description to the control my mother exerted over me. I correlated the 'mini lava flows' of my body aches to hidden stresses in my life ready to 'erupt.'

When my husband complained of swelling in his back, I wondered, 'What causes swelling?' The thought, *Some type of inflammation or irritation,* crossed my mind. I asked myself, 'Are there situations in his life that are irritating him?' (There were.) Even the word 'inflammation' lent to the idea of 'flaming' or 'flaring;' to me, that meant pent-up anger over these situations he needed to release.

Remember, always let your mind take you where it will even if the correlations seem corny or stretched. If your mind brought it forward. . . it might be important.

Step Six—The Connection to Those Around Us

Now, ask yourself:

a. Are there any other occurrences of this malady in my sphere of influence, either now or in my past?

"'What am I feeling? It feels like burning. Burning. . . burning . . . that means anger. What are you angry about? I couldn't think what I was angry about, so I said, 'Well, let's see if we can find out.' I put two large pillows on the bed and began to hit them with a lot of energy. After about twelve hits, I realized exactly what I was angry about . . . When I got through, I felt much better, and the next day my shoulder was fine."

Louise L. Hay,
You Can Heal Your Life

b. Have I seen this malady or something similar in connection with my spouse, children, parents, siblings, relatives, friends, coworkers, or neighbors?

c. Has an occurrence such as this been showing itself prominently in my environment, such as in movies, on television, or in books or magazines I've recently read?

d. Do I see it at the office, at home, or out shopping?

The closer the contact, the more prevailing the occurrences, the stronger and more important the message.

If these situations are as strong in your past as they are in your present, then all the more likely the ailment is tied to a situation that began in the past.

For example, my father had lost a leg. In what some may call coincidence, we later moved next door to a couple where the husband had also had a leg amputated. Our move to this house occurred at the same time I had been hospitalized for severe leg cramps. Legs were definitely a strong *Body Song* for me at that time, and not only were these signs showing strong connections to the present, they were showing visible connections to my past. *(More on this and its full meaning later, in Section III.)*

When you are able to see the connection between your life situations and your ailment, you're ready to move on. You will now need to take action to counter the malfunction mirrored in your life. *(There will be more later in the book to help you with that.)*

In the situation of my cancer, I had to stand up for myself, take back my control, make the decisions and take the actions that were right for me, not as they were dictated to me by others. As soon as I did, my cancer diagnosis and situations changed for the better.

When we react within our environment in accordance with our purpose and counter against those situations which are mirrored by the symbolic messages of our ailments, the symptoms will either miraculously subside or they will coincidentally be brought under control Perhaps:

• *A new treatment or medicine will come to light*

• *A surgical procedure will correct years of hardship*

"When you separate body and soul, you do create an illness of the mind and emotions."
Lynn V. Andrews,
Love and Power

- *A food allergy will be discovered*
- *A vitamin supplement will solve the problem*

The answer will always be in keeping with your beliefs and within the direction that you seek.

> *"I often ask patients to carry out a dialogue with their bodily symptoms or with the organ that is giving them problems, through writing, meditation, or drawing. Sitting with you journal open while being receptive to your thoughts, ask your body what it needs or what it is trying to tell you."*
>
> Christiane Northrup,
> *Women's Bodies,*
> *Women's Wisdom*

STEP SEVEN—SUMMARIZING

Write a brief summary of what you have learned from this exercise and create a list of action steps you can take to counteract any negative or disagreeable situations.

Lastly, ask yourself:

"What actions can I take to improve this situation?"

IF YOU CAN'T FIND THE CONNECTION

Throughout the remainder of this book, you will find more direction on how to dig deeper and find your inner message. In addition, there are three main reasons why you may not yet have found this correlation *(which I guarantee is there)* between an ailment and its underlying connection.

1. If you cannot find the connection between your life situations and your ailment, you may not be looking back far enough into your past.

For quite some time, I struggled to find the meaning of my cancer, which my doctors had diagnosed in 1985. I had a hard time seeing the correlation between my ailment's symbolic meaning and my situations in the mid-1980s. I sensed I'd missed something but had no clue as to what. I eventually remembered my first hint of cancer had actually come in a miraculous and unusual event nine years before my diagnosis.

My mother had an in-home business and a workstation in the spare bedroom on the second floor. We'd been doing some work, and she'd sent me to the basement to retrieve some craft supplies. Downstairs, a full two floors below where my mother sat working, I reached for a box and I heard a voice behind me. *If anyone ever says you have cancer, fear not.*

I turned to see who might be speaking to me, knowing

40

I'd left my mother upstairs, and we were otherwise alone in the house—no one was there. We had no television or radio on at the time, no way anyone could be speaking to me. Yet, this voice sounded as if it were whispering directly in my right ear.

At first, I thought I had imagined it and turned back to look for the supplies. As I reached for the box a second time, I heard the voice again. This time, more distinctly saying, *If anyone ever says you have cancer, fear not.*

I turned again to see who might be speaking. I had no doubt this time that I had heard the voice, nor did I doubt *what* I had heard. The voice was that clear and distinct. Again, no one was there. I remember thinking, *Why would I get cancer? No one in my family has ever had cancer. (My mother later contracted colon cancer.)*

I heard the voice one more time saying, *If anyone ever says you have cancer, fear not, for I am with you.*

As amazing as this may sound, I then turned and went back upstairs as if nothing had happened, and, by the time I reached the top step, I'd totally forgotten the words of the voice. I never told anyone or thought of the incident again until the moment my doctor sat with me in his office and told me that very thing.

So the answer and connections to my ailment were not only to be found in the mid-80s when my ailment became a physical reality, but also back to the time when the hint of them first occurred in the mid-70s. This, at a time when I had not only been warned by what I decided had been an angel but also during the period in my life when my father had died and my mother looked to me to fill his role around the house. I had been put in the position where I'd given over the power of my life to others, something that would later be an important key in my cancer recovery.

I'd found my connection and its deeper inner meaning. I knew that now. Once I found my forgotten memory and its connection to my ailment, its meaning 'rang true.' I uncovered many more understandings about my life at that time—all due to interpreting the symbolic meaning of a symptom.

Another reason you may have not yet discovered an emotional connection to your ailment is:

2. You may have *one symptom* with a *multiple,*

"We are not meant to stay wounded. We are supposed to move through our tragedies and challenges and to help each other move through the many painful episodes of our lives. By remaining stuck in the power of our wounds, we block our own transformation."

Caroline Myss,
Why People Don't Heal and How They Can

"I have come to understand that every time my life goes astray, it's because I'm not listening to my inner voice. That's when I lose my peace of mind, and as a result, I experience intense food cravings. Then I overeat, and it becomes a vicious cycle."

Doreen Virtue,
Constant Craving

complex connection. Sometimes I find that I am 'fortunate' to have one symptom with multiple connections when it's more common to happen the other way around (multiple symptoms with one connection). Weight is often one of those. I find 'weight' can relate to 'waiting.' It can be a 'weighty burden' I've taken on or, just the opposite, a tremendous 'loss' I haven't accepted. Depending on where the weight resides, that part of the body may offer more insight. Are you carrying it in the waist (*waste?*), hips, thighs, buttocks? Just before I 'give birth to an idea' I may gain weight in the stomach. *(See: Appendix B for an example interpretation of an ailment with a complex meaning.)*

3. Another reason for not being able to find the connection between your life situation and an ailment could be due to a *mistaken perception* in your belief system, a belief which may be blocking you from seeing the *Truth*. What is a *mistaken perception*? Turn the page to find out.

CHAPTER SIX: MISTAKEN PERCEPTIONS

6

WHAT IS A MISTAKEN PERCEPTION?

A *mistaken perception* is a deeply ingrained and inappropriate belief about yourself, a particular situation, or another person.

Like a horse wearing blinders, our perception doesn't cause truth not to exist, it simply prevents us from seeing the whole picture and what is already there. Think about that for a minute—what you want might *already be there!*

A friend of mine who teaches journaling and poetry classes taught me the difference between 'Truth' with a capital 'T' and 'truth' with a small 't.'

"Truth with a capital 'T,'" she said, "is what you swear to on the witness stand. It's hard facts. It's the state of how things really are beyond our perception.

"On the other hand," she continued, "truth with a small 't' is the essence of what we remember, clouded by our personal point of view and experience. But truth with a small 't' may not be Truth with a capital 'T.'"

When we become too far removed from Truth, our decision-making process becomes clouded and we no longer

"Defenses are the plans you undertake to make against the truth. Their aim is to select what you approve and disregard what you consider incompatible with your beliefs of your reality."
Foundation for Inner Peace,
A Course in Miracles

see ourselves for who we really are and who we were meant to be. We sidestep our purpose and begin letting go of our dreams. We may make inappropriate decisions or stop moving forward altogether due to confusion and/or fear.

As explained before, doing so causes our innermost core and its purpose to feel threatened. In response, it sends out warning signals in an attempt to regain our attention and get us back on track. These signals may be subtle hints found within our environment or may escalate into more unavoidable warnings experienced as an ailment or 'accidental' injury. Our 'bodies' desperately want us to see the Truth, tirelessly cry out for us to find our way, and offer a means of doing so when we see no other way out.

Let me share a simple example of how finding the Truth within a mistaken perception changed my way of seeing and helped me to instantly find a solution to a problem.

My youngest son is a master of leaving messes. As he left the house one day, I sighed as I noticed a pile of dishes sitting by the sink. I began rinsing them and putting them into the dishwasher. I picked up a blue and white food thermos he'd left behind. I tried to unscrew the blue lid from the white bottom so I could rinse it out, but couldn't get the lid to loosen. I tried with all my might but could not budge the lid.

My other son was in the adjoining room watching television, so I asked him to remove the lid. He tried and tried but he could not get the lid off either. Then, he tipped the thermos on its side holding it up so I could see and asked, "What's wrong with it, anyway?" As he did, something that didn't match my perception flashed before my eyes. Had I been a cartoon character, my eyes would have bulged out of their sockets to stare closely at the thermos. Why was there a huge, gaping hole in the bottom? Because the 'lid' of the thermos was the heat sealed *bottom*, not the lid at all. Since the thermos had been left on the counter upside down, I just *presumed* the thin blue stripe on the top was the lid. My presumption had led to a *mistaken perception*. I had not seen the Truth. Once I knew the Truth, my perception instantly changed. Now I knew why the "lid" wouldn't budge; it wasn't really a lid. The problem had been *instantly* resolved.

Another great illustration of a mistaken perception is the tale of the five blind men and the elephant. Each,

"Truth will correct all errors in my mind."
Foundation for Inner Peace,
A Course in Miracles

"You act, and feel, not according to what things are really like, but according to the image your mind holds of what they are like."
Maxwell Maltz,
Psycho-Cybernetics

44

seeing only with their hands and only that which lay directly in front of them, perceived in truth (small 't') the appearance of the beast. But since none could see the elephant as a whole, none could describe the elephant as he existed in Truth (capital 'T').

WHAT HAPPENS WHEN WE SEE THE TRUTH?

One of my favorite perception stories is about a young wife and a ham. As she prepared the ham for her husband's dinner, she cut off three inches of the end as she had always seen her mother do. But she wondered, why do we do this? So, she called her mother to ask.

The mother stopped to think for a moment and said, "Well, I always cut off that three inches because that's what I'd seen my mother do." They decided to ask the grandmother about it.

The grandmother laughed and said, "Why, that's easy! I only had one pan in those days and it wasn't quite large enough to hold the whole ham. So, I cut off the three inches to make it fit."

Changing your perception changes how you see things and instantly, immediately, changes how you do things. If you are having difficulty dealing with a troubling situation or person in your life, look for a way to change your perception to see the *Truth* of the matter and the situation will change. It's almost magical.

WHY DO WE BELIEVE OUR MISTAKEN PERCEPTIONS?

So, if they are mistaken perceptions, why do we believe them? What causes us to hold fast to something that might not be true? The three main reasons are: *programming* (through education, religious upbringing, and social expectations); *survival tactics* (most often

"And so these men of Indostan, disputed loud and long, each in his own opinion; exceeding stiff and strong, though each was partly in the right; and all were in the wrong!"

John Godfre Saxe,
The Blind Men and the Elephant

"Say not, 'I have found the truth,' but rather, 'I have found a truth.'
Kahlil Gibran,
The Prophet

gained during childhood); and by simply *not having enough information* to make a more educated decision.

PROGRAMMING

My father loved playing mind games. He'd often ask me questions like, "If a tree falls in a forest and no one's there to hear, does it make a sound?"

Sometimes he would ask, pointing to his blue dress shirt, "What color is this?"

"Blue!" I'd blurt out in a hurry. What a silly question. Who couldn't answer that?

His eyes, just as blue as his shirt, would sparkle and dance with anticipation as he would ask his next question. "How do you know it's blue?"

"It is blue," I'd say again, this time not quite as confident. How could it not be blue? What was his trick?

"How do you know it is blue?" he'd ask again, making me rethink my answer.

"But it IS blue," I'd protest.

"You say this is blue because I taught you that it's blue," he said. "Since you were a small child, we pointed to this color and told you, 'This is blue.' In school, your teachers taught 'This is blue.' Your friends, who were taught the same as you, all say, 'This is blue.' You are not saying, 'This is blue,' because you know it to be true, you are merely repeating what you've been told."

"But it IS blue."

Consider for a moment my understanding of the color blue and compare it to this: In 1492 people all over the world believed the world was flat. They believed this with their whole heart and mind and no one could tell them otherwise for they *knew* it was true. . . until Christopher Columbus came back and told of his wonderful discovery.

Imagine how knowing the Truth changed their lives *instantly. . . and forever.*

That's what perception versus Truth is all about. . . it's a powerful magic and it doesn't even require a wand.

SURVIVAL TACTICS

Perceptions don't just happen, they're made. We build them from data we've collected along our life's way. And

"The solution to eliminating unwanted behaviors and establishing personal power which grants control of your life lies first in recognizing that you are a singular example of what you believe."

Nell M. Rodgers,
Puppet or Puppeteer

46

because we've built them through hard work and perseverance, through pain, through suffering, through tears and sweat, we're not readily accepting when it comes time to tear them down. Our mistaken perceptions loom before us like a wall. We begin to fear what we can't see on the other side and, more importantly, we fear what others will think or say or do if we act differently from them. After all, many of the perceptions we hold fast to were established for that very purpose, to protect us in the presence of fear. They were survival tactics.

I can think of no better example of this than in the child's fairy tale about the ugly duckling written by Hans Christian Andersen.

The Ugly Duckling did not know he was a swan. He mistakenly believed he was an ugly duck. He believed this with his whole heart and without a doubt because this is what he'd been taught *since the day of his birth*. His mother told him he was an ugly duck. His siblings said he was an ugly duck, and all the animals on the farm referred to him as 'an ugly duck.' Thus, the Ugly Duckling had no way to see his perception could be wrong because he had no one to show him he might be something other than what he'd been constantly told. Like my father had tried to teach me, the Ugly Duckling had continually been programmed and had his belief reinforced by all those around him.

Why do some countries, religions, schools—even parents—strive for separation from those unlike themselves? Because it reinforces the beliefs they wish to impose. Thus, the Ugly Duckling was not living in Truth nor in doing so was he being True to himself. Alas, how could he when lies were all the Ugly Duckling knew? How can any of us? The Ugly Duckling had yet to learn how to break free from this restrictive mold. He had fallen victim to his own survival tactic.

You see, as long as the Ugly Ducking continued to believe what he had been told, he carried with him a sense of security that protected him from a harsh reality his young mind was not yet able to accept or fully understand. He needed that secure sense, no matter how false it might have been, in order to survive those early, difficult days.

So when he finally fled the farm, he carried with him the seeds they had implanted within him so that even

"We do not like to acknowledge that a situation is other than we would like it to be. So we kid ourselves. . . . and because we will not see the truth, we cannot act appropriately."
Maxwell Maltz,
Psycho-Cybernetics

"Then [he] ran away, flying over the hedge fence, and making the little birds in the bushes fly up in fear. 'That is because I am so ugly!' thought the Duckling."
Hans Christian Andersen,
The Ugly Duckling

> "Cried the Hen, 'You have nothing to do and that's why you have such fancies. Purr or lay eggs, and such notions will pass away."
>
> Hans Christian Andersen,
> *The Ugly Duckling*

> ". . . many of us are living the lives and dreams imposed upon us by our family, friends, and society. Once we understand the fears, frustrations, and loyalties that sabotage our dreams and best efforts at personal growth, we can free ourselves from doubt and defeat and find out what we really want to do with our lives."
>
> Lindsay C. Gibson,
> *Who You Were Meant To Be*

though he had escaped the cruelty of the farm, he had not yet escaped their messages. Those lies followed him wherever he went, sprouting up like weeds because he furthered them. And the more the Ugly Duckling believed those words about himself, the more he acted out his beliefs, thus causing others he met to believe them too.

As part of his journey, the Ugly Duckling came to an old, falling-down shack. Inside lived an old woman, a cat, and a hen. They took the Ugly Duckling in and allowed him to stay with them, but if ever the Ugly Duckling spoke of swimming—the one thing he loved to do more than anything else—the old woman, cat, and hen chided him for wanting to do something so repulsive.

How often in our lives do we hold back from doing the one thing we wanted more than anything else for fear of what others might think or do? This was the case for the Ugly Duckling. He tried to obey the wishes of the old woman, cat, and hen, and held his tongue about swimming as much as he could, but didn't often succeed for his desire was too great.

In addition, because the Ugly Duckling lived under the constant influence of these three non-swimmers, he began to doubt the validity of his desires. He believed their words and, sadly, believed something must be wrong with *him* and his need.

When the Ugly Duckling realized that, right or wrong, his desire to swim could no longer be ignored, he left the old woman, cat, and hen and the safety of the old shack to face the world and a cruel hard winter alone. Eventually, the Ugly Duckling decided he had nothing left to live for. He saw a beautiful flock of swans land across the pond and decided to swim over to them. He believed they would be so repulsed by his looks that they would peck him to death and end his misery.

As he reached the swans and bowed his head awaiting the worst, he saw his reflection in the water. For the first time, he recognized he wasn't an ugly duckling at all but a beautiful swan.

That very second, the Ugly Duckling was freed from his mistaken perception and his life changed instantly and dramatically—forever.

Stop for a moment and think about the powerful impact and change this recognition had on the Ugly

48

Duckling's life. What had formerly been filled with hardship and futility, changed instantly—*INSTANTLY*.

Remember, the Ugly Duckling did not physically change in any way at that moment. What changed was *how he saw himself*.

Make no mistake about it, the Ugly Duckling had been born a swan. He was *always* a swan, but *he never knew it*. He could never have accepted it as Truth before that moment. His mistaken perception prevented him from doing so just as ours prevents us.

Who could we be if we could only see beyond the shroud we've draped around ourselves? What could we accomplish? What goals could we reach?

We need only change our perception to do so. We need only remove the blinders that we wear. Test your beliefs. Are they Truth with a capital 'T' or truth with a small 't'? Read on to learn more!

Our First Glimpse of Truth—A Light in the Darkness

In June of 1996 as I waited to turn into a shopping mall, my van was rearended. After the collision, my injuries seemed to worsen day by day while my sons, who had been in the vehicle with me, had no complaints whatsoever. *Why?* Even my physician could not explain it.

In search of answers and relief from my pain, I read John Sarno's book, *Healing Back Pain*. When I read the following passage, I felt as if an alarm bell had gone off inside me. He simply said:

> *"Invariably those patients who have a gradual onset of pain will attribute it to a physical incident that may have occurred years before, like an automobile or skiing accident. Because in their minds back pain is 'physical,' that is 'structural,' it must be due to an injury. As far as they are concerned there 'has to be' a physical cause. This idea is one of the great impediments in the way of recovery. It must be*

"And the great swans swam round [him] and stroked [him] with their bills. . . . and the old swans bowed their heads before [him]."

Hans Christian Andersen,
The Ugly Duckling

"Seventy percent of all patients who come to physicians could cure themselves if they only got rid of their fears and worries. Don't think for a moment that I mean that their ills are imaginary. . . . Their ills are as real as a throbbing toothache and sometimes a hundred times more serious."

Dr. O. F. Gober as told to Dale Carnegie in *How to Stop Worrying and Start Living*

49

resolved in the patient's mind or the pain will persist."

Could the suffering be all in my mind? I thought about that during my pain sessions. I would ask myself, *"Is this pain from the accident? Or is there some other cause I've yet to see?"*

Though I did not yet know how to change my mistaken perceptions, an enlightening thought had settled into my mind.

I continued to face many difficult days and it took me a long time to totally understand all I needed to know, yet that flash of knowledge became the key I needed to press forward. From that simple discovery, I continued to question my beliefs and to ask if they were *truth* with a small 't' or *Truth* with a capital 'T.'"

"But if you have accepted an idea—from yourself, your teachers, your parents, friends, advertisements—or from any other source, and further, if you are firmly <u>convinced</u> that idea is <u>true</u>, it has the same power over you as the hypnotist's words have over the hypnotized subject."

Maxwell Maltz,
Psycho-Cybernetics

HOW DO WE RELEASE A MISTAKEN PERCEPTION IF WE DON'T KNOW IT'S THERE?

If we totally believe something with our whole heart and mind and have every reason to believe it is true, how do we discover whether or not it is a mistaken perception?

Ask.

Many years ago, I came to a crossroads in my life where I had a desire to know myself and my beliefs better. Over a period of weeks, I wrote them down.

It surprised me to see how many of them were based not on personal experience but on what others had told me—*even if my experience and the belief conflicted!*

Only then did I remember what my father had taught me about the color blue—that many of our beliefs are merely social and habitual programming. They are not Truth with a capital 'T,'" but rather, truth with a small 't.'

By the time I had made these conclusions, my father had long since passed away. I could not call him on the phone and say, "Dad, you were right!" But I could change what I believed, and I did.

We cannot alter who we are, but we can alter what we believe about ourselves and the world around us. As you

"One thought change invites another. A necessary first step to transformation is to do something—anything—different."

Nell M. Rodgers,
Puppet or Puppeteer

can see from the tale of the Ugly Duckling, perception alone can create a powerful and instantaneous change.

Question your beliefs. Ask yourself the questions that follow. In doing so, find out *specifically* what you believe about these things and write them down. Putting a belief into writing forces you to clarify an otherwise vague thought. You will be surprised by how different a belief feels in writing. You will find you have an inner sense while putting your belief into words, allowing you to discern the difference between a belief in Truth (capital 'T') and a belief in truth (small 't'). When you read what you have written, your internal senses will allow you to feel whether what you have written is complete, honest, or still lacking in truth. *(See Section IV, Connection, for more on this feeling sense.)*

You may also be surprised by how vague your beliefs actually were before writing them down even though you may have believed you understood them perfectly while holding the ideas in your mind. This is because the brain has an alternative language that quickly interprets feelings and essences into its own personal code, enhancing our ability to think quickly and effectively. In writing, these coded images and feelings have to be drawn out and defined. They can no longer exist in the brain's code without being fully described. This descriptive detailing clarifies your beliefs.

If, after completing the following exercise, you want to do additional work on your belief system, I highly recommend Dr. Nell M. Rodgers' book, *Puppet or Puppeteer: You Hold the Key to the Life You Really Want.* In addition, you might consider Carol Adrienne's meditation tape, *Overcoming Obstacles*, which directs the listener to visualize a belief and to recognize that it can be released for a new one.

"Consider the fact that every sight, sound, smell, taste, or sensation you have ever received—either consciously or paraconsciously—is like a tiny radiant centre with millions of associations emanating from it. Now think about trying to note down all these associations."
Tony Buzan,
The Mind Map Book

EXERCISE 2–QUESTION YOUR BELIEFS

Ask yourself the following questions. Make sure to answer them in writing. A first set follows for your general beliefs, while the second set focuses in on single, more specific beliefs. Give yourself several days (or weeks) to answer and reflect upon your answers.

PART ONE—OUR GENERAL BELIEFS

When I first started looking at my belief system, I wrote out a general list of beliefs in my journal. I asked myself about the following beliefs:

- What do I believe about Illness? Injuries? Death?
- What do I believe about Education? Government?
- What are my beliefs concerning Religion? God?
- What are my beliefs about Love? Sex? Marriage?
- What beliefs do I have about my loved ones?
- What beliefs do I hold on to about myself?
- How have my beliefs affected my life?

PART TWO—DISPELLING A BELIEF

Let me share another story about a mistaken perception. A few years ago, my husband took the boys on a white-water rafting trip, leaving me home to write. The quiet was glorious. I was thoroughly enjoying my time alone. Mid-week, I made a quick trip to see my chiropractor for a routine adjustment. As he went through the process of realigning my spinal column, he noticed the lymph node on my right arm was unusually enlarged.

As a cancer survivor, I knew that any abnormality in a lymph node wasn't good. I'd been cancer free for a long time. I thought of all that would transpire now. Just for my M.D. to evaluate the problem, would require countless tests, days in the hospital, sleepless nights, and stress for the entire family. As I relived all I'd been through the first time, I couldn't bring myself to call the doctor. In all honesty, I decided that if I'd come this far just to fall down again, I didn't want to go on. I knew at the very least that I didn't want to go the traditional route again, so I didn't make the call to the M.D.

Twenty-four hours passed. I woke to a new day. I felt good, but still noticed the sore spot on my arm. I walked into the bathroom to brush my teeth and hair and that's when it hit me.

Two days before—the day before I had gone to the chiropractor—I had frosted my hair. I'd had a particularly hard time trying to both see and pull the strands of hair through the cap. I'd ended up sitting backwards on the sink, alternating holding the hand mirror and crochet hook in my right hand—the same arm that was sore. All in all, it had taken me quite a long time to get all the hair pulled through. I'd sat there for a couple of hours and, at one point, had even started over trying to get it just right. No wonder my arm hurt!

Suddenly, everything made sense. I had simply strained my arm doing my hair. I wasn't dying. I wasn't facing months of treatment. I'd merely jumped to conclusions and distorted my perception. My beliefs were such that I couldn't see the Truth. My mind automatically just presumed it must be cancer.

A simple question, "Could my lymph node become enlarged for any other reason?" might have saved me hours of worry.

Ask the following questions to clarifying a belief:

- What is my belief?

- Why do I think/fear/do this?

- How did I acquire this belief?

- When did I start believing it?

- Can I disprove this belief? Could there be any other explanation?

- What do others believe about it?

- Do my beliefs match my experience?

- If it weren't for this particular belief, how would my life be different?

Note: Don't be surprised when you discover that one belief often hinges upon another. You will need to explain and define each belief brought forward in order to find the real Truth you are seeking from this exercise. For best results, always write down the first thing that comes into your mind, then ponder it, clarify it, restate it.

"The important thing is not to stop questioning."
Albert Einstein

COULD THERE BE ANOTHER WAY OF THINKING?

In the book *Psych-K: the Missing ~~Piece~~ Peace in Your Life*, Robert M. Williams discusses perception in a story he tells about a fly on a window, trapped, and desperately trying to get out. The fly can see outside, but it can't break through the glass, and it can't see the open door just yards away.

So many times in my life I felt just like that fly. I would try to accomplish something only to be held back. I could feel it right within my reach but couldn't seem to grasp it. Why?

Was I trying to break through glass when an open door lay just yards away? What couldn't I see?

In trial proceedings, the jury is asked if the criminal is guilty *beyond a shadow of a doubt*. Many of our beliefs can be blown full of holes yet we continue to hold steadfast to them. Before we can break free of the invisible grasp they have on our lives, we must open ourselves to new possibilities. We must learn to think differently.

In her book, *Embraced by the Light*, Betty Eadie describes her near-death experience, including a point where she encounters a drunkard. Her angelic guide explains how this man's state of being would indirectly serve an honorable purpose. Later, the drunkard would be seen by an attorney who, in turn, would be inspired to do greater works in helping others. The guide explains to Eadie that the two had made an agreement prior to coming to earth about helping each other in this way.

When we see how other people in our lives, even those who cause us irritation, are there for a reason, they take on a whole new perspective. *We* take on a whole new prospective. Our lives are changed simply because we took one small step in thinking differently.

One of my mentors helped me to see how the people in my life were acting as a mirror, showing me aspects of myself I needed to see in order to improve my life and grow beyond my present boundaries. When I learned how to see myself reflected in others, I started seeing them and their actions differently. How could I condemn *them* when they were showing me something I did myself? I will explain *mirrors* in more detail later in the book. For now, the impor-

"Be not forgetful to entertain strangers: for thereby some have entertained angels unawares."
Hebrews 13:2,
King James Version

"There are angels that walk among you that you are unaware of."
Betty Eadie,
Embraced by the Light

tant thing is to understand there may be another way of seeing, even if the present belief seems obvious and without flaw. There may be an open door just yards away from where you are banging your head on the closed window.

Morty Lefko explains in his book, *Re-Create Your Life*, how, when we form beliefs, we do so based only on the information available to us at the time, particularly when we are children. As we grow and mature, we learn there may have been other explanations for what happened to us, explanations we might not have been able to perceive at the time due to immaturity or a lack of knowledge.

Unfortunately, by now, the long-held belief may be programmed into our subconscious where we no longer see it—just like the horse with blinders or the fly against the closed window. So we don't realize we need to reprogram that belief or, in other words, release the mistaken perception. How can we release it if we don't know it is there?

But this is where our *Body's Songs*, our maladies, offer us a clue. We may not see the mistaken perception, but we will recognize pain. The pain we feel can be an indicator of the error in our belief. Think again of the fly beating itself relentlessly against the closed window. Wouldn't that hurt? And how many times must it suffer that pain before it realizes it should go in a different direction? And won't the pain continue to increase the more it tries to forcefully go about its flight in the same mistaken direction? (I don't know if flies can feel pain, I'm only thinking in terms of if I were continually banging my head against a solid, unmoving pane of glass—doesn't it feel that way sometimes?)

Now, here is where we are often tricked. The symptom of this pain—the pain of beating our head against the glass—is clear to see and understand. We have (perhaps) a headache. We go to the doctor. He gives us a pill. That blocks the pain. But it does not stop us from beating our head against the glass. The only way to truly stop the pain is to stop hitting the glass with our head, and to do that we must think differently, we must go in another direction. We must see through our mistaken perception—the one telling us that the closed window is the direction we want to go—and see, instead, a new way. But how do we find it?

"... *fundamental beliefs about yourself and about life (the kind of beliefs that shape your self-esteem) are usually formed before the age of six, based on early interactions with parents and other primary caretakers.*"
Morty Lefko,
Re-create Your Life

"*He who can believe himself well, will be well.*"
Ovid,
Metamorphoses, 43 BC

Truth in its highest form cannot be contradicted. So, if we can find even one alternative explanation or opposing contradiction to our belief, we have proven that our perception *could* be flawed, leaving room for error. If there is the possibility of error, there is room for change in our viewpoint because we may not be seeing entirely in Truth.

How many murder mysteries begin from the premise of the accused standing over the victim, holding the smoking gun, only to be proven later that someone else had been the true perpetrator? Our belief—our truth—is often witnessing the accused over the dead body. We call them "guilty" without looking thoroughly at the facts.

The book *A Course in Miracles* asks its readers to meditate on the verse, "I see only the past," and teaches that we form many of our beliefs and perceptions based merely upon what we knew or experienced in the past, which is not based on what is happening to us right here and now.

When you analyze a perception or belief and discover an alternative answer, one you had not considered before— maybe even several, remind yourself that you made the best decision possible at the time based on the information you then held. But now, your belief or perception may no longer be useful. It may be time to release it and let it go.

We pick up perceptions like germs. We hear a television commercial and a perception is formed. A friend makes a comment and a perception is formed. We read an article in a magazine or the newspaper and a perception is formed. For every story, there is another side, another point of view. Perceptions have different viewpoints too.

There could be an alternative explanation for the pain I suffered after my automobile collision. The muscle and body aches could have been associated with the found spinal misalignment. They could have been contributed to by a hormonal and low thyroid imbalance. These pains could have been heightened from stress or psychosomatic conditions. They might have stemmed from food allergies. The fact is, there are so many different alternatives, there is no way to really know either through medical or psychiatric means what *actually* caused this pain. The only certain conclusion is there isn't any one conclusion.

So, how can I wholeheartedly believe in any one of them without doubt? And if there is room for doubt, I must

". . . the problem was automatically enlarged and amplified: by going into the library of my mind and retrieving all past experiences labeled 'Rejection,' I was experiencing a lifetime of accumulated events rather than simply the one in the present moment."

Stephen Wolinsky,
Trances People Live

release all beliefs I have held about this pain, for Truth holds no doubt.

Being free and open to not only accepting other explanations, including an underlying emotional connection, I am also in a position to recognize that my pain may not actually have physically existed at all—*except in my mind*.

That's a scary thought, I know. The pain in every sense felt real. For nights on end, month after month, this pain woke me in the middle of the night, robbed me of sleep, prevented me from enjoying simple pleasures in life, blocked me from working, and stopped me from doing even basic chores around the house. The thought that what had totally debilitated my life could be *all in my mind* felt absurd and unacceptable. So, I continued to look for healing from the medical community even though it did no good. The fact remained that until I began to look at what I'd been hiding *within* my body, my body couldn't begin to heal and stop suffering from pain.

EXERCISE 3—DECONSTRUCTING OUR BELIEFS

Our perceptions—beliefs—can be deconstructed, taken apart, analyzed, and rebuilt with Truth. Here's how:

STEP ONE—WRITE OUT THE BELIEF

Write out the belief or your perceived truth. Make sure to both state the belief *and* why you perceive it as truth. For example:

> *Because my pain began in conjunction with my automobile collision, and worsened over the next year and a half, my belief is that my backache stemmed from the accident in 1996.*

STEP TWO—DISPROVE THE BELIEF

You are now asked to find any means where you can disprove this belief. Stephen Hawking and other promi-

". . . my sickness is my belief, and my belief is my mind; therefore all disease is in the mind or belief."

Phineas Parkhurst Quimby,
Is Disease a Belief?

57

nent scientists believe anyone can find evidence to support a belief, but when we find evidence against it, that's when our perception of the situation changes. Remember, Truth (with a capital 'T') has no doubt, no alternative, no other possibility. Einstein knew this and thus in proving any theory, he first attempted to *disprove* it.

Thus I wrote:

> *There could be an alternative explanation for the pain I suffered after the automobile collision. The muscle and body aches could have been associated with the found spinal mis-alignment or they could have been contributed to by a hormonal and low thyroid imbalance. These pains could have heightened from stress or psychosomatic conditions. They might have even stemmed from food allergies.*

STEP THREE—EXPLORE NEW POSSIBILITIES

Did you find any other possibilities? Like the Ugly Duckling looking down into the water and really seeing himself for the first time, you have now come to a place where real growth and change can take place, often instantaneously. And I wrote:

> *The Truth, as I see it now, is there are so many different alternatives, there is no way to really know either through medical or psychiatric means what actually caused this pain. The only certain conclusion is that there isn't any one conclusion. Therefore, my search for Truth continues, but I suspect in knowing this new information that even the collision itself was no accident. Being hit from behind and suffering in all that I did from that point forward, began from an inner emotional connection I had not yet been able to see. Meaning, my pain did not stem from my injury, no matter how much agony I caused myself to feel. Rather the more*

58

intense the pain, the more strongly my Body's Songs were desperately trying to get me to see what I'd refused to see up until that point. I had become as the fly against the glass, fighting to go in a direction closed to me and not seeing a wide passageway open to me.

Keep in mind that we give tremendous credence to our physical pain, we take notice of it, medicate it, cut at it with surgeries. Why then do we not accept that what hurts us emotionally from deep within our core might also create some signal, some sign of its distress? Is it so impossible to believe that what lies in the mind alone can not grieve, ache, cry out in pain? Thus, if we say *it's all in my mind*, that does not discount its ability to cause us real physical pain nor mean in any sense that it is not real.

From a room down the hall, I heard my father cry out in pain from a leg he no longer had. While his doctors tried to convince us that these were merely phantom pains, I assure you that to my father, my mother, and myself, they were very real. And yet, how can a leg that is not there cause pain?

You may not yet know what the Truth is, what you do know is what it isn't. You now must go in search of a new answer and a new belief and in doing so, return here again and again to test that belief until you find the Truth. I will not leave you to wander this journey alone. I have more, much more, to lead you along that way.

In addition to the information that follows in subsequent chapters, remember these points:

1. Recognize your state or condition is only a belief and beliefs can be changed.

2. Separate what you see with your eyes from what you feel within. Understand that your perception has connected the two, but they are not connected other than in your mind.

3. Work with what you feel apart from what you see, interpreting your feelings on their emotional level.

"In some strange way, the limb is still there, still a part of the body, and in a sometimes not-so-subtle way. True, it's gone physically, but the patients remain adamant about one thing: the missing limb is still 'out there,' still a part of their most intimate being. That's why it's called a phantom."

Thomas Walker,
The Force Is With Us

4. Design a plan to counter and balance any negative findings and continue to enhance and support any positive findings based on your interpretations.

SECTION TWO: COMMITMENT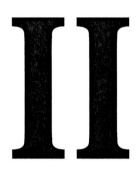

"It is a common belief in many circles that a person doesn't make the necessary changes in his or her life until the pain has gotten so great that they finally have to make the necessary alterations, overcome their fears, and just do so."

Tom Bird,
~~Write~~ Right From God

CHAPTER SEVEN: COMMITMENT, DEDICATION, AND DISCIPLINE

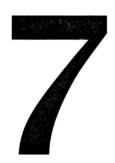

If you have repressed your purpose and desire to the extent that you are now experiencing physical symptoms, then you more than likely have a strong barrier or fear standing in your path. In order to press through to total well-being, you will need a dedicated *commitment* to take action towards overcoming that fear and achieving your goal and purpose.

A dedicated *commitment* is evidenced by a person who presses on towards their desired goal despite the consequences they face. An example of this was shown when the Ugly Duckling left the old woman's shack to pursue his desire to swim. He readily left behind the shack's safety and warmth, knowing the fulfillment of his deepest heart's desire meant more to him.

Without commitment, we quickly turn back when the going gets tough. Commitment propels an Olympic runner to go that extra meter faster and stronger than his nearest opponent. Commitment brings a climber to the top of Mount Everest. Commitment binds a long-lasting relationship, and commitment holds fast the caregiver when their patient dies in their arms. Commitment is also the

"To continue believing in yourself, believing in the doctors, believing in the treatment, believing in whatever I chose to believe in, that was the most important thing, I decided. It had to be."

Lance Armstrong,
It's Not About the Bike

difference between talking about doing some thing and *actually doing it.*

COMMITMENT IS PERSISTENCE AND DETERMINATION

When my oldest son was two, I parked my shopping cart within arm's reach of a large stuffed animal display at a local toy store. In the split second I turned my head, he plucked a large, shaggy lion from the shelf. At first I thought it was cute. He certainly had chosen an adorable animal. But when I tried to make him put it back, he clamped down on that lion with both arms and refused to let go. No amount of convincing, pulling, or threatening could change his mind. The harder I tried to take the lion, the louder and stronger he protested. He had never been an unruly child; his determination caught me off guard. We ended up buying the lion even though in those days it cost more than we could really afford.

That, to me, is commitment defined.

Commitment is about determination, persistence, and, sometimes, strength, but it's also about the choices we make every day—conscious or otherwise—that either enhance the quality of our lives or extinguish them.

Making conscious choices and sticking to them is a difficult, ongoing process. The only way we can remain committed is by first understanding the four vital components involved in such a commitment. Those four components are: *Recognition, Responsibility, Forgiveness, and Discovery.*

RECOGNITION AND CHOICES

Recognize that a commitment is a conscious choice made with our full awareness. Every moment of the day we are making choices for ourselves. We make decisions about what to wear, what to eat, how to face the day. We decide how to respond to our spouse when he or she says, "Good morning." We decide how to react to the neighbor's

"Let's get very clear that we need to pay attention to what we expect, since that's what we're going to get."

Sue Christensen,
Making a Six-Figure Income on Your Terms

64

dog who has once again spilled the garbage all over our lawn during the night.

Before we have gone through even one hour of our day, we have made countless choices—many of which will determine our outlook and expectation for the hours yet to come—never realizing we've done so, never taking the slightest pause to wonder how our lives might differ if we'd chosen another way. In fact, we often make important, life-affecting choices without even recognizing we've made any choice at all.

CHOOSING OUR ATTITUDE

The first time I had conscious recognition that my attitude might be as important as any other decision I made in my life occurred some ten years into my marriage.

One night, six o'clock came and went without my husband coming home from work as he usually did without fail. Of course, this happened before everyone had cell phones so that when people were away from their desks and in their cars, they were truly out of communication. We lived in the country, so finding a phone might have meant quite a walk if he had a flat tire or breakdown.

At first, I became angry. *Why hadn't he called? Where could he be? Didn't he realize dinner would be ruined?* As time passed, anger turned into worry. I fed the boys and sent them to play in their room. Still no sign of him.

After worry, came fear. *What if he never came home? What if I had to raise the boys alone? How would I pay the bills, afford college, just plain survive?* Still he didn't come home. I tried the office line again and again. No one picked up the phone.

By now, nearly two hours had passed without a word. I didn't know what to think. I'd already raced through every emotion I knew. Then I did something I had never consciously done before.

I began to practice what I would say when and if he came home. I played the scenario over and over in my head playing both my role and his and acting out on my mind's stage all I planned to say and his reaction to it.

I role-played first anger, then worry, then fear—then love. I imagined his reaction to each one. And, because I

"Now we have the opportunity to use the conscious power of our minds to create self-love, abundance, freedom, and joy in our lives."

Shakti Gawain,
Reflections in the Light

had plenty of time to think this through, I asked myself what kind of reaction I really wanted from him in return.

Easy! I wanted to know what had happened; I wanted to know he was safe; I wanted to know that he still loved me. It didn't take rocket-scientist thinking to imagine how he would react if I greeted him with anger, worry, fear, or third-degree questioning; I wouldn't get the response I desired. Only by greeting him with love and appreciation would I get the response I desired.

Once I had decided I would respond with love, the universe responded in kind with the sound of the automatic garage door opening. He was home!

I never asked why he'd been late. I just greeted him with my usual hug and "Hello." He looked tired and said nothing while removing his shoes, hanging up his coat, and changing into more comfortable clothes.

I suggested we eat in the sitting room on TV trays where it would be more relaxing and quiet. As he ate, he talked in great detail about all that had transpired, including the unexpected meeting at the end of the day when an important employee had threatened to quit. Obviously, the last thing he'd needed after such a trying day would have been an angry, nagging wife. Instead, we had a very enjoyable evening, perhaps more so than any we'd had in a long time. In fact, after that night, we planned for more evenings where we could share just such a quiet dinner alone. None of that would have happened had I chosen not to respond to the situation in Truth and love.

I learned a great lesson that night and have continued to think out my reactions ever since. I now know I can *choose* how others will respond to me simply by how I respond to them. I find that whenever I choose to respond in anger, fear, or worry, I receive the same type of response in return, and I'm always sorry I didn't stop myself when I knew I had the chance.

PERCEPTION

Our perception of ourselves directs us to find what we *believe* we will find. Think about that for a minute. If I *believe* I am lucky, then I am looking for luck, and I will

". . . because it is your energy, eventually that energy, that negative energy you have been producing, must return to you. This is the law of the universe."
Rosemary Altea,
You Own the Power

"Your focus is your reality."
Yoda,
Star Wars

66

find it. If I *believe* bad things always happen to me, I am looking for them and. . . (See where I'm going with this?) Exactly!

This governs not only how we present ourselves, but also how we perceive our environment and all that is around us. Whether or not we realize it, our perception of ourselves, our choices, and our actions are a reflection of our inner beliefs and that's why our choices play a strong role in any commitment we make.

What we seek, we find. Always. Don Quixote saw raging knights that in Truth were nothing more than rotating windmills. Our perception and our choices color everything we see. Learn to recognize the choices you make on a daily basis. Learn to see how those choices not only affect your physical being but reach down into the core of who you are.

If no obvious choice shows itself to me, I make one up. I ask myself which I prefer. My made-up choices are sometimes harder to decide than the real ones actually confronting me, but they help me see that I *do* have a choice, even if the answer may be obvious to me.

For example, after the birth of my second son, my husband told me he didn't want me to have any more children because he thought I might die if I did. (I'd nearly bled to death both times.) I asked myself:

> *"How much do I want another child? Am I willing to risk dying to have one? What good would that serve? Or, am I willing to relent in order to better assure myself that I will be around to finish raising the two boys I already have?"*

Posing my own choices helped me to see why I made the decisions I did and to understand more clearly who I really am. Recognizing my choices offered me many opportunities to improve my life and to see how many choices were available to me every day.

Through this process, I'm able to see that even if I *think* I don't have a choice, I do. However, some of my choices are more obscure. For example, not every choice is a decision between what's right or wrong. Sometimes I must choose between two *right* answers. I didn't always

"So saying, he gave the spur to his steed Rocinante, heedless of the cries his squire Sancho sent after him, warning him that most certainly they were windmills and not giants he was going to attack. He, however, was so positive they were giants that he neither heard the cries of Sancho, nor perceived, near as he was, what they were. "Fly not, cowards and vile beings," he shouted, "for a single knight attacks you." A slight breeze at this moment sprang up, and the great vanes began to move."
Miguel de Cervantes,
Don Quixote (1605)

recognize that. I would worry about making the wrong decision when really there wasn't one.

Sometimes our choices are limited not by our actions but by our morals and values. I've often committed to a choice that's more socially acceptable. These choices are strongly embedded from our upbringing, such as giving a gift to Mom on Mother's Day or spending Thanksgiving with the family back home. While I may recognize I *could* choose to skip Mom's gift or traveling this year, that choice is considered socially unacceptable to me. It doesn't matter which choice I make as long as I simply recognize that it *is* a choice.

Commitment is a decided choice. I can choose to believe and respond to my body, its reactions, and all the situations around me with an attitude that I will press through, find a better way, and find healing on all levels, or I can be what my one friend calls *"a miserable person who wants to stay that way."*

MOUTH CONFESSION

My oldest son came into my office one day. He said, "Mom, you missed Pink's biography on television last night."

"Was it good?"

He got a puzzled look on his face. He said, "Do you know, she never told her friends 'I *wish* I were a rock star' but always said '*When* I am a rock star. . . .'"

"When are *you* going to start talking like that about *your* dreams?" I asked.

"Right away," he said.

He had learned a valuable lesson about the power of *how* we say things. My father-in-law knew this and had been the one to teach it to me. From the time we first met until his death in 1998, he constantly reminded us about what he called *mouth confession*. He knew how our spoken words condemned or revived us and often caught us in the act of speaking negative statements.

How often have you heard yourself or a loved one say any of the following?

I am so dumb that I . . .

"I saw how a person's words affect the energy field around him. The very words themselves —the vibrations in the air— attract one type of energy or another."

Betty J. Eadie,
Embraced by the Light

"It is very important for all of us to notice how we limit ourselves by limiting the meaning of words."

Stephen J. Wolinsky,
The Dark Side of the Inner Child

Knowing my bad luck, I'll . . .

I will never be that (rich, thin, smart, lucky).

I could never do that.

They would never choose me for . . .

We even wish ill health on ourselves by saying things such as:

I must be getting Alzheimer's, I can't remember anything these days.

STOP IT!

Stop it right now! There might be many things on the road to total well-being that will take time, effort, and even a change of heart. But making a determined choice to speak positively and lovingly is one small step you can take right now that will have a tremendous and immediate impact on your life.

Remember to always keep in mind that what we speak becomes a part of our perception of ourselves—a part of our belief system even if we know on the surface it is not true. Don't fall back into the mistaken perceptions you've begun to shake off. Stop yourself now from making negative statements.

As a people, we have become so accustomed to negative language, we accept it as a kind of love. In the 60s and 70s, Henry Harlow did studies on monkeys, including one study where monkeys did not receive loving affection from their mothers but, instead, shocks and slaps from a mechanical surrogate. The study showed that monkeys accepted those times of punishment as 'love' and taught the same to their children in turn.

We do the same thing with some of the horrible things we say to those we love even though we mean them in jest. We say, "You're so dumb," (or blind, or old). We laugh about these things. They laugh with us—and agree! We accept

". . . whether it's high vibrational joy, or low vibrational worry, what we're vibrationally offering in any moment is what we're attracting back."

Lynn Grabhorn,
Excuse Me, Your Life Is Waiting

"These little monkeys would be frightened away by brass spike mom—and yet it was she they turned to for comfort. . . . No matter how abusive the mothers were, the babies persisted in returning. They returned more often, they reached and clung and coaxed far more frequently than the children of normal mothers."

Deborah Blum,
Love at Goon Park

69

their negative remarks as a sign of their love. We don't see that their words are like a kind of invisible fly swatter that we are constantly whacked with first on the right cheek and then on the left. We accept those stinging blows, we return them with a smile, and add a blow from our own invisible swatter. "Whack, whack, whack." We surely must be scarred by all those 'love taps,' but we keep right on doing it anyway because it's all we know and because no one's ever taken the time to tell us to stop.

The next time you recognize the swatter's blow, take the time to visually see the fly swatter in their hand (or yours). Once you've 'seen' the swatter, you'll stop using it and you'll stop accepting the blows.

In this world, you already receive a tremendous amount of negative energy. Don't add to that negativism by speaking to those you love and care about with more negative words.

Don't tear *yourself* down either, especially out loud. Do you remember the story of Cinderella? When she first heard about the Prince's upcoming dance, she gathered together bits of trim and lace found around the house. She used these bits of forgotten decoration to make herself a beautiful dress. When her evil stepsisters saw the gown she had made, they pulled off the trimmings and trappings one by one until nothing remained of the dress except tatters.

Criticisms and negativity have the same effect on our body's countenance as Cinderella's stepsisters had on her dress. The stinging blows leave us vulnerable and down on ourselves. Only when we begin to build ourselves up and speak positively will we be able to clearly see the choices before us and find our way to total well-being.

If you find yourself frequently saying negative things, I recommend Lynn Grabhorn's book *Excuse Me, Your Life Is Waiting.* Lynn will show you how your negative thoughts and words not only govern your perception of yourself, but actually draw negative influences into your life.

Always remember to recognize your choices both in how you act and how you speak and you will be on your way to keeping a dedicated commitment.

"Look in the mirror and notice what you think and say. Sit down to pay bills and listen to your thoughts then. Go to your job and listen to what you think about your work, abilities, and career prospects. . . . Are you feeding what you want to grow?"
Melody Beattie,
Beyond Codependency

"Start your day with the intent to look for positive aspects about everything and everybody. Then intend to find them."
Lynn Grabhorn,
Excuse Me, Your Life Is Waiting

RESPONSIBILITY

Making a committed choice requires that we take *responsibility* for that choice, and that is the second component of commitment. Accept responsibility for all your choices, conscious or otherwise, as well as their consequences. Stop blaming others for who you are. Instead, take action to change, one step at a time, what you can.

Not long ago, my younger son came home complaining because he'd discovered he would need to complete twice as many assignments for a midterm grade than he thought. He berated the professor and said he hated the class. My son argued, "I didn't know." He still refused to take responsibility for his error even when he learned the assignment's details had been available from the beginning on the professor's website. Instead, he pleaded his case to each family member as they came home, hoping—I presume—that one of us would give him either exoneration or justice, but neither would help his forthcoming grade. He worried himself into a frenzy, unwilling to accept either the responsibility or the consequences for a mistake he himself had made, and in turn, causing himself further delay and pressure. Eventually, and after being offered no consolation or relief from us, he stayed up most of the night so he could hand in the assignments at the scheduled time.

As his mother, I could see how he only needed to admit his mistake and then move forward to do all he could to correct it. Easy. But not so long before, I *myself* had been lax in not seeing how *my choices* allowed me to ignore my own responsibilities.

CLEARING OLD CHOICES MAKES ROOM FOR NEW

For many years, I wore discounted, dated, and worn-out clothing. This was a choice I had made but did not initially see it as one. I had always been surrounded by money-conscious people, and I believed I had no choice but to wear these things because I did not want to be a burden on my family. After all, my husband had to look his best to meet with his clients. The boys outgrew their clothes faster than I could store them away, and I never went

"The more responsibility you take for yourself, the less you will take sides, fight, verbally abuse, pout, withdraw, become depressed, be insensitive, be aggressive, retreat in fear, or have guilt, 'shoulds' and 'oughts.'"

Nell M. Rodgers,
Puppet or Puppeteer

"To be willing to accept total responsibility for yourself put you in a position of being worthy of receiving and attracting the object of your desires."

Wayne W. Dyer,
Manifest Your Destiny

anywhere except the grocery store. Why did I need nice things for sitting around the house?

I did not see how this choice meant that I saw myself as unimportant or unworthy. I believed my sacrifice helped my family and, thus, was a worthy one. However, I had taken it to extremes and became entrapped in a vicious cycle because the less value I saw in myself, the less need I saw in having nice things. The less value I saw in my things, the less I valued myself. The less I valued myself, the less worthy I felt of meeting my own needs, fulfilling my purpose, or seeking the desires of my heart. Someone else's needs always came first.

When I finally confronted myself and sought out the truth about how that made me feel, I realized I felt cheated. I felt bad about the clothes I wore, and I blamed my lack of nice things on my family, particularly on my husband who controlled the purse strings.

Then, one day, my husband noticed me putting on a pair of ragged shoes. He asked, "Why are you wearing those?" and tried to get me to throw them away right then and there. I wouldn't. He didn't understand why I would continue to wear shoes that were falling apart. For once, I could see that he couldn't be held responsible for the condition of my shoes when I had not even once complained nor tried to ask for a new pair. Only *I* could be blamed for that. *I* needed to take responsibility for my choice.

As I began to heal my life, I could see that I *was* important and that I *did* deserve nice things just as much as any other member of the family. I started taking positive steps to change my old behavior. I started taking responsibility for my choices.

First, I cleared my closet of everything I no longer liked, regardless of how much I paid for it or who had given it to me, and without a second thought as to how few times I'd worn it. As my closet cleared, I felt liberated. I felt as if a huge burden had been lifted from my shoulders.

Some of the items I sold in a yard sale for pennies on the dollar. Some I gave to charity. Some, like the pair of shoes I'd continued wearing even though the dog had chewed the heel *ten years before*, I threw away. I did not keep anything I did not intend to wear and wear with pride.

Next, I replaced tattered and worn out items with a few quality pieces of clothing. Having a few nice things

"To discover the truth, I search for the illusion which I want to believe is true, but is not."
Spencer Johnson,
Yes or No

"A person of integrity does not blame others for his failure—or expect others to provide his success. He shoulders his own destiny."
Denis Waitley,
Timing Is Everything

gave a huge boost to my self-esteem. I looked better and felt better too. I decided that I would rather have a few quality items over a whole closet full of clothing that only tore down my self-esteem. I certainly didn't become a spendthrift, but I did recognize that just as we always found the money to meet my husband's needs and that of our boys, we could also find the money to meet mine.

THE EMOTIONAL REFLECTION OF QUALITY

I didn't understand at first how my actions and beliefs about the things in my life reflected on my actions and beliefs about *myself*. As I began to respect myself and honor myself with quality things, the inner parts of my life began to heal. Not only do I now believe 'I am worth it,' I've learned that quality items last longer, work better, and cause less headaches along the way. Most importantly, now that I know my things are a reflection of how I see myself and since I want to be a quality individual, I now purchase quality items for myself. This doesn't mean I stopped looking for bargains or buy above my means. I just make sure I buy items I'm proud to own and that I really want, even if that means having to save for them or pay a little more.

In the past, whenever I had bought a big ticket item such as a car or a computer, I would always 'cheap out' on the extra features. I didn't want to overburden the family with yet another expense. If a four cylinder would suffice, why did I need a V-8? Why buy expensive, name-brand clothes when they went out of style in a week?

A few years ago, though, I traded my Sonoma pickup for a Lincoln Navigator, and when I bought a new laptop computer, I got the maximum memory, speed, and hard drive available. I have never been so pleased with anything as I have with these two items. To me, these small extravagances equaled buying a Bentley or Rolls. Just looking at them makes me smile. What could be better than a daily reminder that 'I'm worth it'? I no longer look at these items, dreaming of the day when I can trade up to something better . . . . I have better—now.

Amazingly, as I started thinking in terms of quality, the whole appearance of my life and home took on a higher quality as well. Many nice things began flowing into my

"Too often, our possibilities were narrowed, by ourselves or by our choice to believe the limiting opinions of others, to the point of our living in stifling rigidity with a tightly compressed self-image. . . . Suddenly, most of the world seemed impossible or inaccessible to us—in our imaginations."

Denis Waitley
Timing is Everything

life. After clearing out the clutter, we decided to do some extensive redecorating. My husband even surprised me with a larger-carat diamond wedding ring. I *am* worth it!

Quality began showing itself in other areas too. My friends became a quality component. Those who I'd allowed to use and abuse me, gradually faded out of the picture while true, caring friends began to replace them.

Perhaps more than any other, this one simple step of making quality, responsible choices, started me on a path of recovery and well-being that hasn't stopped since.

Treat yourself to a few items of quality when you buy for yourself and others. Tell yourself you *are* worth it, and take responsibility for the choices you've made even if you did not previously see that you had made a choice.

EXERCISE NUMBER 4—CLEARING AWAY THE PAST

Here is an exercise designed to help you choose quality for your life:

STEP ONE—CLEAR YOUR CLUTTER

Begin by cleaning out your closet.

> *a) Remove any item you no longer wear or have never worn.*
>
> *b) Remove items you dislike—even if they were gifts.*
>
> *c) Remove items that no longer fit.*
>
> *e) Clear away items that are long outdated or that have aged longer than wine.*

Women in particular keep 'fat' clothes and 'thin' clothes and gravitate back and forth between the two. When I lost 20 pounds, I realized I deserved a reward for such hard work and for achieving the success that I had. I didn't want to wear my 'thin' clothes from three, four, five, even twelve years ago, I wanted new clothes that were in style, clothes that reflected the *new* me. In addition, I

"Stay out of the past; it doesn't exist."

Lynn Grabhorn,
Excuse Me, Your Life Is Waiting

"When you are attached to another person or any thing, that person or thing will, in some way, determine when, how, what and whether you make decisions or take action."

Nell M. Rodgers,
Puppet or Puppeteer

didn't want a reminder of my heavier, three-sizes-bigger days, so out went the fat clothes too. It also meant I had a greater incentive to stay thin with no fail-safe clothes hanging in the back of the closet.

Ask yourself why you are holding on to these things. What attachment do you have to them and why? Your closet is the closest symbolic representation to your mindset. If you own clothing 10, 15, 20, or more years old, then it might be time to pass those items to someone else. Why? Because they are also carrying with them a past energy of your life, an energy of where you were then and not from where you are now. The more items you keep with this past energy, the more you will be stuck in the routines and habits of the past, and the more you will block yourself from receiving new and better things now and in the future.

At one time, I owned a large amount of clothing that had belonged to my mother. They were beautiful things and of a far better quality than I could afford, but after hanging on to them for many years, I decided to part with all but a few items. I needed to move away from the mindset those clothes held over me.

Even more recently, I made a new pass through my closet after completing a very healthy, but cathartic writing session. I decided it was okay to part with several pairs of stretch pants I bought when my son was in the third grade. That was eleven years ago. Not only were they well-worn, I had not worn any of them for at least two to three years. I parted with ten turtlenecks of various colors which I had long since delegated to the 'work clothes' pile. Since I only rake leaves or that sort of thing once or twice a year, I figured I didn't need ten work shirts. Perhaps most significant was my decision to let go of a bathing suit my mother purchased for me around 1988, and a sweater that had been worn by my cousin who died in 1981. I can't tell you how good I felt after releasing those things from my life. Releasing those things went beyond just making more closet space, I had released a long-held burden and attachment. I gained power by allowing those things to pass from my hands.

Clear your closet of old clothing and no-longer-needed attachments. Sell them, toss them, give them away, but clear them entirely from your life. Send your body a

"I needed to shed the old vibrations that were in my dreads, and it was time to grow some new ones."
Lenny Kravitz,
Yahoo online interview

"It's never about the object."
Peter Walsh, Organizer on
TLC's TV show *Clean Sweep*

message that you intend to treat it to a quality life. Empower your life by letting go of the things from the past and move forward into the present and the future you want.

STEP TWO—ROOM FOR NEW AND BETTER THINGS

Replace what you removed with a few quality items. Buying a couple of new outfits every season keeps your spirits high and your wardrobe looking great. Don't forget to clear away the old items as you do. My mother had a rotating system where her dress clothes from the previous year became her everyday clothes. She then donated her two-seasons-old clothing to charity. Wherever she went, she looked fabulous and felt good about herself.

STEP THREE—CONTINUING THE PROCESS

Follow through on this with the rest of your home and life. Clean, scrub, clear away, paint, refresh, revitalize your surroundings and yourself. Clear out the attic, your kitchen drawers, the garage. Honestly ask yourself why you are holding on to the items you have? What makes them important, and are they being *presented* as important where they now sit or are stored?

In one episode of The Learning Channel's series *Clean Sweep*, a show where out-of-control clutter is cleared out and reorganized, one of the hosts (Peter Walsh) pointed out an important lesson about our beloved clutter. The homeowners had kept many items that were linked to the wife's deceased brother. The host delicately guided them into seeing how the brother wasn't the items. They had kept so many more or less useless things—things they couldn't use, things they had no intention of ever using—simply out of sentimentality for the brother. They had so many things, they had lost track of their own lives, their own dreams, their own hopes for the future.

The host helped them see their error, helped them see they needed to separate the love for their brother from the items they had kept. Walsh then guided them in keeping a few of the most treasured things. He explained they could display those while letting go of the other countless items which, in reality, had no real meaning or purpose other than to remind them of the loved one they had lost.

"Your clutter serves to completely block you from letting other things into your lives."
Peter Walsh, Organizer on TLC's TV show *Clean Sweep* (Paraphrased)

Walsh said something else that made a lot of sense to me. He said, the items we have around us should be a reflection of both who we are now and who or where we want to be in the future—not who we once were. (Wow!)

For example, while packing to move into our present home, I found in the basement two oversized boxes full of trophies I'd proudly earned twirling a baton as an adolescent. They held many precious memories for me and, because of those memories, I had moved these two boxes six times. I can admit now, not once in those six moves had they ever been unpacked. Those trophies meant the world to me. Or so I thought. But, you know, it didn't take much for my husband to make me see that the trophies were no longer an important part of my life—now. Not only had I left them packed away, I knew I had no place to display them in our future home—even if I had wanted to. But what can one do with some 60 trophies? I hated to throw them away.

By my good fortune, during our yard sale a woman came through and saw my boxes of trophies sitting there. She asked, "What do you plan to do with all those trophies?" And I said, "Well, I really don't know what I can do with them." So, she began to tell me of a woman who taught baton and how with very little money she had built a small group and liked to encourage the girls all that she could. After talking with her, I happily donated all my trophies to this worthy cause, thus passing the enjoyment and recognition I'd received to others. I have pictures of my mother's bookcase loaded with my trophies if I should ever want to look at them. But for the most part, the memories associated with them are *inside* me where I can look at them anytime, and I no longer need them physically in my life, even though they had been hard won.

FORGIVENESS

The next important component in making a commitment to healing is *forgiveness*. We must learn how to forgive ourselves for any poor or misguided choices we believe we may have made in the past.

Forgiveness is more than forgiving those who have hurt us it's just as important to forgive ourselves for

"A house overflowing with odds and ends and tidbits you've held on to for someday has no space for the things that might truly enhance today."

Julia Cameron,
The Artist's Way

"I can be hurt by nothing but my thoughts."

Foundation for Inner Peace,
A Course in Miracles

allowing ourselves to be hurt. *A Course of Miracles* says we can only be hurt if we allow ourselves to be hurt.

In any commitment, there might be some faltering along the way. There might be days when your best intentions go astray. As I explained before, when I prepared to give birth to my first son, I committed myself to going natural all the way. I had prepared for it, planned for it, and practiced every day. When the first real pains hit, I screamed, "Bring me drugs!"

What good could I bring to myself or others by constantly berating myself for that falter? Yet, many of us do that every waking moment of the day. We beat ourselves over the head with invisible clubs as if our self-infliction will make the emotional pain go away. For some reason, we just don't see that the best way to make the pain stop is to *take away the club*! Unless we stop beating ourselves, how can we make the pain stop?

NO REGRETS

My father first took ill when I was just three years old. For many years, he had periods of ill health. As he neared his final days, my mother chose to keep him at home instead of placing him in a nursing home. She cared for him to the best of her ability.

One day, I passed by his bedroom door and heard him call out, "Jamie! Come talk to me. Tell me about your day."

But I just hurried on down the stairs calling back over my shoulder, "Not now, I can't."

Several days later, my father died.

For years, I blamed myself for killing him, for stealing away his will to live. If only I'd taken a few extra moments to stop and talk to him on that day. All he needed, I reasoned, was a few moments of my time, a few words of encouragement, a word from me to let him know we still cared. Instead, I'd hurried out the door to play.

I learned a great lesson from that mistake . . . *no regrets*. I live my life always trying to fully express myself to others—today, now—because they might not be here tomorrow. I try to make decisions that feel right to me, decisions I won't regret later. I want no regrets haunting me tomorrow. They are too hard to forget.

Even so, there are still life situations that cause me to

"Within you, whoever you may be, regardless of how big a failure you may think yourself to be, is the ability and power to do whatever you need to do to be happy and successful. Within you right now is the power to do things you never dreamed possible. This power becomes available to you just as soon as you can change your beliefs. Just as quickly as you can dehypnotize yourself from the ideas of 'I can't,' 'I'm not worthy,' 'I don't deserve it,' and other self-limiting ideas."

Maxwell Maltz,
Psycho-Cybernetics

"Forgiveness is a releasing of our resistance to positive energy, not the transgressor's at whom we are so benevolently aiming our forgiving smile."

Lynn Grabhorn,
Excuse Me, Your Life Is Waiting

wonder if I made the right decision after all. There are some choices that don't seem to have a right answer.

My mother's weak heart had hindered her cancer treatment. Doctors had postponed surgery, fearing her heart would not endure the shock. But, as she continued to defy the odds against their every prediction, they relented and scheduled her for surgery in one of the top facilities in the country, the MD Anderson Cancer Treatment Center in Houston, Texas.

Around that time, I had many strong premonitions and felt my mother would not survive the surgery. I think she may have suspected it, too, and gave me particular instructions as to what I should do with her things should she not survive. Due to financial constraints, and because I had two small children at home at the time, I decided not to fly across the country[1]. I knew in doing so, I might never see my mother alive again. I accepted that with 'no regrets' because I decided that if I were to lose my mother, I wanted to remember her as the vital and lively woman I'd always known. I did not want to remember her the way I remembered my father's last days where he lived in a hallucinogenic world, unable to comprehend our presence, unable to keep his dignity or presence of mind. I also knew she had both the excellent care of some of the finest doctors in the country, as well as the loving concern and presence of her second husband, son, and grandniece. So, I stayed home.

My mother survived the surgery but died a week later due to complications. Had I made the right decision? Did I have 'no regrets'? I thought I had done the right thing.

Unfortunately, the rest of my family did not support nor understand my decision. Since July of 1990, we've barely spoken. I not only lost my mother that day, I lost the balance of my family as well. I hadn't accounted for that loss in the long-term. I thought my family would remain my family no matter what. I was wrong.

For a long time, I told myself that I had forgiven them for turning their backs on me. I understood their point of view even if they didn't understand mine. But my forgiving them didn't make the situation go away. It didn't make my emotional pain stop. *Why?*

Because they didn't want or need my forgiveness. They didn't feel they were wrong in any way. They didn't

79

have any use for what I had offered them. It took me a long time to see that I did not need to forgive them, I needed to forgive myself.

Forgiving one's self, I've found, is often far more difficult than forgiving others. But then, I feel that many people don't really understand what forgiveness is.

Maxwell Maltz, who wrote *Psycho-Cybernetics,* offers one of the best descriptions of forgiveness I've ever read:

> *"True forgiveness comes only when we are*
> *able to see, and emotionally accept, that*
> *there is and was nothing for us to forgive.*
> *We should not have condemned or hated*
> *the other person in the first place."*

I'd often cried myself to sleep, remembering how my brother and close cousins had forsaken me. I'd frequently called to memory the pain they had caused. I'd never forgiven them—not according to Maltz's definition—and more importantly, I'd never forgiven myself.

Are there events in your life that you need to pass from your memory? Are there situations you dig up time and time again? This is no different than picking a scab off a wound. How is it supposed to heal? Of course, it will scar and that scar will remain a constant and painful reminder of all that befell you.

In the ancient texts of Enoch, as written about by Elizabeth Clair Prophet *(The Hidden Mysteries of Enoch),* there is an interesting account of Cain and Able. Everyone knows that Cain killed his brother Abel. So, as Enoch walked the seven hells as shown to him by an angel of God, one would expect to see Cain suffering there from eternal damnations, right?

But not so. Instead, Abel is the one there, sentenced to cry out, day after day, hour after hour, accusing his murderous brother.

As I read it, I thought, *"How odd; who would have thought those that were murdered would be cast into hell?"* For a moment I was dumbstruck. From that lesson I learned the curse of not forgiving others.

The past is gone. There is no sense in rehashing it. *A Course In Miracles* says, "You see only the past." What that means is, we judge the present based on what has transpired in the past. We become blind to what is

"The true definition of forgiveness doesn't mean that you condone the act. It means that you never mention it again. . . ."

Shemane Nugent,
(in reference to her husband's, Ted Nugent, improprieties during a Fox News 2003 interview)

"This is the spirit of Abel, who was slain by Cain his brother; and who will accuse that brother, until his seed be destroyed from the face of the earth. . . ."
Elizabeth Clair Prophet,
The Hidden Mysteries of Enoch

happening now as we hold on tightly to what we remember from the past.

Whenever I think of my brother or cousins, I first remember how they turned against me and react to each new situation with the old one pinned front and center in my mind. I don't see how they are acting now, I only see how they reacted then. I judge everything that happens between us based on the prerequisite of yesterday. Everything in the now is first whitewashed with the color of then. From that perspective, it is not possible for me to see the present or any change that might have occurred. It is not possible for me to believe they could be anything except what they were then.

In order to forgive them or myself, I must first remove that constant reminder of the past and release the old memory. As long as I continue to view their present actions through the veil of what they did in the past, I will never be able to forget or heal from the pain I feel. And, more importantly, as long as I continue to nurse that emotional pain, it will stand as a roadblock to my forward movement in obtaining my highest purpose. It will become as an open sore and will eventually show itself as a physical ailment.

A good friend of mine is always quick to remind me in the heat of any argument, "Don't forget how I forgave you years ago for . . ." But what she doesn't see is that she never really did forgive me—if she had, the error would have been forgotten. There wouldn't be a need to remind me over and over again of her supposed forgiveness.

What's more, my belief is that she did not need to forgive me for whatever it was that I did. She instead needed to forgive *herself*. She needed to stop beating herself with that invisible club.

So How DO You Forgive Yourself?

Step One—Recognition and Acceptance

Remember, self-forgiveness begins first with the recognition that you are the one to be forgiven and not the other way around. Recognize too that even though you

"I never see my brother as he is, for that is far beyond perception. What I see in him is merely what I wish to see, because it stands for what I want to be the truth."
Foundation for Inner Peace,
A Course in Miracles

may have forgiven others, they might not feel they have done anything wrong nor might not want your forgiveness.

STEP TWO—AN ALTERNATIVE POINT OF VIEW

See how the other person may have viewed the situation. Slip on their shoes, walk a few miles in them. What did they see? What did they feel? It doesn't matter if their perception is right or wrong, as long as you recognize what their perception is or was.

STEP THREE—LEAVE THE PAST IN THE PAST

Recognize that the past is passed, gone, water over the dam, milk that has spilt, cement that's hardened. You can't change it, you can't make it go away. Accept that and move forward.

STEP FOUR—GROWTH

Ask yourself what you have learned from the experience. On her meditative tape *Overcoming Obstacles,* Carol Adrienne advises her listeners to see this aspect of life as a gift.

Visualize yourself as receiving a box. Open it up, look inside. See the lesson materialized as an object. Using symbolism and parallels as you did in 'Interpreting an Ailment,' uncover a meaning for the gift of this lesson.

Understanding the meaning, holding fast to the gift, offer yourself forgiveness, using the lesson to prevent any error of that nature in the future. Use the lesson to prevent others from making the same mistake. Release the past, and let it go. Think of this incident as a burst of fireworks on the Fourth of July. See it scattered across the night sky, lighting up the darkness then dissolving into nothingness.

The next time you think of the incident, remember the gift too. Train yourself to focus on what you've gained rather than on what you've lost. Soon you will find you no longer feel the pain of this once hurtful event.

In the case of my brother and cousins, I visualized myself as a baby in a basket being left on a stranger's doorstep. I'd been abandoned by those who were supposed to love me. For me, the gift was in knowing that the abandoned baby was adopted, taken in by others who loved her and filled her needs in ways those who left her behind might never have done. Knowing these other individuals greatly enriched my life.

In the bible, God gives Job all he had previously lost, I've gained much from the relationships I've had with friends who love me for who I am. They've been there with me to share both in times of joy and sorrow, serving as surrogates in place of my relatives who were not. My life has been filled with surrogates, from the aunts and uncles who stood in for the grandparents I never knew, to my friends who have served as mother, father, sister, brother.

These friends became like precious gems to me, and the gifts I've received as a result are their sincere care and concern. Because of this, I spend a great deal of effort nurturing my friendships and keeping them strong. I know how important these people have been to me in my times of need.

I've gained, while those who abandoned me, lost. They lost out on the chance to know me and to share with me the experiences of my life. When I remember that they have abandoned me, I remind myself again of all that I have gained and of the good people who *were* there for me rather than dwelling on those who weren't.

FORGOTTEN IS NOT THE SAME AS BURIED

Let me inject one last note on forgiveness. Forgiveness requires an acceptance, a realization, and a release. Letting the past go, freeing yourself from the burden, is not the same thing as burying it deeply inside of you. I believe both my parents did this with the loss of their first daughter. I am in no way suggesting that they should have forgotten her. What they buried within themselves and refused to release was not her precious memory but the blame they inappropriately placed on themselves for her accidental death. Planted like a perennial bulb, their self-inflicted blame was sure to grow and raise its ugly head time and time again, showing itself eventually in physical form.

To fully heal your life, you need to allow yourself forgiveness. Do not withhold forgiveness from yourself. Do not force your body to physically manifest your self-berating battle scars into ailments, for this surely will

"'Who is my mother, and who are my brothers?'" Pointing to his disciples, he said, 'Here are my mother and my brothers.'"
Matthew 12:46, New International Version

"To get to forgiveness, we first have to work through the painful experiences that require it. Forgiveness doesn't mean that what happened to us was okay. It simply means that we are no longer willing to allow that experience to adversely affect our lives. Forgiveness is something we do, ultimately, for ourselves."
Christiane Northrup, *Women's Bodies, Women's Wisdom*

83

happen over time if you do not learn to forgive. An ailment can become like Abel's nonending cry in hell, "Who will avenge my blood?"

COMMITMENT AND TOTAL WELL-BEING

In order for you to reach the place I call "total well-being," you must first make a commitment to yourself to do so. Without this self-commitment, you will continue to live within the bounds that others have set for you. You will continue to suffer needlessly within the consequences of your inappropriate choices that up until now have been based purely upon a mistaken perception of yourself.

By making a commitment, you learn the consequences of your actions. You learn the value of your choices. You learn to forgive and to use the lessons of your past as a gift to build on your future. Yet, sometimes, no matter how committed we may be, we come against failure and cannot see why we can't break through to success. The reason lies within the last component of commitment, *discovery*.

DISCOVERY

Discovery is searching out the reason for any faltering of a sincere commitment and understanding that failure means only that you are about to reveal a previously hidden, stronger commitment to *something else*.

This stronger commitment is due either to a mistaken perception or childhood situation that is now no longer appropriate for your life. That's right—faltering on a commitment is a tremendous *opportunity*. It is like a beam of light shining in the mind's dark attic, allowing you to see something you had stored away at a time when that choice provided you with support or security.

In his book, *Re-create Your Life*, Morty Lefko talks about how as children we often adopt strategies that are useful to our survival at the time. He says:

> ". . .they develop survival strategies that
> help them deal with the anxiety that stems

84

from their negative beliefs. As a survival strategy is formed, the child also forms a belief about that strategy. 'I'm good enough because . . .' 'What makes me worthwhile is . . .' 'The way to deal with a dangerous world is . . .' 'The way to survive is . . .'

Later, these survival strategies become negative tapes we play subliminally in our minds and we become enslaved to the now forgotten commitment until we try to counter it with an opposing one. That's when we are alerted that the underlying commitment or strategy exists, and we have the clues we need to uncover and release it.

In the movie *Indiana Jones, The Last Crusade*, Indiana searches for the Holy Grail. When he crosses over the great ravine to the hiding place of the cup, he is met by a 700-year-old knight who has been vigilantly guarding the grail.

This knight represents our hidden commitments. We don't know they are there still guarding us from some long-ago sensed danger or fear, waiting to be relieved from their post by a new sentry. However, like in the movie, the 'knight' (our commitment) must be satisfied that the new sentry will continue to uphold the values and underlying moral fiber that he has stood for all this time. Indiana proved his worthiness by choosing the right cup (Grail). We do this with our commitments by showing our subconscious mind the benefits of our new goal.

When we are struggling, trying hard to understand why no matter how hard we try we can't succeed at losing weight, being drug free, quitting smoking, avoiding abusive relationships, staying well, or countless other resolutions we promise ourselves, it's because we haven't yet seen the *underlying* commitment, the 700-year-old knight still guarding his post.

For me, *food* has always been an issue, and on countless occasions I've promised myself that I'd quit eating sweets or lower my carbs and fats, that I'd lose weight or get in shape, only to soon give up and give in.

Why?

Because beneath my sincerity to lose weight—and previously unknown to me—I had long carried another

"Survival strategy beliefs are based on a child's observation of what it takes to feel good about herself or himself, to be important, to be worthwhile, or to be able to deal with life."

Morty Lefko,
Re-create Your Life

"The first belief that is created becomes a person's point of reference and therefore carries the most power. It becomes the person's standard to measure experience."

Stephen Wolinsky,
Quantum Consciousness

commitment—one far stronger and more diligent than my open decision to eat healthy.

How did I discover this previously unrecognized commitment? By asking myself 'why' in the midst of the act. Catching myself in the act of eating something I'd earlier said I wouldn't, I asked myself, "Why are you eating this?"

When I eat, I have found I have a strong commitment to eat items that are appealing and taste good. If they aren't, I begin to feel uneasy inside, almost panicking, as if I will starve. It's within the panic I might make a choice (and it is a choice) to eat something more fattening or less healthy because I am *feeding the fear and not the need.*

Where the fear stems from, I do not know nor do I need to know. The why doesn't matter provided I can identify the presence of fear. The fear signals that I have encroached on the underlying commitment and that is the clue I need to understand what the other commitment might be.

Discovery is finding the opposing commitment. Once found, it can be exchanged for a new one. It is only in not seeing the opposition that we are unable to overcome it.

Healing on the physical level begins by seeking the underlying connections and healing them on an emotional level. We learned that lesson in Section One. Now we have yet another opportunity to dig beneath the surface and see what some of those connections are.

Buried within our minds lies any number of mistaken perceptions and unrecognized Truths. Until they have been rooted out and sorted through, the body will continue to fidget and complain if not with one ailment then another. "HEAR ME!" it cries out. "I need attention!"

Remember how I said that I must reassure the old sentry that his position will be well guarded? If, when I eat, I recognize fear and see that my fear stems from being afraid that I'll starve, then I must show the old guard that my new way of eating will not allow me to go hungry. I need to prove this through my actions or the old guard will not give way to the new—the old commitment will not give way to the new one.

In the book *Psych-K*, Robert A. Williams says:

> "... *unlike the conscious mind, the subconscious thinks literally rather than*

"A positive thought, decision, or reassociation does not have more mass or power to override a negative thought, decision, reassociation, or creation. The existing thought must be dealt with because it was created first and remains in consciousness."
Stephen Wolinsky,
Quantum Consciousness

"It is almost impossible to really change one's behavior permanently and effortlessly if the beliefs that led to it still exist."
Morty Lefko,
Re-create Your Life

86

abstractly. . . . It is important to define your goal as specifically as possible and to do it in sensory-based language visually, auditorily, and kinesthetically."

Therefore, it is important that we use signals our subconscious mind—the home of this old guard (or outdated commitment)—understands in explaining that our intent is worthy and upholding of the original intent (aka, preventing me from going hungry). Keep in mind, however, that it is the *presence of fear*, discovered while questioning a falter or hesitation, that leads us to the clues needed to unearth this intent.

Fear is a commitment in itself. Think of two strong teams of men pulling on a rope in a tug of war. Who will win? Both are pulling in opposite directions as hard as they can. No wonder we start and stop and falter on what we truly want to achieve! No wonder we pull ourselves in first one direction and then the other!

No wonder the more I try to change the way I eat, the more I provoke the fear inside me that I'll starve and the more the opposing commitment tugs me the other way, convincing me to eat, eat anything, so that I won't starve.

Only by disengaging my fear and removing the opposing force, or better still, by getting both sides to work together, am I able to succeed with my new commitment (to eat healthy). By doing that, I'll have both the old guard and the new guard pulling on the same side of the rope. There won't be a struggle because there won't be anything to pull against my commitment. In other words, if through my actions I can prove to the old guard (the subconscious commitment) that I will not let it starve and that I will be eating enjoyable foods, both the old guard and the new will be satisfied. They will be pulling together as a team. Without opposition, there is no doubt I will win, there is not even a battle. If both teams are pulling together, who can oppose them?

Perhaps then, the hardest part is to recognize *the sense of fear*, the underlying clue that we need because we might have lived with fear for so long that it feels perfectly natural and not like fear at all.

"Once, however, a correct or 'successful response' has been accomplished—it is 'remembered' for future trials. It has 'learned' how to respond successfully. It 'remembers' its successes, forgets its failures, and repeats the successful action without any further conscious 'thought'—or as a habit."
Maxwell Maltz,
Psycho-Cybernetics

"If God be for us, who can be against us?"
Romans 8:31,
King James Version

CHAPTER EIGHT: OVERCOMING FEAR

AND RECOGNIZING TRUTH

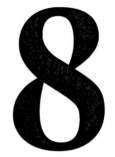

The first step in overcoming fear is *recognizing it*.

However, we often have lived in fear for so long that we no longer recognize it or feel it. Instead of reacting against it, we've become comfortable miring in it. Even though we may feel downtrodden, burdened, or even physically ill, we may not see or believe in the fear attached to it. The fear may have become such a common bedfellow that we actually cling to it. This is because when we know what to expect, the routine brings us comfort even if the situation is ultimately painful, degrading, or dangerous. We feel 'safety' in its familiarity.

So how do we recognize our fears?

Fear can be identified when we catch ourselves holding back from doing something we wanted to do or when we say something we know deep down inside we didn't really mean. By the time we catch ourselves doing this, it may be too late to change it but *recognizing* it is the first step.

When you catch yourself in a personal lie based in fear, you may feel a physical *pulling* or other sensation within your stomach. You may suddenly feel uncomfort-

"By understanding how fear and other negative emotions adversely affect healing, you may more easily identify how you are interfering, consciously or unconsciously, with your own healing process."

Carolyn Myss,
Why People Don't Heal

able, irritable, or develop a headache without knowing why. These subtle *Body Songs* are alerting you to the lie and its underlying fear.

At the time this takes place, you might not be in a position where you can change your decision, although we all have choices as you've already learned. The important thing is to later work through what happened and why it triggered your fear. By doing so, you will gain a new perspective on this fear, thus shining Truth on the lie—which, in turn, will defeat it.

CLARIFYING YOUR FEARS

The next step after recognizing a fear is to clarify it.

There are two main types of fears and the goal is to determine which kind of fear you have just encountered—*Primal Fears* or *Specific Fears*.

PRIMAL FEARS

A Primal Fear is:

- *The fear of separation from a loved one or God*
- *The fear of pain and suffering*
- *The fear of the unknown*
- *The fear of death*

We all have Primal Fears in one form or another, and they include fears of near-and-present danger such as having a gun thrust into your face or as in the case of losing control of your car on an icy road.

Imagine the Grim Reaper and his long scythe. He is the ominous image we've come to recognize in association with the aforementioned fears. Oddly, we seem more readily able to accept and live within the bounds of a Primal Fear since its presence is with us always and can happen at any moment without warning. At least for most of us, a Primal Fear does not prevent our active participation in life or the pursuit of our purpose.

"What aspects of this experience show up in other areas of my life? In what situations, and when, have I felt this fearful before?"

Michael Lee,
Phoenix Rising Yoga Therapy

90

SPECIFIC FEARS

A *Specific Fear* is everything *else* we fear—from being bitten by a dog to being afraid to fly or even the fear of asking for a promotion or a raise. These are the fears we'll address here.

In actuality, none of us are so much afraid of a situation itself as we are afraid of its subsequent consequences. In other words, a person who's afraid of heights is not so much afraid of climbing as they are afraid of *falling*.

For that reason, I see Specific Fears as being like a Mardi Gras clown wearing an oversized papier mâche' head. It is beneath that facade of the mask where the true fear lies and, therefore, *all* Specific Fears can be broken down into their underlying Primal counterpart.

As our Specific Fears are broken apart to see what they are really made of, we begin to see them differently, especially when we look at ordinary, everyday situations. We quickly realize we are not afraid of the Specific Fear at all, but rather it is the underlying, hidden Primal Fear that drives the illusion of our Specific Fear, and that is all fear really is—an illusion.

Fear is the master trickster and illusionist which is why I like the image of the Mardi Gras clown. He builds layers and layers of 'what ifs and 'might bes' over top of our Primal Fears so that we don't recognize them.

Psychologist Stephen Wolinsky *(The Dark Side of the Inner Child)* refers to this as *futurizing*. In other words, we imagine a situation that could happen (or just as easily not happen), and we dwell on that possibility, which causes us to become afraid. This in turn causes us to block out other possibilities, preventing us from seeing what may be a very simple solution.

Another of my favorite fairy tales is about a man in English peasant times who becomes engaged to a farmer's daughter. To celebrate, she goes into the home's cellar to fetch a bottle of wine and finds an axe stuck in the ceiling. She begins to futurize that the axe will one day fall out of the ceiling, hit her husband on the head, and kill him. The whole family becomes caught up in this fear. There is much wailing and crying until the fiance' arrives. Hearing the family's fears, he simply reaches up and pulls the axe from the ceiling.

When we are able to see that we could easily remove

"I love that feeling of having everything in my spirit say 'It's not okay, you shouldn't do this,' and just doing it anyway and being okay afterwards."
Eric Bergous,
U.S.A. Freestyle Skiing

"Fear is a beast which thrives on a lack of knowledge."

Jamie L. Saloff

"... one style of futurizing takes place when a person projects herself into the future and imagines a catastrophic outcome.... The odd part about futurizing is that I feel the pain of the imagined situation 'right now'...."
Stephen Wolinsky,
The Dark Side of the Inner Child

"And ye shall know the truth, and the truth shall make you free."

John 8:32,
King James Version

the axe from our fear, we are usually no longer afraid. We are then able to see the Truth and liberate ourselves. However, because fear is the master illusionist, we sometimes have to dig down through many layers of Specific Fears before we find the true and Primal Fear, and these fears are not always easy to identify.

Once you recognize the Truth, you will be able to easily overcome the fear. The following exercise will help you to peel away those layers and to see your fears for what they really are.

EXERCISE NUMBER 5—REDEFINING FEAR

1. Using index cards and word-association phrases, write down your perceived fear. *(If necessary, review the section, How to Do Word Association Exercises, found in Appendix A.)*

   For Example: I am afraid of dogs.

2. Ask yourself, is this a Specific Fear? Or a Primal Fear? Remember, a Primal Fear is the fear of pain and suffering, death, the unknown, or the separation from a loved one or God. All other fears are Specific Fears.

Keep clarifying your fear. Ask yourself, is this the True fear or could it be something else?

   Am I afraid of dogs? Or am I afraid of being bitten by a dog?

   I am afraid of being bitten.

3. Ask yourself, again and again, no matter how many times it takes, is this the true fear?

   Am I afraid of being bitten? Or am I really afraid of the pain of the bite, the suffering it would cause, the possibility of being maimed or even dying?

   I am afraid of the consequences of a bite.

"Stop thinking the world has to change before you can be safe or happy. You create your own safety through your energy flow."
Lynn Grabhorn,
Excuse Me, Your Life Is Waiting

4. Is this final fear a Primal Fear of a Specific Fear?

I'm afraid of the pain—pain is a Primal Fear.

If your fear is not the fear of separation, pain and suffering, the unknown, or death, continue to clarify and strip away the layers until you find the Primal Fear.

Like the fairy tale maiden and the axe in the ceiling, you can become so caught up in a fear of what *might* happen, you don't see what your fear is really all about, which is typically just an illusion or one of a hundred possibilities. Once you dissect your fears and find the underlying truth about them, you will be able to easily identify how to overcome them. In many cases, you may even end up laughing at yourself when you see how you have tricked yourself with smoke and mirrors.

THE MARDI GRAS CLOWN UNMASKED

Here is one example of how I found a Specific Fear and unmasked the parading Mardi Gras clown to find the underlying Grim Reaper or Primal Fear.

I had been talking about becoming a publisher as I had been helping some authors get into the Print On Demand publishing field. While having lunch with friends, one asked, "Would you be willing to look at my friend's book about blacksmithing? Would that be something you'd consider publishing?"

I heard my mouth say, "Yes, I'll be glad to look at your friend's book," while my stomach contracted and told me, "No, you wouldn't." I had just lied, and I knew it.

It wasn't that I didn't feel blacksmithing couldn't be a viable project for the woman; rather, I wasn't personally interested in the project and wouldn't give her book the time and energy needed to carry it through to completion. Why, then, had I just said yes when I meant no?

I first thought I'd been afraid to say no because I feared my friend might be offended. But why would she be if she were truly my friend? She wouldn't have. So, later on, I asked myself, "Is this the true fear?"

I reasoned, "I'm just afraid of losing a friend. I'm afraid of separation." But as I dug down deeper and

"Am I really telling myself the truth?"

Spencer Johnson,
Yes or No

93

"Become aware of the feeling tones you roam around with all day long; from dawn to lights out. Stay awake. Become aware!"

Lynn Grabhorn,
Excuse Me, Your Life Is Waiting

"The only way to get rid of the fear of doing something is to go out and do it."

Susan Jeffers,
Feel the Fear and Do It Anyway

deeper through the layered fears, I discovered something more important. I had not yet personally clarified my own goals towards the publishing endeavor, and to cover my own self-doubts I had said yes when I meant no to protect myself from having to explain my doubts. In the long run, I still had feared separation as I had feared looking foolish or silly, but now I knew the Truth.

When we lie to ourselves and act out of obligation or fear, our body *knows*. It may send a *twang* of recognition such as a headache, a stomachache, or some other mild symptom. This is why muscle testing[2] works so effectively. Our bodies *know* the Truth, always. However, when we begin to act habitually out of fear over a long period of time, our body may take a more drastic action to get our attention—such as when I contracted cancer.

When I'm able to clarify my fears and see them for what they really are, I'm able to stretch myself beyond them and create new and better situations in my life.

Fear, then, is a sign that we are near to great change. Many of these changes will actually enhance our life, but because we are unsure what lies beyond that change, we hold back in terror. Instead, we need to see our fears as a kind of *deja vu*, a clue alerting us to the possibility that we are in the presence of a great opportunity. Why? Because in order to reach and fulfill our highest purpose, we must first face off against our *innate challenges*.

An *innate challenge* is an inborn struggle we face— oftentimes repeatedly—as a part of what I see as a spiritual evolution. For whatever reason, there seems to exist a universal law which states all life must face challenge in order to improve and enhance its living capabilities and performance.

For now, the important thing to remember is that when you feel the presence of fear, it's probably due to the approach of one of these challenges. Yes, that means that fear is a good thing! All of this will be discussed in detail later as you learn the value of your desires and enter into the pursuit of your goals.

Until then, let's talk about engendering positive change and setting for ourselves a path to make those changes happen.

SECTION THREE: FINDING AND FULFILLING

THE DESIRES OF YOUR HEART

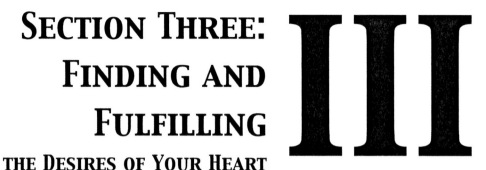

"When it comes to our careers and how we spend our life, there is within each one of us something unique that we have to offer. It is always something that we love doing, and which we do well, because we find it easy and very satisfying. If we can connect with and activate this unique factor, then it seems to me that we must be traveling on the right road, because we are bringing into expression our true self and creating our reality in a way which really serves us."

Suzanna Thorpe-Clark,
Changing the Thought

CHAPTER NINE: MAPPING OUR DESIRES

9

WHY YOUR DESIRES AND GOALS ARE IMPORTANT

In the fall of 2003, song writer–artist Warren Zevon died of lung cancer. When first diagnosed, his doctors predicted he had little time left to live. However, he was determined to create one last album before he died—which he did. In doing so, he tremendously outlasted his doctors' predictions. Many others have done the same, some even finding total healing, merely by activating a *purposeful goal*.

Purposeful goals are like air and water to our spirit. They extend our ability to live and propel us through otherwise excruciating circumstances. Our goals, our dreams, our passions, and our obsessions fuel our joy, our peace, our ability to be well and live well, and our ability to love ourselves and others. Without goals, we have no drive. We have no reason to get out of bed each morning. More importantly, if our goals are tied to fulfilling our

"Three doctors said my case was incurable. . . . When I told my physicians I was going to travel around the world and pump out my own stomach twice a day, they were shocked. Impossible! . . . When I got back to America. . . . I had never felt better in my life."
Earl P. Haney, as told to Dale Carnegie in *How to Stop Worrying and Siart Living*

"Nothing happens unless first a dream."

Carl Sandburg

"Desires can, however, be seen in two ways: (1) Energy to be used or (2) a resistance to rejection or failure."

Stephen Wolinsky,
Quantum Consciousness

". . . we cannot drift aimlessly—hoping to keep every option open—because we will wind up doing nothing in the name of 'being open.' . . . without some kind of focus, you will not be able to engage your life deeply enough to let the synchronicities take you where you need to go."

Carol Adrienne,
The Purpose of Your Life

highest purpose, we'll live our lives with a greater degree of enthusiasm and vigor. Suddenly, life has a reason.

A purposeful goal begins with our deepest heart's desires. Search the corners of your heart. Surely you'd admit to at least one spark within you longing to do this or to accomplish that—a feat you may feel is impossible or silly. And yet, the desire never leaves and persists in tugging at your heart no matter how hard you may try to ignore it or tamp it down, no matter how much you may say it can't be done.

Why *do* our desires persist as they do, constantly fluttering inside our mind and reminding us of our one-day dream? Why do they want acknowledged so much that our physical body will literally break down in pain and cry out when our desires are repressed? Because our desires are one of three components vital to realizing our higher purpose.

DEFINITION BRINGS CLARITY

How will you know you've gotten 'there' or 'made it' if you haven't first defined what 'making it' and 'getting there' is?

When we clearly define something, it becomes visible in our minds. It can live and grow in our imagination. It is that imaginative thread that becomes the beginning weave of reality. From our imagination comes a physical possibility, a hope to hang on to, a dream to reach for. This is the beginning edge of any reality. Without our ethereal imaginings, we have nothing to build upon. Our hopes and dreams are the beginning of all our foundations.

In order to give them credence, spark them to life, and ignite their flame of reality, I use an exercise that is so effective, I must revise my own desires every few weeks. By that time, the majority of them are already complete. Of course, some of my desires take longer to fulfill as I project what I want far into my future, reaching for long- and short-term goals.

This amazing exercise is designed to clearly define your desires and help bring them to fruition. It is based upon the concept that once a desire is known and clearly defined, the doors of opportunity will readily swing open, making the possibility of that desire available.

There are lots of ways to acknowledge our desires and to put them on to paper. Years ago I learned a lot about identifying goals in various aspects of my life from Denis Waitley's book *Timing Is Everything*. Denis recommended setting goals in the categories of: physical, family, financial, professional, community, mental, social, and spiritual. Breaking goals into different categories allowed me to see my life in a different way than I ever had before. Since then, though, I've revised those goal areas to be: *future aspirations, material desires,* and *professional desires* (or work-related) as these are the areas I tend to focus on most.

When releasing your desires and setting goals, define what it is that you truly want. Tap into your heart and write them down. When you write them down you are transferring that magical power from the ethereal essence to the physical reality of this world. You are showing the universe that you mean for this to happen. In a sense, it is a written contract between you, your higher self, and God. By writing them down you are acknowledging to yourself that they can really happen and that you *want* them to.

My favorite and the most effective means for doing this has been through image mapping my desires. I first discovered Tony Buzan's Mind Mapping[1] method while looking for a way to view my writing in a more visible, three-dimensional way and quickly grew to love his mind-freeing technique. I've included a couple of my image maps in this book, but there isn't a wrong way to go about this exercise as long as you follow the tips below. If you need more ideas on how to Mind Map, be sure to look at Buzan's *The Mind Map Book* for more details.

EXERCISE 6—DEFINING DESIRE

For this exercise, I like to use oversized, blank index cards because they are portable, inexpensive, and easy to keep in a visible place, but you can also use large poster boards or drawing paper.

Basically, an image map is used to create memorable and symbolic images representing each desire or goal.

"Remember, even Santa makes a list."

Jamie L. Saloff

"The Mind Map harnesses the full range of cortical skills— word, image, numbers, logic, rhythm, colour and spatial awareness—in a single, uniquely powerful technique. In so doing, it gives you the freedom to roam the infinite expanse of your brain."

Tony Buzan,
The Mind Map Book

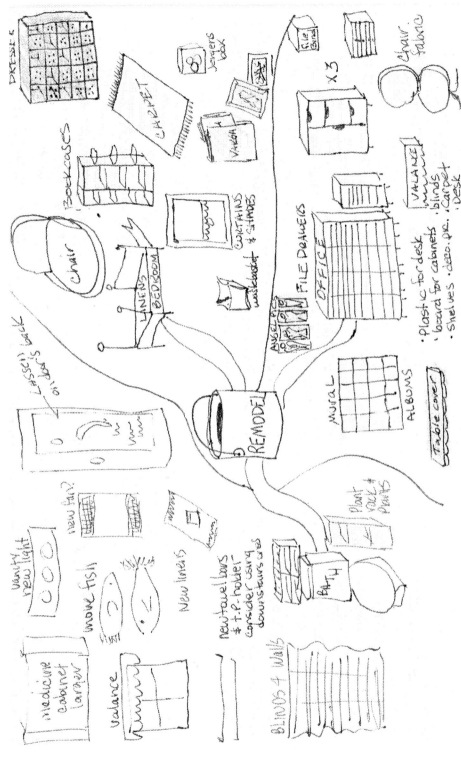

Example image map illustration. Note: 95 percent of this has been accomplished!

Example image map illustration

"I circled 'maze' in the center of a blank page and clustered, electrified by the connections in my head that spilled and radiated outward from its center as I continued to cluster, I suddenly experienced a shift from a sense of randomness to a sense of direction in all this welter, and I began to write."

Gabriele Lusser Rico,
Writing the Natural Way

Many of Buzan's maps radiate clockwise from a central theme in the middle of the map. I recommend you use image mapping sinc the images cause the mind to think in physical (real) terms. Feel free to use stick-figure people or oversimplified images if you're unable to draw. An interesting side effect is that the more maps you make, the better you become at creating recognizable images. However, if you would like more help in creating them, check out *Drawing on the Right Side of the Brain* by Betty Edwards, or try the simplified, anyone-can-draw books by Ed Emberley. Remember, the images are important but no one has to know what they mean except you.

If all else fails, try Inspiration Software[2] available fromwww.inspiration.com. Originally designed for kids, the software is easy to use and contains lots of images for expanding your mind.

Here are some other tips to for mapping your desires:

STEP ONE: CLEARLY IDENTIFY YOUR DESIRES

By knowing what you want, the more likely you are to receive it. Therefore, it is very important for you to detail your desires as clearly and specifically as you can. If you want money, identify what it is for. If you want clothing, indicate the kinds or types of items. Shoes? Jackets? Ties? Blouses? Skirts? Socks? Handbags? Are they a particular brand name or designer? If you want a car, identify a particular model or note key design features. If you desire a new home, what amenities are important? Do you imagine it in a particular neighborhood, a particular city or state?

Even if your desires center around less materialistic goals, you must indicate what those desires, such as peace, love, joy, health, or well-being mean to you. Do these feelings relate to specific situations or types of people around you? Do they instill a certain sensation inside you? Write down a symbolic image to represent each of these things.

Our desires will be fulfilled if we make them known and *believe* in their possibility. Even the American Constitution is written with the words "in the pursuit of happiness."

"Delight yourself in the Lord and he will give you the desires of your heart."

Psalms 37:4,
King James Version

STEP TWO: IDENTIFY EASY STEPS

If the desire is a complicated, multifaceted goal, break it into a series of easy-to-accomplish tasks or steps you can see and accomplish. Map those steps as well.

STEP THREE: BE OPEN TO OPPORTUNITIES

Ask for opportunities and they will come. Be alert for and take advantage of opportunities that coincide with what you've asked for.

When we decided to remodel our bedroom, we needed to sell the dressers. One of my friends had expressed a liking for these, so I called him and asked if he'd be interested in buying them. My husband had some time off, we wanted to start our remodeling right away. So I explained to my friend that picking them up quickly was of the utmost importance. But he didn't pick them up. Our remodeling couldn't start until the furniture had been removed, so after waiting a month, we found someone else to take the items. Unfortunately, my friend and I had words over this. He treated me as if I had stolen something from him. I had a hard time understanding his reaction. I felt that if he had truly wanted the dressers, he would have honored my request to pick them up quickly. For him, the opportunity had opened, but he hadn't reached out and embraced it. The door had opened, but he didn't choose to walk through it.

The universe is keen to fulfill our desires and needs. It provides the opportunities. All we are asked to do is reach out our hand and claim them. However, if we do not take that step, if we do not reach out, the opportunity soon closes to us.

How many opportunities have we missed simply because we didn't reach out and take the options open to us? How much more could we have had, how many desires of our heart, if we had only asked and accepted all we'd been offered?

"Ask and it will be given to you; seek and you will find; knock and the door will be opened unto you. For everyone who asks receives; he who seeks finds; and to him who knocks, the door will be opened."

Matthew 7:7-8,
King James Version

STEP FOUR: SPEAK IN POSITIVE TERMS

It is very important that you speak or write about your desires in *positive* terms. Begin to identify yourself with the trappings of what you want.

103

"It is the job of the conscious rational thought to decide what you want, select the goals you wish to achieve, and concentrate upon these rather than upon what you do not want. To spend time and effort concentrating upon what you do not want is not rational."

Maxwell Maltz,
Psycho-Cybernetics

"Always make your statements in PRESENT TENSE, such as 'I am' or 'I have.' Your subconscious mind is such an obedient servant that if you declare in future tense, 'I want,' or 'I will have,' then that is where it will always stay—just out of your reach in the future!"

Louise L. Hay,
You Can Heal Your Life

Think about it in this way: If you had a child who loved skiing, constantly talked about skiing, read about skiing, watched skiing on television, and searched it out on the Internet, wouldn't you as a parent want to enrich your child's life with a skiing experience? In other words, you wouldn't buy her a motorbike. You would buy her skis. But as adults, we don't always think about what we want. For whatever reason, we focus on what we *don't* want.

Why would our hearts lead us to gain something we appear to not really want? When you give gifts to others, don't you try to find that special item you feel they will love and appreciate? This is true within the universal laws as well. We are given what we are seeking and have buried within the deepest channels of our hearts and minds, even if those desires are not consciously known. More importantly, the desires we receive are a direct reflection of what we have focused on. Look back to the section on *Mouth Confession* and recognize how our words and thoughts create what we will later receive as our thoughts serve as a testament to our desires.

Here's an example of how to speak about our goals. I had been intently focused on a few extra pounds that I had gained. Every time I thought about the weight, I said something to myself like: "I really need to lose some weight," or "I *have* to lose some weight," even, "I want to lose weight!" But none of those statements were as powerful as the day I switched to, "I am going to lose five pounds." Even as the words passed over my lips, I felt a shift, a change in my thinking. I knew that "I am going to lose five pounds," meant I was serious about it and that I intended to take some action. In fact, I found it almost impossible to say "I am going to lose five pounds," if I didn't mean it. The statement carried that much power.

Another important thing to know about speaking positively of our goals is this: On the other side of the universal veil, there is no distinction between a good or bad experience. What we might consider a painful or hurtful situation is just another opportunity for learning and growth to them. Therefore, if we spend our time focusing on pain, distress, chaos, tragedy, hardship, or devastation, the angels and guides who want to help us have everything we desire, will lend all in their power to bring those things to us. They will do so with the same vigor and joy as an innocent child bringing his mother a dandelion from the backyard. For years I kept asking, "Why am I always sick?" I kept focusing on my aches and pains, and what did I receive in return? More illness, more pain, more misery.

STEP FIVE: LET GOD WORRY ABOUT THE 'HOW'

Don't connect desire with outcome. You can choose the desire or choose the outcome, but not both.

One of the first lessons I learned about prayers—which are a simplified form of asking for our desires—was to pray the *need*, not the answer. I had the bad habit of always telling God how to fix things. When I learned to allow God to do the fixing, and to let Him decide the *how*, my prayers were then answered rapidly and effectively.

Once, I desired to have a better car. Chevrolet had rolled the first Toyota-built Novas off the assembly line. I really liked them but knew I couldn't afford one. Months passed. Then, during a visit my parents, my stepfather invited me into his garage. He had lost his prized Cadillac in a collision, and since he and my mother were planning to retire to Florida, they did not see any need to invest in a new, expensive automobile. When the garage door went up, my mouth fell open. There sat my dream car, my-every-desire-fulfilled-in-minute-detail car. I wasn't sure how, but knew that car would become mine.

A couple of months later, about the time my parents moved, my husband received an unexpected bonus and I convinced him to buy their car for me. He did. I loved that car and kept it for a long time.

More often than not, we focus on the *how* instead of the outcome. We are so sure that the outcome can only be achieved by our small-minded, pre-engineered transcript. Thus we place our focus and our expectations on how we want things to happen and then can't understand why we haven't achieved our goal. In the meantime, we are missing opportunities because what we see doesn't fit in with what we are expecting.

In the case of my car, I didn't know or even see a possibility of a *how*. I only knew of my desire. Yet, with a little patience, my dream, in all its splendor, soon sat in my garage.

"Consider how the lilies grow. They do not labor or spin. Yet, I tell you, not even Solomon in all his splendor was dressed like one of these. If that is how God clothes the grass of the field, which is here today, and tomorrow is thrown into the fire, how much more will he clothe you, o you of little faith?"
Luke 12:27,
King James Version

As a child, I longed to be a teacher. I had spent many happy hours envisioning what teaching might be like. As I grew older, my dream became shrouded by others' opinions, as well as a lack of time and the proper education. It took me years to see that my preconceived means of teaching had blocked me from realizing that I had already become a teacher. Not only had I taken advantage of opportunities to teach young people, I'd also taught adults, even those older than myself. I'd done so without taking the path I thought necessary. I had received the dream (the desired outcome) through other means.

Learn to recognize the difference between asking for the means versus asking for the outcome. Keep your focus on the goal, not the pathway leading there. Many surprises, open doors, and unique opportunities will come your way and show you how to acquire all that you want. This, in essence, is what *synchronicity* is all about.

STEP SIX: FOCUS ON ONE DESIRE AT A TIME

Focus on one major desire at a time. While I usually have anywhere from twenty to thirty desires on my maps at any one time, I typically focus on one major goal. When I try to actively pursue more than one intense goal at a time, I only end up fumbling them all. If, instead, I focus my energy on one pursuit at a time, I find all my goals falling into place synchronistically. For example, trying to start a new and rigorous exercise regimen while also trying to remodel the house, is not a good idea.

STEP SEVEN: BRING YOUR GOAL TO MEMORY OFTEN

Most importantly, follow the keys I've given you and keep your desires map in a prominent place so you will see it often. Use a brightly colored highlighter or crayon to add a 'glow' around each desire as it is fulfilled to remind yourself of how many desires you've obtained.

If I get down, reviewing my image maps is a quick way to boost my ego. I love going back to my cards and seeing how many good things have come into my life—things I asked for and received.

"Desires are seeds waiting for their season to sprout. From a single seed of desire, whole forests grow."

Deepak Chopra,
The Way of the Wizard

"Put all of your attention on today's agenda—not next month's. Put all your energy into this workout—not the workout you hope to have six months from now."

Denis Waitley,
Timing is Everything

STEP EIGHT: CREATE NEW DESIRES FREQUENTLY

When you find many of the desires on any given map have been fulfilled, create a new one which serves to inspire you toward new endeavors.

I am constantly amazed by how many things I have accomplished in so short a time. Sometimes I even have a hard time thinking of what to do next as, suddenly, my possibilities have no bounds.

WHAT HAPPENS NEXT?

What will happen to your goals now? First, you will find many little goals you would like to fulfill. As you focus on each one and define what it really is, you will accomplish it. In most cases, you will complete these first goals very quickly, even if you've believed they were unlikely or impossible.

Your next set of goals will be larger and more complicated. You'll have the confidence to reach for these goals because of the success you had with the first set of smaller goals. Like before, you'll know to clarify them and break them into easy-to-accomplish ministeps. These goals will materialize quickly too. So fast, in fact, the power might scare you. There may be a period where you hold back because you feel you don't deserve all the good things coming your way.

Whenever I doubt I am worthy to receive any of my desires, I think of my children. I remember how I expend great energy to bring them every good thing possible, and then think, how much more would God do for me? I do not know any loving parent who would wish ill on their child. How could God offer any less to me?

Reading this book, and some of the books recommended along the way, will help you work through those issues and soon you too will be reaching for loftier goals.

Eventually, your goals will be focused on your highest purpose. The goals you accomplished in the beginning will seem silly now. Understand that those goals were important in order for you to reach this higher point. At this level, your goals will require diligent effort, focus, and clarification. At first, you might be surprised you are even considering imagining something that is seemingly so

"Set your goals high, and don't stop 'til you get there"
Bo Jackson

"Which of you, if his son asks for bread, will give him a stone? Or if he asks for a fish, will give him a snake? If you, then, though you are evil, know how to give good gifts to your children, how much more will your Father in heaven give good gifts to those who ask him!"
Matthew 9:11,
King James Version

impossible, while at the same time knowing confidently within yourself that this is indeed what you are meant to do. When you first started reading this book and working through this exercise, you would have never dared reach this high or believe this far beyond possibility. At this higher level, you know nothing is impossible to you other than your own self-limiting beliefs.

These highest of goals will redefine who you are. They will change your life in ways you never expected and they will inspire you to continue reaching for all you desire.

. . . all in all, life is good.

CHAPTER TEN: ACKNOWLEDGING YOUR SKILLS

10

Your goals, dreams, hopes, and innermost, heartfelt desires will lead you to your highest purpose and to a place of great fulfillment. If you ignore these inner-built dreams which propel your purpose, your body will resist and fight back, urging you toward that innate core objective—your highest purpose.

It may be that you already understand this, perhaps you once attempted to pursue a goal only to be thwarted. Try as you might, you found your goals blocked or lost in "maybe someday" limbo. *Why?*

WHEN YOU FALTER

There are several reasons why you may feel as if you have faltered in achieving your goals: You may feel uncomfortable or fearful; you may feel lacking in motivation or energy to complete a goal; you may feel blocked or prevented; you may feel you don't have enough education or money or that you are too old, too young, or too physi-

"You are never too old to make significant contributions in life, and if you have to do something to make people sit up and take notice, then by all means, do it."
James Colt Harrison,
writer reviewing the movie
Calendar Girls

cally challenged; you may not know where to begin. While all these excuses sound legitimate, the heart, which tugs relentlessly at your soul, cannot be wrong. That implanted desire has a purpose and requires some means of fulfillment. If so, then how can we overcome these barriers?

FEAR

Feeling uncomfortable or fearful is usually a symptom of one of the other reasons listed below, masked by the fear of the unknown. You may find it helpful to reread the chapter on fear *(See: Section 2)* and to do the fear exercise detailed there.

MOTIVATION

If you lack motivation or energy, it may mean you have not totally clarified your goal. Either you don't have a clear image of what the goal is, or you have not truly accepted its possibility. It may also mean you are not sure how to proceed or lack the needed information to do so. *(More on this follows.)*

TOO OVERWHELMING

If the goal is a large or overwhelming undertaking, you may not know where to begin or how to prioritize the various tasks into an appropriate order.

My youngest son does not work well in situations where he is given too many tasks to complete at once. Sometimes, it helps to give him a list, but often he will absentmindedly scratch items off before they are done. In the long run, if I just give him a few tasks at a time, he is more likely to complete them. When he is done with those, I give him a few more. I keep them simple. "Clean your room," is a complicated, multitask job. "Put your dirty clothes in the hamper," is clear-cut and easy to accomplish.

Sometimes, we need a starting point, a place where we feel safe testing the waters. One friend of mine longed to 'one day' move to another state. She often talked about doing so but never did anything about it. I encouraged her to begin by just looking at possible cities and to get a sense of the places she might want to consider. Once she did that,

"I worked with and felt my fear daily for weeks. If I could change how I felt on the inside, I knew something would change on the outside. This has always been a part of my belief system."
Christiane Northrup,
*Women's Bodies,
Women's Wisdom*

"Pat yourself on the back for every perceived obstacle you've created. Without them, you cannot know what you want."
Lynn Grabhorn,
Excuse Me, Your Life Is Waiting

her plans quickly took shape and, within a year, she had moved. In the beginning, she'd felt overwhelmed by the many obstacles blocking her way. She soon found that as she strove toward her goal, all the necessary elements fell into alignment one by one on an 'as needed' basis.

Our life's path is such that we are often shown only the beginning stages of a goal. In this way, we are not overwhelmed by receiving too much information at once. But sometimes even one simple goal may feel over-whelming. As with my son, redecorating my bedroom was a complicated, goal. When I began to count up the many things I would need to do in order to complete that goal, I dragged my feet in completing the job. For times like this, I find it helpful to create a list of minigoals, then prioritize them in order of importance.

When I'm working synchronistically, my first, second, or third priorities may not be in tune with the universe. As in the case of my bedroom remodeling, I found myself midway though the project and halted. The bookcases I'd ordered had yet to arrive and nothing else could be completed until they were installed.

Coincidentally, the opportunity for me to acquire some items for my bathroom became available. I had not planned to start my bathroom redecoration until I completed the bedroom. Nevertheless, the timing fit together so well that I could not ignore this minor side-step. Working in this synchronistic manner allowed me to purchase, at a discount, out-of-season items that greatly enhanced my bath's decor. Had I waited, I might have searched endlessly and paid a higher price for their equiv-alent. Amazingly, the bookcases arrived the next day. I was back on track with the bedroom, a few steps ahead of my original plan. Working synchronistically and being open to change allowed me to make the most of my so-called delay.

When working towards your desires, you might not always be able to *see* all that is coming together on your behalf. While on a diet plan, I watched as some weeks the scales would show my weight dropping; during others, nothing appeared to happen. I learned that sometimes our bodies lose in different places and ways. By taking my measurements, I had visible evidence of the inches coming off even when pounds hadn't. Something invisible to my

"Each life goal must be broken down into bite-sized pieces. Each small task or requirement on the way to an ultimate goal becomes a mini goal."

Denis Waitley,
Timing Is Everything

eyes had been taking place. Remain diligent. Keep thinking positively. Keep moving forward. All will work out as it should.

BLOCKED

You may feel blocked or in some way prevented from achieving a goal either by another person (or persons) in your life or by your circumstances. Understand that when another person or circumstance appears to prevent our completion of a goal, this is a *perception* and a *choice.* Re-read the chapters on these concepts and allow yourself to accept this fact. *(More information on overcoming this blocked feeling is in this section.)*

NOT 'ENOUGH'

You may feel you don't have enough money or education or you may feel you are too old or too young to reach your goal. You may feel you are too ill or physically challenged. I often felt these things myself because I'd yet to experience the miracles that occur when pursuing a goal.

It is true, though, that some goals require preparation before they can be accomplished. For example, imagine being thrust behind the controls of an airplane while in the air and having never had any instruction, maybe never even having ever flown before. Wouldn't you feel intimidated? You would be destined to fail simply because you were untrained to do this task. Yet think how much more confident, even excited you would be to sit in the pilot's seat knowing you'd earned the right to be there. Flying would then be a pleasure and a tremendous privilege.

If you lack training or the proper tools, then make those things your first goal, the first step on your path to the desired result.

WHEN YOU LACK THE SKILL

Desire and skill are partners. Each time we take action towards our desires, we are rewarded with skill. That skill may be an ability to do something better or it

> *"Any of us can perform little suicides all day long by not speaking up for our needs or waiting for permissions that never come."*
>
> Lindsay C. Gibson,
> *Who You Were Meant to Be*

may be a greater understanding of how things intrinsically work. Some skills we learn though training, practice, and education. Some skills we learn through life experiences.

Skill is not just learning how to fly a plane, write a book, play a piano, or build a house, it's also learning how to teach, how to forgive, how to love, how to grieve.

Before I could write the book that burned inside my soul, I had to learn how to form words, how to put pen to paper, how to clearly state my opinions. But I also needed experiences and values to form the viewpoint from which I would write. I had to suffer through cancer and other ailments so I would know how it felt to be seriously ill and could relate to others who had experienced suffering too.

Skills are something we need to enhance, appreciate, and acknowledge. They are an important aspect of who we are and all we can be. But we cannot gain skills by hoping they will one day fall out of the sky into our lap or by complaining that we don't know how to do something. We have to take some action toward our desires in order to obtain the necessary skills. The skills learned are a part of the reward we gain for moving forward toward our goals.

Skill is a tool not unlike a hammer or a screwdriver. Ask any woodworker and they will say that in order to create a quality product, whether building a birdhouse or a fine dining room cabinet, having the proper tools is a must. For any goal you want to accomplish, you may need to enhance your "tools." Your tools might be a physical item such as a scroll saw, an artist's pallet, a printing press, or a computer. Or "tools" might be wisdom gained from a book, a workshop, or a knowledgeable professional.

For me, makeup had always been something I hurriedly applied in less than five minutes before running out the door. I admired women who were born with the great looks and beautiful skin I didn't have. Then one day, while my husband and I were sitting in a waiting room, I picked up a magazine featuring women's makeovers. Neither of us could believe the amazing transformations in these women with just a change of their hair and the application of the proper makeup. I decided I wanted a makeover too. From looking at those women's photos, I realized the makeup style I'd learned in the seventh grade no longer worked for me as a middle-aged mother of two.

"The only barrier to the expression and application of all our mental skills is our knowledge of how to access them."
Tony Buzan,
The Mind Map Book

"Are you doing the work you like best? If not, do something about it! You will never achieve real success unless you like what you are doing."
Dale Carnegie,
The Dale Carnegie Scrapbook

My makeover amazed me. Not only did I find an outer beauty I hadn't known I possessed, I discovered why they call these special designers makeup *artists*. The woman who applied my new look patted, daubed, smoothed, blended, to create a natural-looking yet greatly enhanced me. I learned that the right makeup made me feel different about myself, more confident, enabled. I also became more aware of my eyes, my lips . . . my smudged mascara. I learned that for a price, I could learn a new skill, create a better me. Beauty wasn't something others were born with (or not); it was a skill.

Often we feel incapable of reaching our goals because we haven't realized the missing skill isn't something learned as much as it is a matter of habit and practice.

Years ago, I had a great friend and one-time coworker who often complimented me on my organizational abilities. She claimed she didn't have the skill herself, though she'd never taken the time to learn what being organized meant. She'd never really tried to be organized. She learned that with very little effort she could choose to be organized just as easily as she had chosen not to.

LOOKING AT THE PARTS TO FIND THE WHOLE

Why is it we sometimes have to do what feels meaningless to learn a skill? Why do typists perform drills, pianists practice scales, skaters trace figure eights? Because in all we do, we build on foundations and rise from humble beginnings.

Skill is a vital component and the second of three keys necessary in finding and fulfilling our highest purpose. As each day passes, we learn something more, we add another piece to the whole. We might not see how flipping burgers for two months lends to our one day being a great ballet dancer or how a rainy weekend camping trip translates to our being promoted to CEO twenty years later. But they do. Our lives are an intricate puzzle with each organic shape interlocking with the others to form the whole of who we are.

A common, funny skit is for a person to take apart a complicated piece of equipment such as an automobile motor and then put it back together only to discover several parts are leftover. These they throw away as unim-

"Wax on, wax off."
The Karate Kid

114

portant even though the viewer of the show knows the parts are important and that some chaos is about to happen for the lack of those parts. Although we can see the obvious outcome of the skit before it happens, we seldom see this in our lives. We have a hard time making sense of the parts we don't know how to fit into our purpose.

In a vision, I saw a labyrinth made of lush green shrubbery and manicured grass. At first, all I could see was the maze of twists and turns, dead ends, and circlebacks. But then I saw how those things fit into the pattern of my life. In the labyrinth, no matter how many choices were available to me, I only had one entrance and one exit. The whole of my life consisted of all that lay *in between.* I had been given the freedom to explore my life as much or as little as I chose. I discovered that what might seem like a dead-end passage—a job that abruptly ended or the loss of a loved one—did not mean this part of the journey or exploration had been wasted—not in the least—because whatever I'd discovered in that passage *added* to the whole that I am and to the knowledge I would carry with me down the next turn.

Think of life as a video game adventure where the traveler seeks out hidden clues and keys they'll later need to win the game. We need to experience those so-called dead-ends in order to be successful in other levels of our lives. Somehow, and as impossible as it seems, all those memorable bits of information scattered over the whole of our lives are important to who we are to become—even if we can't see them as such now.

"The labyrinth governs (and also constitutes) man's circuitous windings through space and time, by ordering, guiding, checking and growing him both from and to his source. It is not other than a model of existence as we know it, a mandala, and a two-dimensional version of the spherical vortex."

Jill Purce,
The Mystic Spiral

TAKING CREDIT FOR YOUR SKILLS

As we live and grow, we collect a variety of skills and experiences. So many, in fact, that we might not even realize just how many skills we actually have.

For a period of years, I homeschooled both of my boys. (Both have since graduated.) Our evaluation system for credit was as follows:

One credit equals –

- *A completed textbook*
- *Taking a college class*
- *Writing a ten-page (or more) paper*
- *120 days of focused activities*

One afternoon, while evaluating their credits, I thought about all the books I had read, all the pages I'd written, and I started to wonder what *my* evaluation credits would look like. Going back to post-high school, I summarized them using a similar point system.

As I noted these credits, I charted them on an image map in clusters according to category, trying to think along the lines of college curriculum. I put them in clusters relating to:

- *Social studies*
- *Math*
- *Political science*
- *Fine arts*
- *Science and technology*
- *Language arts*

I'd written stories, articles, and books. I'd created countless artistic projects. I also had child rearing, home economics, and teaching skills. I found I had multiple credit clusters in areas such as psychology, metaphysics, language arts, and nutrition, areas where I had read a lot of books, done a lot of personal research, or simply had a lot of life experience.

While these 'credits' didn't gain me an official college degree, they did show me where my skill strengths were concentrated, as well as how those clusters intertwined themselves to bring me to who I am now.

These skill clusters showed me how to move forward. They paralleled and enhanced my desires and showed me open doors in my life I'd yet to see. The information also revealed many skills I didn't realize I possessed, since many had been earned in nontraditional ways.

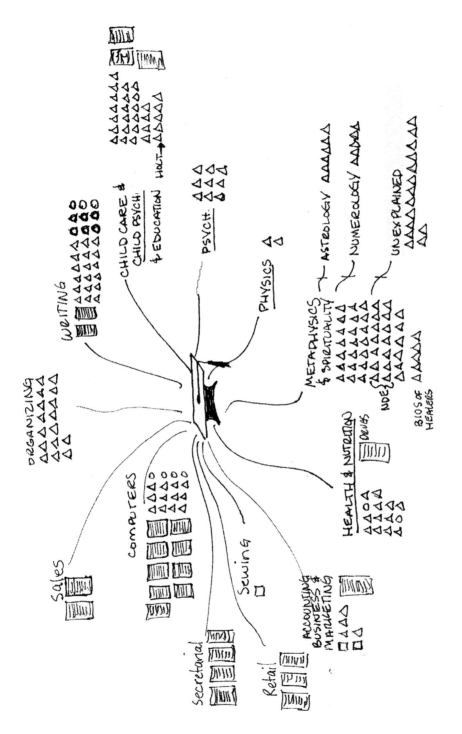

An example of giving myself credit by quickly summarizing on a large index card symbols to represent classes taken, books read, papers written, etc.

EXERCISE 7—SKILLS CREDIT

Create an image map using symbols to equal books read, classes taken, degrees acquired, life experiences, and so forth, as detailed in the list below. Remember to double-count credits when learning and acquired skills are integrated together. For example, writing a science paper is two skills—English and science, so record credits in both areas. Keep this exercise in a safe place as you'll need it later.

"Make a list of every talent you have, however small, and every goal you accomplished that has been important to you."
Denis Waitley,
Timing is Everything

One credit equals –

- *A completed textbook or any nonfiction book*
- *Taking a college class, or any class offering how-to instruction (regardless of length)*
- *Writing a ten-page (or more) paper (each topic, essay, report, or book equals one credit)*
- *365 days of focused activities (i.e., child rearing)*
- *Work or volunteer experience (each type of skill times one year equals one credit. Half credits given for under one year.)*
- *Honors or awards in any given area (one credit each.)*
- *Membership in an organization (one credit per organization, per year)*
- *Travel—especially when doing so includes an understanding or enriched experience of the culture (one credit per trip, per culture experienced)*
- *Fluency in a foreign language (one per language)*
- *Hobbies and focused interests (one credit per interest)*

PURPOSEFUL CHILDHOOD MEMORIES

All my life I had certain recurring memories that seemingly had no significance. These memories were unique because they were not connected to any major or traumatic life event; they were not a part of any celebration, family gathering, or holiday. They were just snapshots of my life. They were often brought to mind for no reason. I couldn't understand why I'd continually remember these particular aspects of my life.

When I created my skills map, I discovered these unique memories served as sign posts of skills and directions I later took. In essence, these memories were confirmation of my being on the right track.

In one such memory, a girlfriend and I had hand-copied story books to sell to friends and neighbors. I could not have guessed then that between the technology skills passed to me by my father and my love of books passed to me by my mother that I would one day play an important role in helping others produce and publish their writing.

In another of these memories, I remember a large bulletin board I'd cocreated with a classmate and friend. The bulletin board won several awards and went on to a national competition. It was not the awards that I remembered or cherished but the board's sense of marketing and design that came to mind—the same sense I would later use to design visual cues for my web pages.

In yet another memory, I am on my front porch playing teacher to the neighborhood kids, using cast off textbooks and outdated worksheets I'd gleaned from past years. I didn't know then I would be both mom and teacher to my own kids, as well as a teacher and mentor to others—both adults and children.

"There is not a single way, but a variety of possibilities within each person."

Philip Burley,
Saint Germain

Chapter Eleven:
The Spiral
of Life

When Desire Creates Skill

11

Purpose is something we gain as we learn, grow, and acquire skills. Purpose is driven by desire and desire by purpose. We don't really know where our desires come from, we only know they seem to live in our hearts and play in our minds. No matter how hard we might try to deny them, it seems nothing can squelch our desires.

In one of my endless endeavors to understand my desires, my purpose, and my life, I covered the floor in index cards, each showing a step in my life's progression of desires, skills, and experiences. A pattern emerged.

Desires created a spiral-like pattern with one of two destinations always recurring, yet building on all that had already transpired

I found that a desire propagated a goal. The goal led to a skill. The skill, in turn, created a new enhanced desire. The cycle then began again—desire, goal, skill; desire, goal, skill; desire, goal, skill; on and on and on. But if I blocked my desire, eventually an ailment arose and created a different destination, one that brought the desire back into focus. I could then choose to further the desire and reach for the goal, or face another ailment. In this

"With each turn man completes a stage in his evolution. In the centre of the spiral he meets himself; this is his higher or complete Self, symbolized by Christ."

Jill Purce,
The Mystic Spiral

scenario, the cycle limped along as such: desire, ailment; desire, ailment; and so on until I acknowledged the desire and worked toward bringing my desire to fulfillment.

This cycle is the spiral of life. For each round we make in the spiral, we gain insight into our experience. The insight might change our perspective and point us in a new direction as we take the next go-round in the cycle. After all, it is our *perception* of any given symptom that gives it any validity or credence.

Remember, ailments are merely symptoms. We can treat the symptoms and make them subside, but if we don't address the underlying emotional connection, new symptoms will appear.

Think of symptoms as if they were dandelions. Unless you remove the root, the flowers continue to sprout, generating seeds for more plants and more flowers. In order to eradicate the symptoms and prevent further ailments from occurring, we must get to the core of the problem by finding the symptom's emotional connection.

My own spiral looks something like this when summarized:

- (Desire) At three years old, I attempted to write words.

- (Goal) Learn how to write words.

- (Skill) My mother put me in preschool and bought me word flashcards, giving me a head start on learning.

- (Desire) Finding my deceased sister's diary empty, I longed to leave some record of myself.

- (Goal) To write about myself.

- (Skill) At age eight, I wrote my first autobiography using a typewriter, a step up from the hand-writing I'd already mastered.

- (Desire) A teacher read *The Diary of Ann Frank* to our class, giving me a new understanding of how one's writing allowed others from all over the world to learn more about a time, a place, a person. I wanted to do that too.

- (Goal) To touch the world with my writing.

"Do not hesitate to do that which you have been called to do for fear of being unworthy for it is in doing the thing that you will be made so."

Jamie L. Saloff

- (Skill) I learned to touchtype and began typing the short stories I'd written.

- (Desire) My father's illness and eventual death, along with the loss of other important family members, led me to want answers for their illness and suffering.

- (Goal) Find answers.

- (Skill) Succumbing to illness myself, I gained a better understanding of what an ill person faced, feared, and allowed to happen. I took notice of wellness strategies and learned what worked, what didn't.

- (Desire) I began writing a book about my cancer experience but found it lacking universally effective strategies that could help larger groups of people, and so I set out to find one.

- (Goal) Seek out more effective strategies.

- (Skill) I worked with various writing mentors, honing my writing knowledge, and learned a means for answering the questions I had about my own illness.

- (Desire) In finding the answers I sought, I looked for ways to present them to the world through writing, the Internet, and other means.

- (Goal) Learn marketing strategies.

- (Skill) I learned to create web pages, utilize print-on-demand publishing, utilize marketing and mentoring techniques.

Of course, the spiral goes on and on, always heightening the desire and skill to a greater level and higher purpose. First, as a child, my desires were singular, simple, and self-focused. As I grew, my desires expanded to include family members and more complicated goals, finally culminating with desires for reaching out to people across the globe and encompassing multilevel goals and technologies.

". . . first teach individuals, then groups, and finally the masses."
Edgar Cayce, as quoted by Harold J. Reilly,
Edgar Cayce Handbook for Health Through Drugless Therapy

CHAPTER TWELVE: WHY YOUR HERITAGE IS IMPORTANT

AND HOW IT CAN BENEFIT YOU

12

Whenever I talk to people about the interconnection between their life purpose and their heritage, they balk, they disagree, they become defensive. Some people react this way because they have no interest in being like their parents. They also immediately tap into that tangled web of emotions created in having lived through the rules, regulations, and expectations put on them during their childhood. Some people react negatively because they feel they're done with all their parents have been to them. They've moved out and moved on. Beyond a basic concern for their parents well-being and occasional visits for holidays or birthdays, they have no interest in returning to the past, particularly if their relationship included abuse, abandonment, or dysfunctional circumstances.

Nevertheless, and despite any objections, our heritage plays an important role in the equation of our higher purpose. Until now, your ideas and sense of purpose may have been driven merely by instinct. You may have walked blindly into opportunities, struggled with life decisions, and just "hoped" you were doing the right thing.

Clarifying your purpose will give you direction in your

"The truth is there are many outside factors that attempt to influence your free will, but you are the only one who can keep your dreams from becoming a reality."

Tom Bird,
Releasing Your Artist Within

life, make it easier for you to look for opportunities, and make effective decisions. However, before, I offer an exercise on identifying and clarifying purpose, there are some important issues to discuss. As I explained earlier, once you commit yourself to pursuing a purposeful goal, you set into motion a series of coinciding events of which I want you to be aware.

So many times before, you may have tried to move toward fulfilling a goal and stopped. Something or someone may have stood in your way—or so you perceived. What you may not have realized is that when these challenges arose, they were evidence that *you were on the right track*. That's right, those hurdles or roadblocks that stood between you and your goal were all part of a larger, purposeful plan. They were designed to reveal an innate challenge and release you from its hold. When we pursue our goals—goals that are our deepest, most heart-felt desires—we set into motion a predestined series of events which are vital to our fulfilling that purpose.

The completion of these events will virtually guarantee the acquisition of your desired goals. Therefore, the presence of these events is a sign not to turn tail and run but to press on, for you are about to witness miracles. Doors will be opened. Persons with knowledge or needed material goods will appear in your life, and the seemingly impossible will occur. You might see a dramatic change in your life circumstance or perhaps find a previously critical person has a reversal in the way they speak to you. These are typical of the kinds of things that happen when you press through barriers to reach your desires and goals.

Yes, there will be consequences. They are a part of the challenge. And yes, you may have to accept some changes to your life. Nevertheless, know that fulliling these deeply ingrained goals ultimately offer you a more rewarding life.

"You are in a very powerful place right now."

Tom Bird

WHAT OUR PARENTS OFFER TOWARD OUR PURPOSE

We have already discussed skill and desire. They are the easiest two of the three purposeful components to understand. But, despite a tangled web of fears, conflicts and social expectations, *our heritage* is perhaps the most vital element necessary in fully defining and understanding our higher purpose.

Carol Adrienne writes in *The Celestine Prophecy Workbook* that we can discover our purpose by "recognizing what our parents accomplished and where they left off." It is this aspect of our heritage that we want to focus on most. We want to take a closer look at the challenges our parents faced because it is their challenges, which they either left incomplete or brought to an inappropriate conclusion, that we might face in some form ourselves.

Our upbringing, particularly our adolescence, acclimates us to our inherent challenges. Our adolescence is the training ground where we gain the information we will later need to understand our innate challenges. As one friend put it, "Perhaps we have parents simply to hand us our purpose."

In adolescence, our parents pass to us the mantle they carried. We learn firsthand of their successes and of their failures. In adolescence, we learn by experience what is socially acceptable and what is not; we learn about our heritage by living within it, and we learn how others before us and within our sphere of influence have faced the same challenges.

It is in adolescence that we begin to gather an understanding of the tools and desires we will later use in our attempts to overcome the challenges we see and live in around us. None of these challenges are new, they have all been present before—though played out in different lives and different situations—by our parents and theirs and theirs before them.

During our adolescence, we begin to relate to individuals whose methods we will one day adapt as our own. As adults, we might find ourselves facing similar situations or making the same mistakes our parents once did. This is a natural progression since the best way to learn how to overcome a challenge is to be thrust headlong into it.

> *"If you can find the higher meaning of their [your parents'] lives, you will be more inclined to see how their lives prepared you for your life mission."*
> James Redfield, Carol Adrienne,
> *The Celestine Prophecy: An Experiential Guide*

> *"So do you figure that the reason we're children is not because we're worthless but because we need time to get that information, and get taller, and when we're grownups we're going to feel just the way we do now except we'll know more nuts and bolts about how to get along?"*
> Richard Bach,
> *Running from Safety*

FAMILY THEMES

Every family member has a story. Every family unit has a theme. Dig deeply both laterally through your family (aunts, uncles, cousins, siblings) as well as backwards (grandparents, great-grandparents, and farther, if possible) looking specifically for common themes—even if all you have to go on is myth and hearsay.

One of my friends, who suffered from breast cancer, had a common breast cancer theme in her family; another found the family's theme to be incest.

My family's theme stemmed around grief and loss due to illness, tragedy, and death. My maternal grandfather had died when my mother was just six months old, my paternal grandmother died after my father turned twelve. One relative committed suicide, leaving three young children behind. Another took both her own life and that of her daughter. My parents lost not only my sister, but also another child, a son who died three days after birth from a congenital heart defect. These deaths left an emotional scar on those left behind, a scar they passed on to me.

A family's theme will be focused around recurring events, illnesses, or family dynamics that directed their lives, their health, and their well-being. This theme is more obvious in some families than others. In the case of my friend with breast cancer, she hadn't recognized the theme until I brought it up, even though three or four of her relatives had died from breast cancer before she contracted it herself.

Some families might have multiple themes. In any case, it is not the ailments, situations, or tragedies themselves that are the themes as much as the families' *reactions* and *beliefs* surrounding those situations. Remember to always look for an underlying emotional connection to these things.

EXERCISE 8—DEFINING YOUR STATEMENT OF PURPOSE

You may find within your family lineage both a main, core theme, as well as several secondary threads that help you understand the means in which you will project your purpose. For example, my mother's family hosted a long line of teachers and preachers.

Sometimes you will find a thread that you can't make

"I didn't know how I'd feel being a mom—it makes me feel as though I somehow have a purpose."

Angelina Joliè
During a televised interview
with Barbara Walters

128

sense of. It could be a thread picked up by another sibling or one that has yet to play a prominent role in your life. In my family, transportation is a major theme. My maternal grandfather worked for the railroad. My two uncles owned a car dealership. My paternal grandfather also sold and manufactured automobiles. Perhaps this is why my brother has worked in the airline business for so many years. He even sold cars for a while. He is furthering the transportation aspect of our common heritage while I pursue others.

Looking ahead at the lives of my own children, I can already see the patterns forming in their lives, readying them to pick up the family's mantle. And when I see my life reflected in theirs, I am reminded of other issues I've yet to work through. Amazingly, as I work through my issues, I see them walk clear of them too and move on to others.

Using family clues and themes, combine your desires, skills, and heritage together, continually refitting and reorganizing the puzzle pieces until the statement of purpose you define feels right. It's not an exact art but one that will help you find direction.

In my own life, my desires and skills cluster in the areas of psychology, health, writing, computer technologies , and communications. I was raised in a heritage of pain and suffering. My skills and heritage have led me to define my statement of purpose as "communicate to others solutions for inner healing."

This is the first of two exercises on finding purpose—so don't struggle over it too much. Once you have a purpose statement, you can begin to act on it, plan goals around it, and move toward obtaining it. As you acquire the different aspects of your purpose, you'll see results from your walking toward it; you'll notice other aspects of your heritage, desire, and skill that are evolving into what you are reaching for.

"Many people have confided in me that they don't have the vaguest idea about their purpose in life. They lack a spiritual connection and are not open to looking beyond their mortality for meaning. For them, I simply offer the idea that they can begin to discover their purpose by learning the most, experiencing the most, and sharing the most value they possibly can with other human beings."

Denis Waitley,
Timing is Everything

"Automatically, as we shine who we are, asking ourselves every minute is this what I really want to do, doing it only when we answer yes; automatically that turns away those who have nothing to learn from who we are and attracts those who do, and from who we have to learn, as well."

Richard Bach,
Illusions

Chapter Thirteen: Bringing All the Pieces Together

13

I am about to share with you an exercise that provides obvious clues to who you are and why you are here. This exercise points out the challenges that were of the greatest significance to those in your ancestry and, in turn, of great significance to you.

Until now, everything we've talked about has been important, but maybe didn't feel as defining for you as you would have liked. This is because as you focused on your personal collection of eclectic family stories, you weren't seeing anything you didn't already know. You wanted to see some significant revelation, something that would clearly define why all of your family situations were important. The exercise I want you to do next is designed to explain why your heritage is important to you; however, it was necessary to look at what we have examined so far in order for this particular exercise to be effective for you.

Just as you learned how your own body creates ailments when you repress your purpose, then it makes sense that by interpreting your *parents'* ailments—and their parents—that you will find significant challenges in your parents' lives. And because we are also looking at the

"From our parents' strengths and from particular growth issues they didn't complete, we can derive our life question and our work or 'mission' in the world."
James Redfield, Carol Adrienne, *The Celestine Prophecy: An Experiential Guide*

emotional connections in these ailments, maybe for the first time, you'll see your parents' ailments from a new perspective. You'll understand why they are important to *your* life.

YOUR INNATE CHALLENGES

In the same way you may have acquired an appreciation or skill from your parents and/or caregivers, you were also given another 'gift.' *Innate Challenges.* An Innate Challenge is *a hurdle or struggle passed from your heritage to you for you to resolve.*

From the wealth of family stories and culture, to the trials and errors your family faced, all this played a role in who your *family* is and was. Your family heritage plays a role in who *you* are.

It doesn't matter if what you remember about your family and heritage is "truth" or "Truth." Much of what you might know about your ancestral past may be only myth, hearsay, and legend. What matters is your *impressions* and *interpretations* of those events as it's your impressions of them that have colored your life.

But how do you sift through decades of life experiences and heritage stories to find those elements that are particular and important to you?

For one thing, you are already familiar with many of your innate challenges, if not by clear definition then by experience, since the same challenges loom before you time and time again until you find some way to bring them to a resolution.

A friend of mine once told me the story of how his ex-wife always knew how to "push his buttons" in order to make him react in a particular way. Over and over, she successfully used those means against him. Near the end of their marriage, he found he no longer reacted to those button-pushing antics and no longer felt bound by their pull. He had found resolution within himself for those fears, challenges, and knee-jerk reactions. In that same way, you will know you have found a resolution to your challenges when you no longer react to their presence.

As previously noted, for this process you are not concerned with the facts in Truth as much as what you personally remember. You are interested ultimately in using this information to benefit your own life. Because of this, it's important that each individual do their own interpretations since each has their own understandings of the deduced symbols or archetypes. What might be the right answer for you may not be the right answer for your sister, your brother, your mother, or aunt. While you may find parallels and similar understandings because of your common heritage, the differences in your individual paths will cause your interpretations to vary. This is the grand gift of this process, since the variance is what creates the particular and individualized answer required. It gives to you the unique insight you so deeply desire.

"Then I began to piece together the scraps of stories my parents had told me of their own childhoods. I started to see a larger picture of their lives. With my growing understanding, and from an adult viewpoint, I began to have compassion for their pain; and the blame slowly began to dissolve."

Louise L. Hay,
You Can Heal Your Life

EXERCISE 9—FINDING MEANING IN YOUR PAST

To do this exercise, use the steps given in *Exercise One: How to Interpret an Ailment*, with the following added considerations:

STEP ONE: YOUR CAREGIVERS

Begin with your main caregivers, your mother/father, guardian, or other figure(s) whose role was most prominent in your upbringing. *(As you feel comfortable interpreting the information, you may add other persons from your sphere of influence, such as your grandparents, aunts, uncles, cousins, siblings, even your spouse, children, or in-laws.)*

STEP TWO: IDENTIFYING YOUR PARENTS' AILMENTS

Working with one individual at a time, make a list of this person's major ailments, those requiring stitches, casting, hospitalization, surgery, long-term medication, or care. Include disabilities and chronic ailments, life-threatening and life-ending situations (even if accidental). And just as in your own interpretations—the more major the ailment for them, the stronger the message for you.

STEP THREE: OUR PARENTS' EMOTIONAL CONNECTIONS

After you have compiled their ailments list, work through the ailment interpretation exercise found on page 31 for each noted symptom, looking for the underlying emotional connections—as *you* see them. Again, you are interested in the meanings to you; however, if this person had some interpretation of their condition, that also plays a role. So, factor in your feelings of their interpretation as well.

For example, my aunt believed that her brother's ailment, a recurring cyst on his neck, was cancer, despite the doctors repeatedly saying it wasn't. She would tell us, "Once you have cancer, you're gone." This statement, based on what had been true in her younger days, proved untrue in the case of her brother. However, her words often haunted *me* after *my* cancer diagnosis.

STEP FOUR: YOUR PARENTS' INNATE CHALLENGES

Of course, the hardest part is translating this person's underlying emotional connection into an appropriate innate challenge statement valuable to *you*. But doing so is not as hard as you might think.

INTERPRETATIONS

My father suffered from hardening of the arteries (arteriosclerosis). This is a debilitating disease in which cholesterol particles collect along the artery walls, eventually blocking them or creating balloon-like pockets that could burst. Interpreting my father's underlying connections gave me the impression that he was holding back particular life pressures—like the expanding air in a balloon—and allowing countless daily annoyances to collect inside him without letting them go. Just as the particles of cholesterol blocked his arteries, the feelings he didn't release blocked his flow of life and love.

Eventually, my father's arteries deteriorated until he lost a leg. In a sense, "he didn't have a leg to stand on" or "couldn't stand on his own two feet." He had lost the ability to "stand up" for himself.

Standing up for myself is one of *my* major innate challenges and doing so was never so important as during my

134

battle with cancer. It was in standing up for myself that I initiated healing into my life.

Analyzing another of my father's ailments, I considered the loss of his teeth. At the age of sixteen, my father had all of his upper teeth extracted. (I never knew why.) I considered losing one's teeth at such a young age as a major and perhaps traumatic event. At the same time, he had suffered from an allergic reaction to penicillin. For this interpretation, I asked myself what teeth represented and determined, in this case, teeth related to one's ability to eat and to smile. For me, food issues have always been a major challenge, as has joy, though I'm often told I have a beautiful smile, and I use it often.

Ulcers to me are an inner sore that eats away at the stomach's lining, so in interpreting my mother's ulcer attacks, I asked myself, "Was something eating at my mother?" My mother also suffered from heart blockage (like my father) and colon cancer, perhaps an inability to release. While there might be countless insignificant reasons emotionally causing these ailments, I deduced that the ailments stemmed from the loss of my sister who died at age nine after having been hit by a car.

My parents rarely spoke of my sister, who died three years before my birth. They hid her pictures in the bottom drawer, as if by not remembering her their pain would also disappear. They buried their grief within their hearts instead of releasing it. Obviously, neither parent dealt well with their grief and, ultimately, I believe it killed them both.

And what of my sister's death? Her passing certainly had an impact on my life. The most significant interpretation I extracted from her death had to be the sudden and unexpected impact of the car that came from nowhere. The true challenge for me has been my own unexplained fear of a sudden and unexpected death of either myself or a loved one. This fear, which began haunting me when I turned nine, intensified after I had been rear-ended in 1996 and has been one of several challenges in my life I've yet to overcome.

Some of these interpretations contain a bit of "tongue in cheek," a little humor never hurt anyone. Besides, no one ever said that interpreting a life challenge couldn't be fun. Sometimes it is by remembering the comical side of

"My grandfather killed my father in my mind. I know he died of cancer—but it was because of what my grandfather did to him."

Lacey Ford
on Henry & Edsel Ford,
The Men and the Machine

135

these interpretations that you can overcome them. Ultimately, just knowing the challenge exists is the all-important first step in overcoming the challenge and bringing it to resolution. Therefore, the goal of this exercise is simply to define as many of those challenges as you can by looking at those who came before you and interpreting the challenges they left incomplete or that were never brought to an appropriate resolution. The more often you find a similar challenge entwined throughout your heritage, the more likely that challenge plays a prominent roll in your life.

FINDING YOUR HIGHER PURPOSE—PART TWO

Remember back in the opening when I talked about purpose and the difference between trying to navigate your way down a ski slope with and without skis? Well, now you have the opportunity to put on those skis (Purpose) and glide down the slope of life with ease. Now you have the opportunity to gather the pieces together and make sense of it all.

One breakthrough for me came when I looked at my skills cluster map. I found it amazing how I had unknowingly gathered all the skills I could want for the desires I had and for the purpose I now know. Another came, as I described in the opening of this book, when I learned to use word association to uncover the meanings of my ailments.

There is a great relief in knowing our ailments have a purpose. We haven't been subjected to meaningless suffering. The pain and grief we feel has been an inner guidance system designed to assure us of finding and fulfilling our life's purpose. All this is based, not by some dogma or fear, but on the deepest, most dearest desires of our heart. This means that the more we walk toward fulfilling our purpose, the greater joy we'll find in our lives, because we'll be doing the very things we want to do most.

I will never forget my shock, now years ago, when a good friend and I talked about God's purpose for our lives. She said she didn't want to know what purpose God had for her. She felt it held something for her to dread. How

"Go confidently in the direction of your dreams. Live the life you have imagined."
Henry David Thoreau

136

could she not want to know all that God and life had in store for her?

What she didn't realize then was the dread she felt was not a fear of God's disapproval or dislike of her highest-most purpose. The dread she felt stemmed from her inner knowing that she had not done all she could to find a way to fulfill her purpose. She had instead repressed her desires and purpose because of fear. This left her feeling guilt and shame, further convincing her to hold back from what she wanted most.

Now you have the opportunity to bring your purpose into view. By working through the heritage exercise for each significant person in your life, your innate challenges will become clear. By seeing your innate challenges, in combination with your desires and your skills, a pattern and a map will emerge.

Although, I located the three components of purpose—*Desire, Skill*, and *Heritage*—one at a time and over long years of trial and error, you have the opportunity, with this book and a few hours of time, to glean the same life-changing information. Don't become frustrated if at first you can't find the meaning of your life. Keep thinking about all you've read herein. Go back and review, if necessary. Keep checking to make sure you've included all that you should in each of the three component areas.

If I can heal my life from cancer and the other many ailments that attacked me, so can you. This is typically what your ailments are about, your body's unbreakable determination to fulfill your deepest heart's desires. Our lives are filled with many choices, but no matter what choices you make, you have not failed your purpose and you have not 'missed the boat.' No matter how sick you may be, no matter how deep within the hole you may have fallen, you still have time to pursue your life's purpose.

EXERCISE 10—REDEFINING YOUR GOALS

Now that you have a clearer picture of who you are and what you want to pursue in life, it's time to go back and reevaluate the goals and desires you created at the

". . . fear, shame, the henchmen of failure. . . Surely you can see how these feelings have never been about you—but other people's reactions to you."
Lindsay C. Gibson,
Who You Were Meant to Be

beginning of this section. You may need to add to what you've written down or you may need to create a new and separate map dedicated solely to your purpose.

Let's go back to the beginning of this section and quickly review the steps necessary to finding our purpose.

Remember:

DESIRE + SKILL + HERITAGE = PURPOSE

The key to overcoming your innate challenges is to follow through on your desires.

Amazing isn't it? The very thing you've pushed aside, tried to forget, buried deep within your soul, is the one thing you need to dig out and pursue since:

1. Purpose is the key to overcoming your innate challenges.

2. By finding resolution to your innate challenges you move closer to your highest, most important purpose.

Start with the desires of your heart. If all else fails, follow those and you can't go wrong. Desire is the number one key component in both finding purpose and crashing through your most difficult innate challenges. Even if you knew none of what I've written here, you would have the illuminating fire of desire inside you.

Time is not hinged on the clock and its minute hand, but upon events. To move your life forward through its labyrinth, create a new event, a new happening. Reach for a new goal—a purposeful goal.

Throughout this section, I have presented a series of exercises which when combined give you a clearer definition of your life's purpose. Using what you learned earlier in mapping and charting your desires as goals, make a new image map based on what you've learned about your purpose. Unlike your desires map where you could list anything you desired, this new map should focus on those goals that will further your higher purpose.

Now is the time to go back, review, and fully clarify what you have learned. Before we continue, here are some general tips to help you.

"Pulling back the bow is a metaphor for doing the work, engaging in the movement and the flow that leads us to our goal."

Lynn V. Andrews,
Love and Power

STEP ONE: RELAX

Before making any considerations, relax fully and deeply. Take relaxing breaths; listen to a meditation tape or do some other activity which will allow you to consider the found information from your highest perspective. (You may want to first review the Section on *Connection*.)

STEP TWO: NO DISTRACTIONS!

Make sure you do the exercises during a time when you won't be distracted or interrupted.

> *"We are all called. We are all chosen. But so very, very few of us have the courage to follow our dreams."*
> Agnes Whistling Elk,
> as told to Lynn V. Andrews,
> *Love and Power*

STEP THREE: GIVE YOURSELF TIME

Give yourself several chances to think through all the information you have gathered from the previous exercises before writing down your final purpose statement. Take time to sleep on it. If you are one of the lucky individuals who feels you already know your life's purpose, allow yourself the opportunity to add to that statement, realign it, or change it altogether if the information revealed points in a new or different direction.

STEP FOUR: IT'S NOT JUST A JOB, IT'S A WAY OF LIFE

Consider that *purpose* is not necessarily a job title or a position of employment. Too often people find themselves in a mundane job feeling that if only they could find a better position, they would feel more fulfilled and have purposeful lives. Purpose does not necessarily equal employment, but it could. Wasn't Jesus a carpenter? Paul, perhaps the greatest of the New Testament writers, made tents. Yet both found their purpose by other means. While our purpose might lead to joyful and gainful employment, it might also be a fulfilling hobby or charitable endeavor. Purpose can be the way you encourage those around you, like your favorite grandmother, it can be some financial backing that you offer, or it can be hundreds of other things as purpose cannot be defined by what's on your paycheck or in your job description.

> *"You will know when you are doing your specific work when there is a deep resonance within your being. The ease and grace with which your life flows is also a clear indication that you are aligned with your true function."*
> Zoeu Jho,
> *E.T. 101*

STEP FIVE: TWO MAPS ARE BETTER THAN ONE

Please note that the purpose map does not cancel out the desire map. Both are important and show you things about yourself. Keep these maps in a visible place and watch for miracles to occur.

What's Next? Now you are ready to move on to something really fun. . . .

Section Four:
Connection
Communicating With God and Our Higher Self

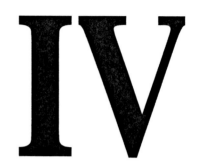

"You don't have to wait to see an angel reader or locate someone with special talents and abilities to receive and benefit from heavenly advice. These messages are meant for you, and God designed them to be easy to receive."

Doreen Virtue,
Divine Prescriptions

CHAPTER FOURTEEN: ARE YOU FULLY PLUGGED IN?

14

WHY YOU NEED CONNECTION

WHAT IS CONNECTION?

Connection is about communicating with yourself and God on the deepest and highest possible level. Depending on your beliefs, you may have previously referred to this connection by one of the following means:

- *Having a hunch*

- *Tapping into your higher self and super-consciousness*

- *Communing with God through His intermediary, The Holy Spirit*

- *Reaching across the stream of consciousness and connecting with the universe*

- *Having a 'gut' feeling*

- *Being one with the Source*

- *Being in tune with self*

- *Hearing from God*

- *Women's intuition*

"What we lack are not ideas but a direct means of getting in touch with them."
Gabriele Lusser Rico,
Writing the Natural Way

"Your intuition is your unconscious knowledge based on your own personal experiences. It is what you somehow sense is right for you."

Spencer Johnson,
Yes or No

Any of these definitions are suitable because it's not the definition that matters, it's the act of making the connection and its resulting evidence that is important. Therefore, in order to avoid confusion and for the sake of these texts, I have referred to the process simply as *connection*, but feel free to substitute whatever personal reference you prefer.

WHY IS CONNECTION IMPORTANT?

Like the wind, *connection* is best known and understood by its results rather than of its presence. When we make and maintain this connection—and maintaining is the key to obtaining its highest benefits—we open our lives to tremendous possibility and potential. Connection brings:

- *Knowledge (on how to do something)*

- *Direction (where, when, how, or with whom)*

- *Inspiration (encouraging us over the rough patches and increasing our passion)*

- *Balance and Flow (opening doors of opportunity, meeting the right people at the right time, synchronicity)*

- *Joy*

- *Peace*

- *Unconditional Love (the highest form available)*

If you are not yet utilizing this simple-to-access gift, you are in for a dramatic and wonderful change in your life. With connection to self and to God you gain the knowledge you need to accomplish your most sought-after goals and to achieve your highest purpose. That's pretty significant, so let me say it again, *connection is the key to obtaining the necessary knowledge and guidance we need to accomplish our deepest heart's desires.*

Connection is also a vital key in obtaining and maintaining total wellness—body, mind, and spirit. It is the ability to tap into a higher consciousness, to gain access to the throne room of our mind. Connection brings us the

144

means and power to overcome difficult emotional and physical barriers. It allows us to see the Truth of a situation and to set our feet on the right path. Connection is of a very personal nature, innate to all we know, love, and require. It is the means to tap into wisdom greater than any known by our conscious mind for:

- *Problem solving*

- *Creating new ideas*

- *Finding new and better ways to do the usual, the typical, and the mundane*

And connection is love to the nth degree.

But if this connection is so awe inspiring, so powerful, so life changing, why don't more people speak of it? Why don't more people show evidence of it in their lives?

WHY WE HAVE PUT CONNECTION ON 'HOLD'

How many of us make time to meditate, contemplate, or spend time in deep thought on a daily basis in this rush-and-scurry world? Something more important always takes precedence, like editing a report for work, taking the kids to soccer practice, making the weekly grocery run, or yet another doctor's appointment.

Another reason we don't take time for connection is that we haven't yet recognized the tremendous power and success we would have in our lives from doing so. If we did, we would immediately make connection a top priority. And since connection is something ethereal, defined mostly by feeling rather than logic, we have a hard time justifying giving an intensified connection a chance. Why?

Because we've all been programmed through our upbringing to disassociate from our connection. How many businessmen are willing to commit to a large contract based on intuition? How many people accept a job on something as flimsy as a feeling? We're taught instead to believe in all that is logical, rational, and practical. We're taught, "Don't believe it unless you can see it." "Don't trust what you feel." "Take no thought of what may be too far outside the lines." So we don't. In addition, we have also been lied to—yes, *lied* to.

How many of us as children knew something—

"Harvard Business School doesn't teach you how to feel something in your gut."
Robert Kraft,
New England Patriots
NFL team owner[1]

145

anything—that we knew-knew-knew to be true, yet we were told we were wrong, that we didn't know what we were talking about. Years later, we may have been able to prove our truth, but because we were so often told as children we were wrong, or simply ignored when we tried to speak up about what we believed, we began to doubt ourselves and to feel as if there were something wrong with us. How else could we explain the strange contradiction between what we were being told by those who claimed to love us and what we were feeling within our hearts and minds?

To cope with this contradiction, we stopped relying on what we felt, as we assumed that our feelings couldn't be trusted. Instead, we relied on others to tell us what to do, what to think, what to believe. We felt safer that way. We felt more accepted. And by doing so, we didn't have to make sense of the inner conflict we felt inside.

Unfortunately, the more we relied on others, the more our inner connection faded. Worse yet, something within us began to die. Our lives no longer felt purposeful, enlivened, or fulfilled. As children, we didn't recognize we had a choice, and by the time we reached adulthood, we had forgotten how to connect, delegating the memory of it to the far reaches of our minds.

"No matter how strong the connection, you were undersized, outnumbered, and out-positioned, and so you had no other choice than to give in as the first wave of severing criticism descended upon you from those who loved you and whom you depended upon the most."

Tom Bird,
Releasing Your Artist Within

WE WERE BORN WITH THE ABILITY TO CONNECT

Making this connection is highly innate to our inner being. When it takes place, we don't recognize it or think about it just as we rarely give thought to the regulated beat of our heart, the intake of our breath, and the rush of blood through our veins. Connection is second nature to us. We were born with the ability to receive this information, thus many of us receive it and use it without even realizing it as such. Communicating on this level takes place anytime, anywhere, every moment of the day.

Okay, if it's that simple, why pay any attention to it at all? Why not just keep on going the way we have, laughing at the funny coincidences, trusting ourselves to somehow get us where we belong without any conscious knowledge of what we are doing or why? Because by working cooperatively with this guidance system we can enhance it; we can raise it from a trickle to a massive flood. We can revitalize our lives and empower them. Perhaps, most importantly, we can induce positive change into our lives with *very little effort*.

Think of connection in this way: Imagine the force of water that flows from a fireman's hose. When aimed on a raging inferno, the power of the water suffocates the fierce flames. But allow the hose to lie on the ground unattended, and the hose becomes a wild snake. Nothing but chaos ensues as the water's flow splashes all around. Now think of your connection as this force of water. Which one do you want in your life? The directed stream or the chaotic splash? Go back to the list of qualities this connection can bring. If you are lacking in any area, know that all of these—*knowledge, direction, inspiration, synchronicity, unconditional love, joy, and peace*—can be brought to a higher level in your life *simply by enhancing your connection to self and to God*.

No matter who you are, knowledge of this type is available to you. But—*how?* What are you listening for? What are you supposed to feel? How will you know the difference between receiving great wisdom that will empower your life from the drivel your mind is just making up?

> *"Trusting yourself is trusting the wisdom that created you."*
> Wayne W. Dyer,
> *Manifesting Your Destiny*

WE CONTROL THE FLOW

My father-in-law used to say, "I know that I know that I know." He didn't know how he knew, not technically or specifically. He would simply say God told him. Yet he had perfect confidence in that knowledge from years of trusting and relying on his connection. Part of his assurance came from a feeling sense, a knowing inside, while another part came from stepping out in faith, learning to rely on his feelings through trial and error, through practice, and through trust. That is what you must do too. You have to experiment, be open, be aware of the results.

One day I prayed asking, "How do we connect?" In response, I received a vision. The vision showed me a child's science experiment: a wooden board set up with a simple electrical circuit of wires, an on-off switch, a

> *"Our communication with you is composed of the sum total of sensing. Though intrinsically you know this, you doubt it at times. But doubt is gradually replaced by knowing, by experience."*
>
> Saint Germain (Spirit),
> Channeled by Philip Burley,
> *To Master Self Is to Master Life*

147

battery, and a light bulb. In the vision, the switch turned on, the electricity flowed through the circuit, the light bulb lit. After a moment, the switch turned off, the electricity stopped flowing, and the light bulb went out.

I understood by seeing this vision that *we* control the on-off switch, but also, *we* control the flow through the wires. If, for example, one of the wires were to be cut or blocked or disconnected from any of its components, the light bulb—or idea—would not illuminate. It's up to us to both throw the switch to the 'on' position and to make sure the connection remains strong by keeping all the circuitry in good working order. Of course, our bodies are not as easy to understand as this science experiment. We can't see any of our 'wiring,' and we don't have a visible on-off switch attached to our brain.

In the chapters that follow, I will give you the means by which you can do that. I will explain, based on my own experience, how you can learn to recognize and enhance your own connection in order that you might empower your life. But first, I will give you a means to feel it for yourself.

"Manifesting requires allowing your beliefs about reality to flow FROM your inner mind's eye and TO the outer world. As you are manifesting, pay no attention to the seeming obstacles that may pop up or else you will reverse the manifesting direction and flow."

Doreen Virtue,
The Lightworker's Way

CHAPTER FIFTEEN: A MUSICAL CONNECTION

15

Music has always played a significant role in my family's life. Even my grandmother, who died in the mid-1920s, had a great affinity for music. She once wrote in a letter:

> *"Yes, dear, we all miss you, it is like a morgue around here. Have not played the phonograph once until today and then John did it. The music didn't sound right at all."* [1]

More than just background noise, music shaped who we were and wove itself through our significant memories.

My mother loved to dance and performed in local productions as a teen in Salem, Illinois. My father proudly played the clarinet in the East Lansing Central High School band and played saxophone in a 1930s garage band when my parents first met. By the time I came along, almost twenty-five years later, my father had long since given up his musical aspirations, but would sometimes play for fun. [2]

My father had such a passion for music and a great appreciation for the quality of sound. He built his own stereos from Heathkits in order to have the latest and greatest equipment available. I couldn't have been more than six years old when

> *"Music, often bypassing the conscious mind, works its magic directly on the rhythmical heartbeat of our inner being."*
> Anodea Judith,
> *Wheels of Life*

my father showed me the virtues of stereophonic sound produced by his latest HiFi set. We stood in the living room where he'd placed several home-built speakers, including a large, table-sized woofer. He excitedly pointed first to one speaker, then to the other, as the separated drum and piano sounds leapt from one side of the room to the next.[3] I remember most how his blue eyes lit up as he shared his musical adventure with me.

A NEW LEVEL OF CONNECTION

Connection for me means music. That is not to say I cannot connect without it. I can. We all can. But, while others are touting the need for meditative silence, for me, music has always led the way.

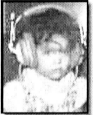

My mother claimed my brother, eighteen years my elder, would cancel a date rather than let a stranger baby-sit me. He says that he would take me into his bedroom, put his headphones on my tiny head, and let me listen to whatever music he was playing at the time. He said I seemed to like it and the music kept me calm.

Maybe even then I was connecting.

Like my father before me, I acquired the habit of listening to my music—loud. My parents didn't share my taste in music. My father said it sounded somewhat like a screeching cat. So one day he came into my bedroom holding an old pair of headphones. That meant that if I wanted to be where my music was—and I did—I had to stay in my room attached to my stereo by a twenty-five foot extension cord, my musical life support. I didn't mind. Plied with rampant teenage hormones and a raging attitude, I found it more desirable to stay in my room as much as possible anyway.

My teen years were perhaps some of the most difficult days in my life. My father's health declined until he became bedridden and eventually died. I didn't have many friends and didn't spend much time out of the house. Instead, I spent hour after hour lying on my bed listening to music, reading books, and writing in my journals.

On one of those days, I fell into a kind of mystical

"You live your life in the songs you hear on the rock and roll radio. And when a young girl doesn't have any friends, that's a really nice place to go."
Alan O'Day,
Angie Baby

150

trance. I remember that although I had my eyes closed, I could see lights and colors, but I had temporarily forgotten about the music playing in my head. It was as if the music had disappeared—it was as if I had disappeared. My only awareness was of light and color, and it wasn't so much that I was looking at light and color as much as I was *a part of them.*

After what felt like a few minutes, I rolled over on the bed and sat up. I couldn't explain how, but I knew I'd just been given an important message, perhaps the most significant in my life. So valuable was this information that I wept, and yet I understood none of it.

I knew with my whole being that what I had been given held great importance for me and for the world. Yet I felt troubled and at a loss as to how to share this information since I had no means to explain it or even describe what it meant. I remember feeling disappointed as I knew I had been given a tremendous gift but lacked the understanding to utilize it. I wrote in my journal how I wished there were some type of machine I could plug into my brain allowing others to understand my thoughts.

I'd have to wait twenty-five years before I'd learn how to unlock the message I had received, but unlock it I did, through music and connection. Today I believe the knowledge I received was the information for this book. After all, I'd known since age three that I would one day write a book, I just didn't know what type. So, perhaps at sixteen, God had given me a taste of what would come in order to keep me plodding forward.

Over the years, my use of music and headphones evolved. I would later come to call what I did *stationary dancing.* My husband and kids have other—let's call them pet names—by which they refer to my method of connection and prayer. I admit, the technique isn't exactly pretty. The one thing I can say for certain, it works.

WHY MUSIC FACILITATES OUR ABILITY TO CONNECT

I knew music inspired me and helped me make the connection that I sought. But why? How?

"There is another, more ancient language, more conducive to discourse on this level but you have forgotten it. It is the universal language of light."
Kenneth X. Carey,
The Starseed Transmissions

This isn't something I made up for the sake of self-gratification. Man has utilized music for connection and inspiration for thousands of years. Tom Kenyon *(Brain States)*, psychotherapist, teacher, and musician, writes:

> . . .*using instruments such as the human voice, drums, flutes and percussive instruments have been documented to alter brain states (i.e. the neural activity within the brain itself). These studies have shown, for instance, that certain drumming patterns increase theta activity within the brain, a state known to be connected with hypnogogic states of awareness, dream-like states of mind, as well as states of high insight and heightened creativity.*

So, depending on the patterns and frequencies, music enhances one of the four brain states—beta, alpha, theta, or delta—opening our minds to creativity, helping us to relax, or allowing us to access higher thought. Because of this, schools are using the knowledge of music's brain-enhancing features to encourage learning, and corporations use music to spur creativity and reduce stress in their workforce. Joshua Leeds, author *(The Power of Sound)* and corporate sound consultant, explains how something called Binaural Beat Frequencies (BBFs) interact with our brainwaves to create these desired states. He explains that BBFs occur when "two minutely detuned sounds create a third sound in the brain." Because of this, "our brainwaves slow down or speed up to match this natural third sound."

In fact, according to sound guru Anna Wise *(The High Performance Mind)* who has been measuring the brain-wave patterns of the spiritually enlightened and highly creative for nearly three decades, the perfect state of mind is a combination of all four brain states, something she refers to as *The Awakened Mind.* She says:

> *The AWAKENED MIND . . . is a brain-wave pattern shared by people in higher states of consciousness regardless of their philosophy, theology or meditation technique. This brainwave pattern can be*

"Music will be the informational medium through which the Totality of Consciousness informs each individual cell of its specific functional duties within that Totality."

Kenneth X. Carey,
The Starseed Transmissions

found during "peak experience" and in all forms of creativity and high performance. The awakened mind is also the "ah-ha," appearing at the exact instant of solving the problem, or getting the insight.

While many recordings specifically designed to enhance your desired mind state exist, you are tapping into the same technologies whenever you listen to music you enjoy. I believe that connecting via music makes perfect sense since those who created the music were typically connected when they wrote the song. Because of this, I have used a wide variety of music for the purpose of connection, not just those scientifically created.

You can use music in the same way to jumpstart your connection, to access your higher self and tap into the deeper recesses of your mind. The following exercise will show you how.

EXERCISE 11—STATIONARY DANCING

Warning #1: When in this near-hypnotic state *you will not hear most outside noises*. This is good for the connection, bad for emergencies. You might want to warn others in the house. You might want to avoid doing this exercise while alone.

Warning #2: Not moving your feet is *very important*. If you have your eyes closed and you move—you could run into something, trip, or fall. Check yourself from time to time and choose a safe place. Stay away from areas with stairwells, dangling lamp cords, and other dangers. Use good judgment as neither I, nor my publishing company, are liable for any injury you might sustain if you don't follow this warning.

Recommendation #1: My iPod ear buds fit comfortably in my ears and work pretty well for this exercise. However, optimum results are obtained from a quality set of headphones[4] that fit snugly against your head and over your ears.

"Those who danced were thought to be quite insane by those who could not hear the music."

Angela Monet

153

Recommendation #2: Sound quality is *very* important. Static or other noises will distract you from your connected state. If you find an odd noise within the music continually distracts you from connection, discontinue using that particular music.

Recommendation #3: We have a rule in my house that my sons will clap their hands if they need me—touching me is very startling. I also warn them not to disturb me unless it is a matter of importance. There's nothing more disappointing than leaving the bliss of a connected state to help a teenager locate their lost shoes or to explain you are not interested in speaking with a phone solicitor.

Recommendation #4: For best results, set your CD or MP3 player to *continuous play* on a single song. I have used hundreds of songs from classical to rap to country to rock and roll. There is no right or wrong song to use. However, I would highly recommend the following song as the one to begin with since it's been known to work well for a wide variety of people. The song is on Paul Oakenfold's *Perfecto Presents Another World* CD, disc two, track two: *Salt Tank - Eugina 2000 (Progressive Summer Mix.)* More choices are listed in End Notes.[5]

Recommendation #5: Try this exercise for a *minimum* of twenty minutes. Longer periods will offer you more of an opportunity to relax, connect, and receive. I typically use this exercise for a period of twenty to forty minutes. The more often you use this method to connect, the better your experience will be.

Here's how the exercise works:

1. Put on headphones to block out distracting noises. Set the music loud enough to be comfortable, and absorbing, not too soft, not too loud *(always be cautious and protective of your hearing!)*. Adhere to all the warnings above to avoid injury or danger.

2. *Plant Your Feet!* Your feet should not move for any reason from the spot where you start. You can move any other part of your body, including: legs, arms, hands, head. You should not move from this initial spot—thus the name, *stationary dancing.*

"Music expresses that which cannot be put into words and cannot remain silent."
Victor Hugo

"Anytime you wish to tap into the landscape of your intuition, turn off the phone, get comfortable in your favorite chair, and turn on some uplifting, instrumental music."
Carol Adrienne,
The Purpose of Your Life

154

3. Close your eyes and begin to sway and move along with the music. Think of yourself as a kind of metronome. Pick out the different instrument sounds and try to follow along with their rhythm. Listen for the music's "heartbeat." Sometimes I try to see the instrument itself, such as a piano or guitar, and visualize the musician playing that instrument. Sometimes I just let my mind flow free and wander wherever it wants to go.

5. Relax. Let go. Shut out everything going on around you except for the music. Use transitions in the music to change directions in your thoughts. It's okay if, from time to time, you open your eyes to check yourself.

6. Have conversations with imaginary friends, visit exotic places, set your mind free. Ask questions. Consider possibilities. Visualize talking with the people in your life.

7. Feel free to stop to write down important insights.

8. If you have been standing for a long period of time and start to get tired, it's okay to sit on the floor or a bench provided you keep your eyes closed and stay with the flow of thoughts. I sometimes continue the motion by gently rocking back and forth or lower my head and cover my eyes with my hands to block out distractions.

9. Don't try too hard. If you're waiting and watching for something to happen, it won't. The more you try to focus on the experience, the more you'll block the connection you're trying to create.

You have succeeded in making a connection if any of the following apply:

- *You have periods where you forget the music is playing*

- *You receive answers to questions you've asked or gained insight or understanding about a problem at hand*

- *Particular words (in lyrical music) seem to leap out and grab your attention and become an answer or inspiration to you*

"Dance is the hidden language of the soul of the body."
Martha Graham

". . . the key to traveling through time is to free yourself from your everyday concerns."
Fred Alan Wolf,
The Yoga of Time Travel

155

- *You feel relaxed and happy or inspired afterwards*

- *Time passed either slower or faster than the expected speed, (See: Chapter 16)*

- *You sense you're facing in a different direction when your eyes are closed than the one that appears when you open them (and you haven't moved your feet)*

Music is not for everyone. We each connect in a way that is in keeping with our beliefs and ideals and by a means that is natural to our way of learning and understanding. In the chapters that follow, I've explained other means of enhancing your connection. Find the one that feels right to you and then use it on a daily basis.

"Music is invaluable in supporting discharge and venting of old hidden emotions which block or impede progressive change or daily function."

Nell M. Rodgers,
Puppet or Puppeteer

Chapter Sixteen:
"Hello? Central!"
Other Ways We Connect

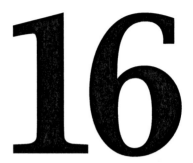

Connecting can be as easy as picking up a pen, reading a book, molding moist clay, listening to music, or simply taking a quiet walk through the park. Here's a short list of some activities we do on a regular basis that lend to connection:

- *Reading*

- *Exercise*

- *Meditation*

- *The Creative Arts*

- *Music*

- *Dancing*

- *Monotonous Activities (washing dishes, mowing the lawn, driving a vehicle, showering)*

- *Writing*

- *Praying*

But how will you know if you've connected by doing these things?

"The arts . . . precisely by their non-regimented, nonconformist character are able to reach into the vast uncharted realm of the future and illustrate ideas and concepts in a way that affects consciousness on an immediate and whole brain level."

Anodea Judith,
Wheels of Life

STEPPING INTO A TIME WARP

The first thing you need to know about connection is that you have experienced its feeling before, even if you didn't pay much attention to it. The ironic thing about being connected is that you are so caught up in whatever it is you're doing that you don't take time to notice you're caught up in whatever it is that you're doing—until you stop doing it, take a break, and look at the clock.

Suddenly you discover time has passed at a different rate of speed than you expected. Either hours passed without your noticing, or the opposite may have happened. You may feel as if you've been hard at work doing something for a long period of time only to see the clock and find mere minutes have ticked by.

Betty Edwards (*Drawing on the Right Side of the Brain*) describes this unique passage of time in association with connection as:

> . . . *Artists speak of feeling transported, 'at one with the work,' able to grasp relationships that they ordinarily cannot grasp. Awareness of the passage of time fades away and words recede from consciousness. Artists say that they feel alert and aware yet are relaxed and free of anxiety, experiencing a pleasurable, almost mystical activation of the mind.*

You don't need to be an artist to feel this way. Any one of those aspects by itself would be a tremendous enhancement to our lives today, especially the feelings of being:

- *Relaxed*
- *Anxiety free*
- *Alert*
- *Aware*
- *At one with our work or purpose*
- *Joyful*

Not to mention the freedom of being separated from the passage of time as so many of us are driven by the passing minutes of a clock.

"My instincts seemed sharpened and finely tuned; my senses heightened. Reality was shiny and new like a freshly washed window. I heard even the faintest sounds, felt changes in temperatures, and was acutely aware of people and objects nearby. In several instances, I felt I had the ability to anticipate what was going to happen next."

Michael Lee,
Phoenix Rising Yoga Therapy

Since losing track of time is something we are all familiar with, *time* is the best reference you have as a meter when evaluating your level of connection. As you experiment with the following activities, take a moment afterwards to ask yourself, "Did time pass more quickly or at a different rate than I expected during this activity?" From your answer, you'll know just how connected you were. I will give you additional means to test your level of connection as we go along, though you'll also know you've been connected by the manifestation of the connected traits in your life *(knowledge, direction, inspiration, synchronicity, unconditional love, joy, and peace).*

> *"It's really great fun to go someplace where there are no timesaving devices because when you do, you find that you have lots of time."*
>
> Benjamin Hoff,
> *The Tao of Pooh*

READING

Read. Why read? Because reading gives your mind a starting point. It offers your brain information to process, to think about, to expand on. Reading fires the synapses in your brain and, in firing them, forms connections to existing thoughts. These reorganized thoughts then become the springboards to new ideas and alternative avenues of action for your life.

When we read in a connected state, words seem to leap off the page and grasp our heart and minds. They inspire us, spur us forward, and provide us with knowledge we can use in pursuing our goals.

Reading is a vicarious experience. In seeing how others survived, lived, loved—whether fiction or not—we activate our hope in finding a better tomorrow and offer ourselves subliminal encouragement to pursue our goals. Those we read about may become our mentors. They serve as role models and as an example we can use in making our own way. *(See: Section V)*

> *"You can do it with any book. You can do it with an old newspaper if you read it carefully enough. Haven't you done that, hold some problem in your mind, then open any book handy and see what it tells you?"*
>
> Richard Bach,
> *Illusions*

Reading may provide us with knowledge or direction that we've sought, or may offer us comfort during a difficult time. But more importantly, reading takes us away from the present and into a higher, inner realm.

In the second and third grade, I changed schools twice. Finding myself alone in a new element, I turned to reading books as a form of entertainment. The stories I read became a form of escape. I didn't understand why back then, but books were a way to disassociate from the pain of being in a new place. While living within the pages of books, I wasn't living in a new town and school where no one understood me. Reading transported me to a faraway, magical land where the meek and mild overcame adversity and lived happily ever after. Once transported there, time passed more quickly. Soon, I passed that awkward stage of my life.

Over the years, I would turn to the magical power of reading time and time again, changing the kinds of books and their topics, but always for the same underlying reason—while lost in books, I wasn't trapped in reality. I was released into a connected, transformed state of being where my thoughts bloomed and my imagination flourished.

PASSIVE EXERCISE

On an annual visit to my endocrinologist, I learned I needed to start exercising in some way to avoid becoming a diabetic. I dutifully followed his advice, eventually even pulling out my inline skates.[1]

I have to admit, the first time I dusted off my skates and put them on, I had my doubts. It had been several years since I'd used them. Having avoided any kind of exercise whatsoever after my auto collision, I gasped for air, my legs ached, my lungs burned. I barely managed to make a few circles in front of the house. But I kept at it, and in about two weeks, I could skate a circuit of six to eight *miles*. On a couple of occasions, I even did ten—not bad for an unathletic, sedentary couch potato.

I was able to accomplish this because once outside amid the sunshine, the songs of birds, and the gentle rippling of the lake, my mind made the switch to the connected mode. I lost track of how my legs felt, forgot about the pain, and instead became one with my environment. I made it a rule not to wear a headset on these outings as I didn't want to block out nature, I wanted to become one with it.

Unfortunately, this is a great form of passive exercise on a pleasant day, many of which abound in the spring, summer, and fall months where I live. But once winter comes to Northern Pennsylvania, that kind of activity

"Exercise is often the going that moves us from stagnation to inspiration, from problem to solution, from self-pity to self-respect."

Julia Cameron,
The Artist's Way

160

becomes impossible. In the past several years we have received record snowfalls in our area amounting to over two hundred and fifty inches of snow a season. So, come winter, I had to find some other form of exercise.

When my husband's back surgery and subsequent physical therapy required that he join a gym, I joined too, and we worked out together. I found I could walk a surprisingly long distance on the treadmill or pedal far longer than I would have ever imagined on the stationary bike by distracting myself with music. *(See: Chapter 15).* The part of my mind that monitored all the pedaling or walking was too preoccupied to notice the aches and pains. Shifting into a connected mode, I lost track of what my body might be doing on the equipment and felt free to move on to higher thoughts.[2] The connection allowed me to think of other things rather than the monotony of walking or riding in place.

EXERCISE 12—MEDITATION

I do not claim to know anything about meditation other than what I've read and heard others say as I've always relied on music to give me the deep connection that I desired. However, I recognize that my method may not be the best for everyone, and I do believe that meditation is an effective way to connect. So, by all means, use meditation as an outlet for connection if you're practiced in it, or seek out a qualified teacher if you're interested in learning more about how to meditate correctly.

I can offer a simple relaxation exercise as recommended to me by Joey Korn *(Dowsing: The Path to Enlightenment)*, author, teacher, and dowser extraordinaire:

1. Take twenty minutes a day, typically after lunch, to relax and meditate. Whether on the floor or on a bed, lie flat on your back. Do not lie on your side or stomach as you will signal the body that you want to sleep.

2. Tell yourself you want to relax for twenty minutes. Your body will automatically alert you when the time is up.

"Meditation is simply the act of being quiet with yourself and shutting down the constant monologue that fills the inner space of your being."

Wayne W. Dyer,
Manifest Your Destiny

161

3. Joey enhances his experience with the use of gentle, instrumental music. You may want to pre-record selections that last twenty minutes to remind you when to stop, but that's not necessary if you program your mind as in Step 2.

4. Close your eyes and take several deep cleansing breaths, breathing in through your nose and out through your mouth.

5. Begin to relax your body, from your toes to your head.

6. As you reach your final stages of relaxation, think briefly of your dilemmas of the day and ask for guidance in finding a solution.

7. Unless you are ill or overly tired, you will not fall asleep. You will more or less zone out. After twenty minutes, you will suddenly return to an alert, conscious state. You will know you haven't been sleeping because you will not feel groggy or slug-gish. Rather, you will feel revived and alert.

8. Rise slowly. Think again about the questions you asked while beginning to relax. You may find you now have a new insight as to how to solve your problems of the day.

This type of meditation doesn't have a voice or any internal dialogue associated with it, rather communication takes place on a level beyond a physical connection. The answers just appears to "be there." In fact, maybe the answers were there all along. We just needed to relax in order to access them.

THE CREATIVE ARTS

In 2001, I attended a retreat co-hosted by Carol Adrienne *(The Purpose of Your Life)*. Carol used a variety of visual objects as part of her work with us. Through her exercises with the class, she showed us how our creativity could be used to switch into the connected mode.

None of what she said or did sank in for the first few

"By using meditation and yoga techniques, though it may not seem to be so, you are freeing yourself from time."

Fred Alan Wolf,
The Yoga of Time Travel

162

days of the retreat. I had been so caught up in just surviving my life that I had totally discounted the value or purpose of anything creative. I had little free time, and creativity had taken a back seat. I'd long since given up my evenings of needlework and other crafts. I'd delegated these items to the back of the closet, moving them farther and farther back into the catacombs as the years passed.

On the third day of the retreat, Carol asked us to create collages from old magazine pages. As in many of her exercises, Carol recommended we sift through the photos, advertisements, and articles she'd thrown haphazardly in a huge pile on the floor and to pull out any items that grabbed our attention—even if we didn't know why. We were also given a theme for our collage.

Something came over me as I began to create a meaningful, self-message from all the pieces I'd collected. Sitting on the floor, carefully trimming and placing my chosen words and images, something inside of me broke free. Creating my collage, I *felt* something . . . a kind of pure love and joy pressed through my constricted veins. I felt . . . *happy*. I enjoyed this creative process so much that I didn't want to stop at the end of the session. I continued to work on it back in my hotel room as if I were driven by some unseen force. I felt compelled, as Roy (Richard Dreyfuss) did in the movie *Close Encounters of the Third Kind,* where he became obsessed with a message he didn't yet understand and resorted to creating a giant clay mountain in the center of his kitchen table.

By creating the collage, I'd opened up something inside of me, something I couldn't yet explain or understand. I only knew it felt good and I had to keep doing it.

I created several more collages after I arrived home, and then shared the activity with several friends, who created collages with the same passion and fervor I had.

> "Survival and health in the 21st century will require innovation and flexibility. Creativity is the key to unlocking these qualities."
>
> Anodea Judith,
> *Wheels of Life*

> "Creativity requires activity, and this is not good news to most of us. It makes us responsible, and we tend to hate that. You mean I have to DO something in order to feel better? Yes."
>
> Julia Cameron,
> *The Artist's Way*

EXERCISE 13—CREATING A COLLAGE

Here's how you can create a collage. This is particularly fun with a group of friends.

1. Gather five or six old magazines (or, with friends, ask each person to bring several). Separate the

"The process of creation is a process of inner discovery. In creating an art form, in abandoning our former modes of operation, we open ourselves to the very mysteries of the universe."

Anodea Judith,
Wheels of Life

pages from their bindings to allow the images and words to slide freely for better viewing.

2. Create a theme. Try making a collage based on your purposeful goals identified in the previous section, or use healing as your theme.

3. Spread the images on the floor or on a large table and mix them up.

4. Begin selecting images and headline phrases that attract your attention. You may or may not know why. Don't over think the process. Grab items quickly. Spend no more than ten minutes doing this. Don't try to figure out how you will use them, just grab the items that stand out to you.

5. In collage style, cut and glue your chosen images to a piece of poster board or large sheet of heavy paper. You may find some items don't fit, and you're free to add more as the collage begins to take shape and form.

6. Hang the collage in a place where you will see it often. I place mine under glass on my desktop so they're always in sight, even if only subliminally.

CREATIVITY CAN MAKE A DIFFERENCE

Creativity is important. Mastery is not. The Creative Arts encompass any activity where you use your hands and imagination to create something new from raw or recycled materials. Whether being creative means painting a magnificent picture or sewing some drapes, chipping out a wood carving or coming up with a new recipe for dinner, it doesn't matter as long as the mind is able to release itself from the mundane and tap into the connected state.

If you have a ready talent, set aside time to do it. Make an appointment with yourself and honor that scheduled time as if it were as important as a doctor's appointment or meeting with your boss. If you are at a loss as to what your creative talent might be, don't be afraid to take a class, learn something new, or explore different avenues of expression. If you need more help, try the exer-

"Never be afraid to try something new. Remember that a lone amateur built the Ark. A large group of professionals built the Titanic."

Dave Barry

164

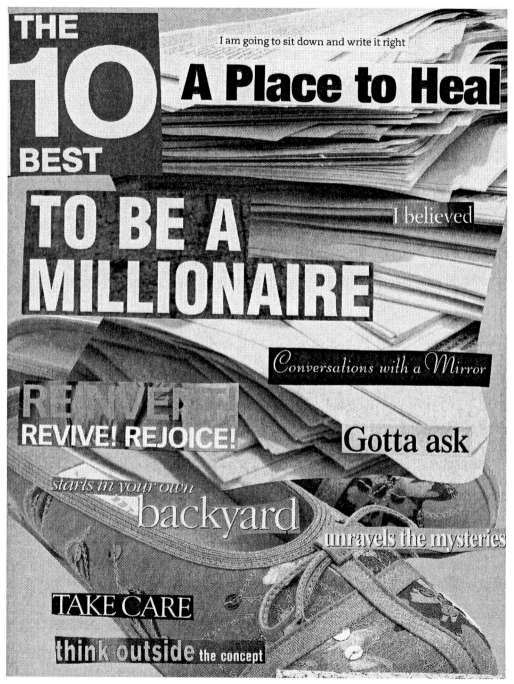

Collage Example

165

cises in Julia Cameron's *The Artist's Way* (which isn't just for the artistically minded).

Tapping into your creativity might be the key you've needed to activate your connection and to open your heart, particularly if you've closed off this area of your life for a period of time.

THE CONNECTIVITY OF MOVEMENT

In Section I *(Relief)*, I explained how directed movement, such as that found in yoga, tai chi, or qigong, could help you release hidden tension and emotional pain. In Chapter 15 *(A Musical Connection)*, I showed how the rhythmic movement of stationary dancing to music could open a connection to the higher mind. But other forms of movement too, whether dancing, exercise, or even yard work, can lend themselves to connection as well.

For example, weightlifting or body shaping, which utilizes free weights, requires a strong focus on how each muscle feels in the process of the lift. This focus on the body removes our attention from problems of the day and other mind hindrances that block our connection freeing our mind to tap into a higher realm.

Movement, even that of walking, creates a flow of energy as it gets the blood moving and the heart pumping. This energy, in turn, cranks up the brain and the creative mechanisms that reside within.

Even if your ability to move is restricted by age, weight, or disability, find some way to move, even if only on a limited basis. By doing so, you will enhance your ability to connect and create.

"Kinesthetically, dance can reflect movements and passions we have long since silenced in our own bodies."

Anodea Judith,
Wheels of Life

CREATIVE IMAGINATION

Creative imagination is the magic beans of possibility. It is the pixie dust of a blossoming invention. It is the golden thread in a new idea. As children we're told that make-believe and imagination are just kid stuff, but put a bit of that magic dust alongside a solid connection and, Mabel, you've got an atomic reaction.

Creative imagination is perhaps the most powerful

gift ever given to us by God. Not only does it require very little skill (if any), it can be used by anyone, even a kid, and, by gosh, it doesn't even require batteries. Best of all, its free.

Imagination is said to be a non-material essence, just make-believe. But I disagree, for how can something immaterial become the greatest inventions and innovations of our time? Within imagination a man dreams up a wheel, a motorcar, a rocket ship; a zipper, a staple, a paper clip; a sewing machine, a personal computer, an assembly line, mass production. From this so-called nothing, the idea becomes a goal, a plan, a project in the works, *a reality* that changes the world as we know it. I would even go as far as to say that the world of imagination is far greater in size than our world of reality, for within imagination's world there are no boundaries, no restrictions, no impossibilities. And so we take from our wanderings in the wilderness of this often-forgotten frontier a bit of essence, and with a bit of cunning, hard work, and some financial backing, we turn that essence—which is something very real and material—into something we can see, smell, touch, and hold.

You can create in imagination, but you cannot erase. If you create an idea or concept for a material object, that concept or object remains. In the future it can be used in conjunction with other like ideas or goods, but the idea itself now lives and cannot be eradicated. The idea can be bettered or improved and eventually outmoded, but never erased. It might be forgotten or lost, but it cannot be eradicated since it could be found. The idea will always exist having been created from, what? The fabric of our imagination. The stuff they say doesn't exist.

What I'm talking about is simply this: In our mind's fluff, in the place where we believe we have nothing material, nothing real, nothing but child's play, there *is* something real. While our ideas are made up only of invisible-to-the-eye energies, something scientists call *vital force energy,* they *are* real and it's this piece of reality in our imaginations that makes it possible to bring what is created in the imaginary world into the physical one.

"Imagination is more important than knowledge."
Albert Einstein

". . . what is revealed by spirit is brought to action in life."
Michael Lee,
Phoenix Rising Yoga Therapy

EXERCISE 14—THE REALITY BOX

Creative imagination is a kind of bank. Not one that holds money, but one that holds an endless depository of ideas. Tapping into this bank and withdrawing from its holdings is the closest we get to being with God and like God, while living on the earthly plane.

Think of it in this way, no matter what you need, the means to get it are within the imaginative part of your mind. You merely need to reach into the ethereal ooze of thought and pull out a handful.

There are two realms that we accept and understand. One is the realm of reality, the here and now, in this physical world. The other is the realm of our imagination.

For a moment, I want you to think of the here and now, all that's real and in the world, reality as we know it, as fitting into a large, but ordinary, cardboard box. Anything that you know of as real is now in that box. I want you to see the box in your mind as if you are on the outside of it looking at it. You can view it from any angle, turn it in your mind. Just know that all reality, the world, the planets, outer space, everything, fits into that cardboard box.

First, notice that "reality" has boundaries. Nothing "real" can exist outside of that box, so reality can only exist inside the box.

Now, as you look at the box, realize that you are not inside the box (or at least, the thinking part of you). You know that you are not in the box because you are looking at the outside of the box. You can imagine yourself inside the box, but the *observer* you is not bound by those cardboard box sides. Therefore, you, or the observer you, are existing in a space that is not real (as we define reality).

Secondly, anything you now see existing outside the box is existing in the realm we refer to as our imagination. Whether you imagined your box in a totally blank space, or a white, heaven-like room, or any other countless creative existences, you still know that all reality is in the box and imagination is outside the box.

Play around for a moment with your imaginary realm. Add anything you like to it. You can place your observer self in a room with furniture, you can see yourself standing beside a magnificent mountainscape, or standing in a windblown wheat field. You can add flowers, rain, moon-

"You can't depend on your eyes when your imagination is out of focus."

Mark Twain

"The problem that faces most of us in becoming manifesters and learning to manage the circumstances of our lives is that we have forfeited our ability to oscillate between the world of form and the unseen world."

Wayne W. Dyer,
Manifesting Your Destiny

beams, flying pigs, unicorns, bugs that talk. There are no limits, boundaries, or morally accepted rules because, in this space, it is only imagination.

Continue creating whatever you would like in this space. Even erase it and start again. Feel free to talk to whomever you want, do whatever you please, you are in an imaginary realm. It's kind of like an awake dream. Create art, fly through the air, talk to dead presidents, be wild, be brave, be boundless. Just remember that wherever you are, the box is also there with all of reality tucked inside it. (I prefer to see my reality box as open, with items haphazardly thrown in like a child's toy box and with items coming in and going out of the box, but feel free to simply imagine your box closed if you prefer.)

Now ask yourself one simple question. What if everything were somehow reversed? What if everything in the box, that which we think of as "real," was the dream and everything in the imaginary world was the true reality? By that, I don't just mean the imaginary things you created now, I mean the whole ability to create what you want, the feeling of freedom, of peace, of unbound possibility. Think about that for a moment.

Wouldn't this also mean that whatever was in the box, whatever you put in there as "real," was also a part of your imagination? What if everything you thought of as "real" were part of your imagination? Now, suddenly, "imagination" is not just a child's toy. Suddenly imagination is a kind of nuclear power.

"But wait a minute," you might say, "if we are this being (the observer) who is in charge of our imaginary realm, then how is it we are living in the cardboard box ruled by the limits of its sides and stuck with its physical pain? Why don't we erase all of our hardships and physical limitations?"

Because it is a choice you made, a kind of game you agreed to play when you came here. The only problem about this game is that you are so good at playing it, you have forgotten it is a game. You see, it takes a very strong connection and focus to play at this level. In fact, just being here in the "real" world means you are a master at playing the game, what we might call a professional, a person envied by those who are not able to manifest themselves at this level of reality.

"Because every person on earth exists as a spirit within a physical body, each dwells consciously and unconsciously in both worlds."
Saint Germain (Spirit),
Channeled by Philip Burley,
To Master Self Is to Master Life

"Jesus said, 'When you see your likeness, you rejoice. But when you see your images which came into being before you and which neither die nor become manifest, how much you will have to bear.'"
Gospel of Thomas,
Nag Hamadi

"Every game we play, we slip into a role, a game identity with which to play. We decide we're rescuer, victim, leader-with-all-the-answers, follower-without-a-clue, bright, brave, honorable, crafty, dull, helpless, just-trying-to-get-along, diabolical, easy-going, pitiable, earnest, careless, salt-of-the-earth, puppetmaster, comic, hero . . . we choose our role by whim and destiny, and we can change it anytime we want."

Richard Bach,
Running From Safety

However, in keeping your focus on the game and on reality, you've forgotten about all the abilities and powers you have when you're not in the box. You've forgotten that you can be pain free, that you can have whatever it is that you want, that you can *be* whatever you want.

My purpose in telling you this through a simple, philosophical exercise, is not to stop you from playing the game, because, after all, we have all chosen to play it and enjoy doing so on another, higher level of our being. My purpose is merely to remind you of the power you have available should you choose to use it. A power that allows you to put into your box of reality anything you need to play and "win" your game.

Here is something to get your mind thinking more along these lines and on how to get items from your imagination into your reality box.

What is a rocket ship made of? It is made of imagination. "But how can that be?" you ask. "I see it on the launch pad. I see it in the sky. I know it's made of metal and plastic, tile and wood, painted and molded, bent and smoothed, polished and honed to perfection by countless people over years and years, some who gave their lives so it might be made possible."

But how did it all begin? Someone thought of it in a dream or in a flash of insight. It lived in their imagination. And how did they bring it into reality? They took the idea they saw in their imagination and they wrote it down on paper. They drew pictures of it, first as a whole, then later as pieces and parts that would go into building the rocket. They talked about it to others and shared their vision in such a way that others saw the vision too. Some laughed, but others believed and pitched in to help. There were trials and errors, there were other new inventions brought into being as they were necessary to make the original idea real. And then, there was a rocket ship flying into space as real as anything else in this world.

In this same way, you can make your imaginative ideas real.

1. Write them down or draw a picture of them

2. Share them with others

3. See them in detail with all their parts

4. Act on them to build them or make them happen.

As long as you only dream of your ideas and hopes, and do not carry them any further than that, they will remain in the other, "imaginary" realm. In order to exist inside the reality box, you have to draw them in.

"Everything that you can imagine is real."
Pablo Picasso

Chapter Seventeen: Writing

The Connection of Words

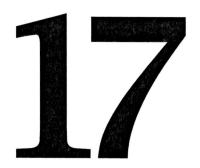

Writing

I have learned several forms of connected writing, all of which have been useful in my life at one point or another and each in their own way. The different types include:

- *List making*
- *Journaling*
- *Marathon writing*
- *Fiction writing*
- *Word association (which is used extensively throughout this book and described in Appendix A)*

Authors Tom Bird *(Write Right From God)* and Julia Cameron *(The Artist's Way)* maintain that staying connected comes from disciplined daily writing.

Bird writes:

The real reason so many of us seek to write

"Even though this connected state is relevant in all areas of life, nowhere is it more common and accessible by anyone than in the world of writing."

Tom Bird,
~~Write~~ *Right from God*

"As a result of either consciously or unconsciously making this connection, we come back in contact with our true selves. You know the one I am referring to; the one that lived, loved, and expressed so openly and freely before the innocently misguided rules of life stepped in and cut us off from the innate purposes and the genuine happiness, peace of mind, and soul fulfillment that awaits us all."

Tom Bird,
~~Write~~ *Right from God*

"During a lecture about goal-setting, our professor had asked each class member to write ten specific five-year goals. At the time, I didn't see how I could possibly achieve them. Yet I had accomplished each one. . ."

Doreen Virtue,
The Lightworker's Way

has nothing to do with writing a book. Way down deep at the base of all our souls we realize the potential of writing. We realize that when approached properly, the most divine of all connections can be made through this art form.

Cameron adds:

It is impossible to write morning pages[1] for any extended period of time without coming into contact with an unexpected inner power. Although I used them for many years before I realized this, the pages are a pathway to a strong and clear sense of self. They are a trail that we follow in to our own interior, where we meet both our own creativity and our creator.

What follows are brief descriptions of several different types of writing and how you can use them as a means of connection.

LISTS

Making a list is an easy way to quickly move your mind through one thought and on to the next. If you take the time to write out your thoughts in complete and correct sentences, you slow your thinking down while it remembers grammar rules, spellings, even proper letter formation. Lists are a fast, simple way to break away from all that is bogging down your mind.

Ira Progoff, Ph.D., *(At a Journal Workshop)*, capitalized on the simplicity of lists in his deep, mind-delving journaling book. Denis Waitley *(Timing Is Everything)*, utilizes lists to help his readers organize their lives and to allow them to recognize their accomplishments. Keith Snyder *(Show Control)* uses lists for organizing his thoughts in order to breakthrough the mundane and to create unique, bestselling novels. And Mind-mapping created by Tony Buzan *(See: Section III)*, is a form of graphic (image-based) list making that releases ideas and connects them to other thoughts stored in the mind offering a kind of supercharged creative thinking process.

Lists, which are a close cousin to word association, can be a means of connection for writing your varied responses to a particular question, for creating ideas for a new project, or for quickly reminding yourself of your accomplishments. According to Keith Snyder, making a list reveals the most common responses first while the middle of the list moves into a more ridiculous zone. Towards the bottom of the list, your mind accesses the more creative and unique ideas, and possibly, the answer you've looked for all along.

In making such a list, the key is to write quickly and avoid censoring any of the items, no matter how foolish or impossible they may sound. The goal is not to judge each entry as it is written, but rather to cause the mind to leap through as many different options as possible, thus tapping into a larger bank of brain memories and possibilities. *(An example of list making was used in Section I, Exercise 2.)*

"... very few words are sufficient to indicate the quality of the experience that is taking place. . . . brief entries enable us to record the largest range of material, so that we can then have a greater flexibility in choosing the subjects and the directions in which we shall proceed . . . ."

Ira Progoff,
At a Journal Workshop

JOURNALING

Journaling allows our thoughts to spill onto paper, releasing uncensored just how angry we were at the waitress who spilled coffee in our lap; our frustration at not being able to complete a task; our fear of tomorrow's job interview; or our pain from a past, hurtful situation. In doing so, we are not only allowing these emotions to move out of the body's cellular level into the conscious level of thinking, we are also providing ourselves with a means to recognize our true feelings on any given issue.

Writing has a way of acting as a kind of truth serum that works in this way: First you write down what you are feeling on a surface level. Your subconscious mind interprets what you've written and provides a response. On the surface, you might respond by writing faster, angrier, or with more passion. The subconscious might also provide subtle hints through body language—a sudden need to rub your head, twiddle with your hair, bite your fingernails, or smoke a cigarette. Along with the subliminal response, you might also have a physical sensation *(a Body Song),* such as a stomach knot, a lump in your throat, or a headache.

In sensing your emotional reaction, you know to continue looking at the words on the page and consider the thoughts in your head. You can't stop now, you are driven by some unseen force dragging you toward the Truth.

When journaling, the interpretation of these actions and feelings happens without thought from the moment you see the words on the page. You know—even if you are not ready to admit it as so—that you have not yet written the Truth and thus must continue on. The physical signals indicate you must dig deeper, even though your ego may be screaming at the top of its lungs for you to run away.

Why would your ego do this? Your ego does not want you to see the Truth. In seeing the Truth you will have the evidence you need to defeat whatever lie or mistaken perception you have told yourself. With Truth, you will have the possibility of instant relief from whatever situation is plaguing you or, at the very least, the knowledge from which you can begin reversing its effects. When you continue on, your writing will bring you this Truth. *(See also: Section I, Mistaken Perceptions)*

MARATHON WRITING

Marathon writing is writing practically nonstop for an extended period of hours—usually over several consecutive days. A fifty-thousand-word draft of this book was written in five days, about ten thousand words a day.

The key to successful marathon writing is two-fold. First, you must keep the pen moving as much as humanly possible, allowing whatever comes to mind to flow on to the paper. Even if your writing degrades into "I don't know what else to say" or "Why am I doing this?" keep writing because the next thought that comes through might be another flood of cleansing words.

The second key is to sustain this diligent pace for several consecutive days. During times of marathon writing, I find some means of seclusion, whether at a retreat, our cottage, a hotel room, or by sending everyone out of the house for a few days. During those days, I wake early, take care of any basic needs, and then begin writing.

". . . it is possible to write for long periods without fatigue, and that if one pushes on past the first weariness one finds a reservoir of unsuspected energy . . . ."

Dorothea Brande,
Becoming a Writer

I will write all day, stopping only to go to the bathroom or to eat. I eat light meals and drink lots of water, always returning to my writing as soon as possible. I'll write until after dark and sometimes late into the night.

This type of writing can be used for several purposes. Of course, it's a great way to write a book—or at least to start one. However, that's not the only reason to use marathon writing.

Writing continuously in this manner is a kind of mind enema. It cleanses the brain of anything and everything that has been stuck in there and that is blocking the flow in other areas of your life. Doing this mind cleanse will move you into the next stage of your life like a dynamite blast. And I guarantee, while sustaining this type of writing level, you will definitely be connected. Just as in making a list, your mind will first dump whatever it is that has piled up in front of your higher mind's door, and once that has been cleared away, will reveal what lies beyond, including information on your life's purpose and how to successfully pursue it.

FICTION WRITING

I'm a writer, I have a lot of friends who write, many who make their living writing fiction. Many more make a *hobby* of writing fiction. In fact, "writing the great American novel" is something almost all of us fantasize doing. There are lots of reasons for writing fiction but here is a very connected one.

When you write fiction, you are giving yourself permission to say whatever you want without having to be polite, politically correct, or morally sound. With fiction writing, you allow yourself to feel and release things you might not otherwise even speak of. This allows the higher mind to release information about you that you don't even realize you are revealing. After all, you know you aren't the serial killer in your suspense novel, the rejected lover in your romance novel, or the bratty child in your young adult novel. The idea that these characters might be a reflection of you never even crosses your mind. In fact, you tell yourself you know the heroine is based on a combination of your best friend and the apartment super-

"The simple reason that this form of communication may not have worked for you as well as you have wanted up to this point, comes directly as the result of not understanding, and thus, not being able to give into that which came pouring through you so naturally."
Tom Bird,
~~Write~~ *Right From God*

"In fictional fantasy, the world of make-believe becomes the testing ground for future lifestyles."
Anodea Judith,
Wheels of Life

177

intendent, Mrs. Constantine. The villain, you contend, is a pseudocombination of your father and your seventh-grade history teacher, Mr. Strem. Not to mention the fact that you would never harm another living being, cheat on your wife, or steal your company blind. So you know these characters are in no way a reflection of you. Or are they?

In 1990, I met author Tom Bird at one of his local seminars on writing. I joined his intensive writers' group that met weekly around his dining room table. Although I had never attempted to write a book-length work before, I suddenly found myself pouring out fictional tales ranging from near-to-real life to far-out fantasy. Tom caught me off guard one evening when he suggested he could see me between the lines of my characters. I seriously thought he'd lost his mind for a moment. But over the next few days, I considered what he'd said and reread, again and again, what I'd written until I could see it too.

During the next five years, I wrote ten more novels. When I went back and considered them later, I saw myself in every one, regardless of the type of character. Moreover, I then could see this phenomenon in the stories I read by other authors.

What you will find, if you go back later and look at your own stories, is that you are reflected there in your character's *motivations*. For those of you who are non-writers, a character's motivation is the *underlying reason* the character chooses the actions they do. For example, I had nothing in common with my young adult male character who lived in poverty painting pictures *except* for the fact that his *motivations* were based on the unfinished business between him and his deceased father—a characteristic of mine I'd not yet seen in myself when I wrote it.

Later, I will write more about these reflections of yourself. For now, understand that writing fiction provides connection because of the release and the ability of the writer to step into this imaginary realm.

"When at its best and most deep, our writing is autobiographical. . . . we realize that if we are successful in releasing that which is in us, others will know how we really feel, or even more frightening is the fact that we, ourselves, will actually know how we feel. That is what truly scares us."

Tom Bird,
~~Write~~ *Right From God*

CHAPTER EIGHTEEN:
THE PRAYER
CONNECTION
AND USING IT EFFECTIVELY

18

TALKING TO GOD THROUGH PRAYER

Prayer is a great means of connection because it's something anyone can do without any training. There is no wrong way to pray, no prequalifications for doing so. A child can pray as easily as an old man.

My first conscious recognition of prayer began back when I was seven and invited to attend vacation bible school with some friends. I remember sitting in the front row of the church with a matronly woman who had just taught our class. All the kids had gathered in the church for the day's closing prayer.

As the reverend spoke, he taught us about the importance of prayer and showed us how to hold our hands in one of two ways. The first, he said, holding his two hands together flat, represented praying with the body of the church. At seven, I didn't understand what he meant by "praying with the church." I thought of "the church" as boards and windows of the building. Praying with "the church" didn't make much sense to me at the time. Then the reverend said that if we interlocked our fingers and grasped our hands together, we were interlocking our hands with God's.

"Is it possible that God wants you to be 'selfish' in your prayers? To ask for more—and more again—from your Lord?"
Bruce Wilkinson,
The Prayer of Jabez

Holding God's hand while praying certainly made more sense to me since it was God I expected to talk to and to answer my prayer. However, as I made this internal decision, I looked around me. Almost everyone in my line of view had placed their hands flat to flat, including the woman sitting next to me. For a moment, I hesitated. *Should I fear holding God's hand?* But still not understanding the concept of the "praying with the church" idea, so I chose to hold God's hand.

From that day forward, I prayed in that way, knowing I could talk directly to God and didn't have to go through the church (even though I later understood what the pastor really meant). Since that time, prayer has been an important and powerful form of connection for me.

I've learned much from my years of prayer and gained many beneficial answers in reply. In the passages that follow, I've detailed some of the important points I've learned.

THE FINER POINTS OF PRAYER

WHEN NO SOLUTION IS IN SIGHT

For many of the problems you face in your life, you can see no way out. In times like these, it is best to pray the problem and allow God to find the solution. God's reply may be far better than any answer you might create in your logical mind.

When you pray the problem, you are unchaining God's hands and allowing Him to free you from your situation in ways you might never have imagined on your own. You are opening your life to the possibility of tremendous miracles.

I will never forget the day a family friend actually *gave* a car to my father-in-law. None of us had ever considered that solution. We were all in awe at the time.

Sometimes when you pray, you might receive an answer, but not necessarily the one you expected. This doesn't mean you prayed the wrong thing. It may mean, however, that you didn't properly identify your problem.

When you clearly define the problem, you are causing yourself to face the truth of a situation. In that sense, you

"Fynn, there ain't no different churches in heaven 'cos everybody in heaven is inside themselves."

Anna as told to Fynn,
Mr. God, This Is Anna

"I'm convinced that when people say their prayers as rote, not praying from the heart, nothing happens. You have to believe. The stronger your faith, the stronger the results of your prayers."

Joey Korn,
Dowsing: A Path to Enlightenment

180

are already on the right track of receiving the answer to your prayer because you'll have gained a clear perspective on what the problem is. Learning to pray the problem forces you to see what you are asking for in a new way, and when you see the problem in a new way, you allow your mind to see new possibilities. So, for example:

Don't Pray: *Lord, I need money to fix my car.*

Pray: *Lord, my car isn't working. I need reliable transportation.*

(Because the problem isn't the lack of money, the problem is the car.)

When I had cancer and my doctors told me I would need extensive chemotherapy, I was filled with a lot of fear. I had heard stories of what people suffered when they were given chemotherapy, including violent episodes of throwing up, hair loss, or other severe side effects like damage to the heart or other vital organs. I greatly feared what lay ahead of me. I felt I could not survive such a caustic form of healing. In fact, I truly believed that if it were administered, I would die.

I prayed, *"Lord, I am afraid of this treatment!"* Since I prayed the problem and did not try to figure out a solution on my own, an amazing thing happened. My doctors *changed* the treatment. Of course, it would have been wonderful to have a miraculous healing with no treatment at all, but that was not in keeping with my belief system at the time. My beliefs were such that I needed to see something physical happening to me in order to believe that I could recover. So the answer to my prayer not only resolved my problem and relieved my fear, the answer also addressed my personal beliefs and needs.

The great thing about praying the problem is that you don't need to worry about the solution. You don't need to lay in bed all night trying to figure out how to "fix" things. All you have to do is state the facts of the problem.

- *I am far from home and my car won't start...*
- *I've just been laid off...*
- *I'm pregnant and unmarried...*
- *My credit card debt is more than I can pay...*

"When prayer doesn't seem to yield desired results, it is usually because the recipient is unable to release fear long enough to restore health and harmony."

Doreen Virtue,
The Lightworker's Way

181

- *I have just been diagnosed with cancer...*
- *My child is severely ill.*

After you have prayed about your problem, step back and let God take control.

OUTCOMES

When we are pursuing a new goal and purpose, we might have no idea what problems we may encounter. We only know what we're reaching for. In those cases, our prayers should focus on the outcome we desire. Then after we have prayed, it's important to keep our focus on the outcome we want and not the *means* by which it will transpire. So often we have an expected script in our mind of how the answer should occur. We are so busy watching for signs that our script is falling into place, we might totally miss a door of opportunity that has opened or miss seeing an answer has already arrived in some unexpected means.

In order to receive our desire, we might journey along an unexpected path or engage in situations we would not have thought would lead us where we want to go. In order to reach the fulfillment, we must be open to these alternative routes. We must trust that God will take us to our desires by the shortest, easiest means, no matter how unlikely they might seem.

Let me share an example that involves how I met my husband. At age fifteen, I prayed I would find a new boyfriend. I wanted a boyfriend (and eventually a husband) who would care for me and about me above any other. I wanted our relationship to be special, to be a friendship and a partnership. I wanted, more than anything, to find someone who enjoyed spending time with me regardless of what we might be doing—if anything at all. What I didn't know was how I would find this person or how I would know he was "the one."

That prayer and desire set into motion a chain of events that were seemingly unconnected and unlikely to fulfill my desire. In fact, I didn't even know they would lead to the answer of my prayer because, as far as I knew, I was simply living my life on a day-to-day basis, knowing God would find a way to fulfill my desire.

As it happened, a girlfriend of mine asked my mother

> *"So, remove any and all demands from your desires, and shift to the inner, knowing that you are bringing the universal intelligence into your life, and that you will leave the how and when up to that intelligence, without judging, demanding, or insisting upon your own personality's prerequisites."*
> Wayne W. Dyer,
> *Manifesting Your Destiny*

and I to stop by a new restaurant where she had recently been employed. However, she miscommunicated the directions and my mother and I went to the wrong restaurant. As far as we knew, other than not seeing my friend, the meal and the day were uneventful. I had no clue I had just changed my life forever.

In a wonderful twist, my soon-to-be boyfriend worked at the "wrong" restaurant. He saw me there and mentioned to a co-worker that he thought I was cute. The next twist came when he saw me with one of his friends just a few days later at school. He asked his friend to introduce us and our path together had been set.

THE MANY PATHS YOU TAKE

Keep your focus on your desired outcome and do not worry about how it will be fulfilled. Take each day and opportunity as it comes. It is unlikely you will make a "mistake." What would have happened if I had not decided to visit my friend at the restaurant? Would I have missed meeting my husband? I don't think so.

I don't believe we can take a wrong turn and miss our calling. What we later view in retrospect as a missed opportunity or wrong turn would have had its own twists and turns, joys and woes, so don't believe those ego-based misconceptions you hear in your mind saying you've lost your chance. New opportunities open up every day.

When you come to a fork in the road, who is to say the smooth road will be the easiest? Who is to say the gravel road will be rough? All you can do is make your decisions based on the information you have at hand and move forward with the best of intentions while continuing to focus on the outcome you desire. In the end, they all lead to the same destination.

In the case of my husband, I would have met him somewhere else along my way. We went to the same school, so some other door of opportunity probably would have opened. How many times had I walked by him in the hall in the three previous years and never once noticed him? Any one of those opportunities could have been *the* opportunity. So don't fear that you will miss whatever it is you most need or desire. Trust instead that your desire will somehow be fulfilled.

"Every decision you make will lead you to a better place if you keep choosing things that make you feel good."
Carol Adrienne,
When Life Changes or You Wish It Would

183

One of my favorite prayers to pray in such a case is "Make a way where there is no way." I have seen tremendous miracles by praying in this way. For example, in one job I held, the manager and I had a personality conflict. This man was a relative to the aging owner and would soon take over the company. I did not want to quit my job, but I did not know how to overcome this hurdle. I prayed, "Lord, make a way where there is no way."

About a week later, I went to work and found the man's office empty. He had quit, foregoing his inheritance, to start his own company. Who could have expected that?

In another situation, my husband's supervisor continually stole his ideas and took credit for my husband's work. I prayed again, "Lord, make a way where there is no way." A few weeks later, the man accepted a job in another state.

In my journey to write this book, I have taken left turns and I have taken right turns. All have still brought me to this point where I am sitting here sharing with you the guidelines to make your life healthier and more productive. My choices may appear to have caused me delays, but who is to say another path wouldn't have offered its own setbacks? No matter what choices I made, I would more than likely still be here at this very moment writing these words to you. The best that any of us can do is to keep moving forward.

"... whether or not it is clear to you, no doubt the universe is unfolding as it should."
Max Ehrmann,
Desiderata

PRAY WITHOUT CEASING

I've encountered many situations where I prayed without ceasing. I've walked the floor hour after hour repeating my prayer, standing in the gap for loved ones and friends. It always seems to make a difference.

My feeling is that God hears my prayer the first I speak them, but the hours I spend praying bring me hope and strength while waiting through a difficult situation.

God does not need any convincing as much as I need the faith to believe. For God, I said it, he heard it, and it was done. It is only my lack of belief which keeps the answer at bay. It is for this reason, and no other, that we have taken to wanting some physical object to look at or to hold as a reminder of our faith and belief. Whether a cross, a rosary, a tailsman, or even a rabbit's foot, these objects remind of us the power of our intention and our prayers.

"Pray without ceasing."
1 Thessalonians 5:17,
King James Version

184

The more science learns, the more we understand the significance of our prayers. This means it isn't just foolishness to pray over our food, our circumstances, our health, or our loved ones. In this sense, we are praying without ceasing and causing the energies and benevolent forces around us to converge on our behalf.

PRAYING ON THE GO

There have been many times I needed a prayer on the go. I might find myself in a situation where I only have time to whisper a quick prayer under my breath or where I want to remain discrete.

Friend and author Joey Korn, who taught me how to relax, also taught me the following little prayer. *(You can learn more about his prayers at www.dowsers.com.)* I have found it useful in countless situations where I need a quick word on the go and use it in a multitude of ways, filling in the blank with any appropriate statement:

> *Dear God, create a unique energy configuration specific to this need by balancing any detrimental energies and enhancing any beneficial energies in order that _____ . For now and for as long as it is appropriate, Amen.*

For noisy restaurants:

> *. . . the area surrounding us might be filled with peace.*

While driving on icy and snow-covered roads:

> *. . . we are able to drive home safely.*

During an argument:

> *. . . we might find a calm resolution.*

Flying in an airplane:

> *. . . the plane might have a safe and smooth path to follow to get us home safely.*

"We can call in the energies we want, whether they be for healing, for problem solving, for raising our spiritual awareness, for bringing abundance into our lives, or for whatever we want to accomplish."

Joey Korn,
Dowsing: A Path to Enlightenment

185

PRAYERS ARE LIKE GOALS

Sometimes we are looking at too big a piece of the whole picture. We might need to break our desires into smaller ideas or thoughts in order to better express them to ourselves and to God. For example, when I had cancer, I separated my hopes and desires into several categories. I prayed about the type of treatment, I prayed about the care of my two-year-old son, I prayed about my husband and how my illness might affect him and his life. There were many small prayers offered up about whatever test or trial I faced on any particular day.

When you are praying for something large in scope, try breaking it into smaller parts and praying for each one separately. You will likely see quicker, more visible results.

WHEN YOU PRAY FOR OTHERS

When you pray for others, don't put *your* desires on them. Pray for their well-being and for their known troubles. Don't spend time trying to "fix" others. Leave the "fixing" to God. In this life, we can only change ourselves. Those who are around us cannot be changed by our manipulation of them. To change others, the best that we can do is to change the way we react to them and, by doing so, they will change how they react to us.

"When you pray for anyone you tend to modify your personal attitude toward him."
Norman Vincent Peale

THINK OF GOD AS A LOVING, EARTHLY PARENT

If my children want something and there's a way to get it for them, I do. I might want them to work for it, I might want them to appreciate it, but I definitely want them to have every good thing they desire. It's in my nature as a parent.

I meet so many people who feel that God would be bothered by their requests and heart's desires. God is not an official of the government sitting behind a desk, inundated by paperwork, phone calls, and nonsense requests. God, in whatever form you believe Him to be, is like a parent wanting to do anything he can to help us succeed and be independent in our lives. I recognize that not every human parent is a good and loving person, but I hope that you will recognize the difference and know that God *is* a loving parent. He wants us to have all we desire.

God answers all sorts of prayers for all types of people, good, bad, young, old, rich, poor, ugly, clean-cut, rough around the edges, and everyone in between. Prayers are not answered on the basis of goodness or deservedness. Prayers are answered on the basis of your beliefs and perception.

WHEN YOU PRAY, EXPECT AN ANSWER

If you turn on the switch, you expect the lights will come on. If you sit down at your computer and start typing on the keys, you expect words to appear. If you get in your car and start driving down the road, you expect you'll soon arrive at the grocery store, gas station, or your place of work. So why should you pray and not expect an answer to your prayer? Why pray at all if you don't want what you are praying for? If you don't expect an answer, how can you receive one?

One thing I know without a doubt, no matter who you are or where you've been, no matter what you've done, if you offer up a prayer and do so sincerely, it will be heard. The answer you receive will be in keeping with what you believe within your innermost heart.

If you pray following the guidelines I've given you here, you will see more answers to your prayers than you ever imagined because you will have removed the countless stipulations and impossible conditions you previously had placed on them. This, in turn, frees the hand of God and His holy hosts to help you in miraculous ways. So expect God to answer when you call on Him.

PRAYER'S LITTLE SURPRISES

Never doubt the power of prayer. Prayer can truly move mountains and call forth miracles. But not every prayer comes to fruition as expected. We have all heard the phrase, "Be careful what you pray for, you might get it."

My father-in-law was a wonderful spiritual teacher and healer. He enjoyed going to prayer meetings and being with like-minded individuals. He loved praying with them

"Expect a miracle, make miracles happen."
Norman Vincent Peale

"Immaculate faith happens in a moment. Immaculate curing, healing, restoration happens in a moment. And the reason it takes so long for most of you? Because the road is paved with doubt and disbelief."
Ramtha (Spirit),
Channeled by J. Z. Knight,
A Beginner's Guide to Creating Reality

"I tell you the truth, if you have faith as small as a mustard seed, you can say to this mountain, 'Move from here to there' and it will move. Nothing will be impossible to you."
Matthew 17:20,
New International Version

and for them. He deeply wanted to have freedom from his job in order to do his spiritual work full time. He began to pray he would no longer have to work.

One day that prayer was answered. He nearly lost his life when his oxygen mask malfunctioned and fed him deadly carbon monoxide instead. True to his prayer, he never worked again. However, he suffered from countless side effects and disabilities which prevented him from doing all he'd hoped in the spiritual community. He often said before his death, "I never thought to ask God for good health."

Why is it that our prayers sometimes come with odd twists and hidden surprises?

In one of my favorite *X-Files* episodes, Mulder (David Duchovny) meets a *jinni* (a female genie) who enjoys playing games with people's wishes. She twists them so that the wish is what the person asked for, but not as they expected. When Mulder wishes for "peace on earth," he finds himself alone amid the empty cars and buildings of the city. In effect, he is the only one on earth, and with no one else to make noise or war, there *is* peace—just not in the form he expected. Mulder then takes to writing a contractual-like wish, filling pages and pages with conditions and stipulations, until he realizes even that is useless, there is always some loophole. So instead, he uses his last wish to free the *jinni*.

These odd little twists in our prayers remind us that we are playing with a tremendous power that we do not fully understand, a power that can, indeed, alter our lives. I think the twists are a warning and a reminder to use that power with care. So pray without ceasing and ask for all your heart's desires, but do be mindful of what you pray for—you just might get it.

"God's bounty is limited only by us, not by His resources, power, or willingness to give. Jabez was blessed simply because he refused to let any obstacle, person, or opinion loom larger than God's nature. And God's nature is to bless."

Bruce H. Wilkinson
The Prayer of Jabez

Chapter Nineteen:
A Compass, a Sextant,
a Topographical Map:
Your Internal Guidance System

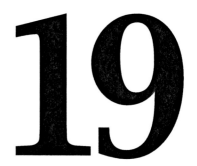

Secret Messages

Up until now, we have talked about connection as something you actively pursue—listening to music, reading a book, driving a car, praying, meditating, or writing down words. But there is another more subliminal level of connection, one that we have access to every moment of the day if we only know where and how to look.

These aspects of connection are sometimes referred to as "dark language" because the information received reveals itself through means of communication other than those we are most accustomed to such as writing, talking, or listening. Instead, the messages appear to us in a kind of code entwined throughout our environment, a code that we must first interpret before the message's meaning can be understood. If you can learn how to find and interpret these "secret" messages, you'll tap into a form of connection that offers you additional direction. Just think . . . you have a built-in Global Positioning System (GPS) always at the ready to answer your questions and guide you whenever you can't find your way.

Throughout every moment of the day, whether awake or

> "We all have access to information about ourselves, much of which we don't even know exists."
> Michael Lee,
> *Phoenix Rising Yoga Therapy*

> *"We need to attune to our inner voice and listen with our whole being rather than just our mind."*
>
> Michael Lee,
> *Phoenix Rising Yoga Therapy*

asleep, our magnificent bodies are receiving and interpreting all that is going on around us. We do not fully understand how this analysis works. We do know the body is capable of reading and interpreting information we might not have even seen or noticed on a conscious level. Most of this data is stored for our later use without any action on our part. Much of it we will never consciously utilize at all. This means we have a huge storehouse of information available to us that we are not using, information that could make our desires and goals easier to achieve. All we need to do in order to access this information is learn how to interpret the signs and symbols that take place in the world around us and inside of us.

INTUITION

You're watching television. On the screen, two stakeout cops sit in a late-model car several hours after dark. All is quiet. The driver stares out the window at the house they are watching. The passenger is eating a drive-through burger and fries. The driver says, "I've got a bad feeling about this." The passenger continues eating. Suddenly all hell breaks loose. The chase is on. The cop with the gut feeling was right. How did he know? *Intuition.*

What is intuition and how does it work? Intuition is yet another level of *Body Songs*. It is one more way for your body to clue you in on what is about to happen or why.

Our body has four main ways it communicates these messages to us: *clairaudience, claircognizance, clairsentience,* and *clairvoyance.* Although these look like large, confusing words, they represent the four simple awarenesses we all experience in one form or another. While it is likely you are more receptive to one over the others, no doubt you have received input on some level from them all—you just weren't aware of it because these are inborn, automatic traits that your body naturally performs. You don't have to think about intuition; it just happens.

The prefix "clair" refers to "clear" so the four types are: clairaudience (clear hearing), claircognizance (clear knowing), clairsentience (clear feeling), and clairvoyance (clear seeing).

> *"Ask your intuition to work for you and then let it. Follow your hunch. Even when the action or decision seems less than obvious or optimal, pay attention."*
>
> Nell M. Rodgers,
> *Puppet or Puppeteer*

CLAIRAUDIENCE

Clairaudience is "clear hearing," which relates to all kinds of sounds. Any type of sound might be heard through this form of awareness, anything from someone speaking, to the sound of a bell ringing, a train's whistle blowing, a baby crying, music playing, screaming, laughing—anything.

Earlier in the book, I told of encountering an angel in the basement. *(See: Chapter 5)* On that occasion, I didn't see anything but heard a distinct voice as clear as if someone had been standing next to me. At first, my senses were confused. How can I hear a voice if there is no one there to speak? But I could not deny I heard the message that came through precise and clear.

On two other occasions, I heard a similar voice. Each time, I heard it as if someone were standing behind me whispering in my right ear. Were these real, audible voices? Or had I received a telepathic message that I *perceived* as audible? I don't know for sure. I only know that I felt as though I had physically heard something.

When my boys were little, I would sometimes walk through the house late at night while everyone else was asleep. On several occasions, I heard quiet voices in conversation coming from the vicinity of the boys' room. I knew it wasn't the boys as the voice reminded me of an adults' conversation such as you might hear around a campfire. I would stop to listen in order to make out what they were saying, but the conversation always stopped. I could never quite make out what was being said, but come morning, I would tell the boys, "Your angels were talking again last night."

"[Archangel] Raphael helps healers by whispering guidance and wisdom in their ears."
Doreen Virtue,
The Lightworker's Way

CLAIRCOGNIZANCE

Claircognizance, or "clear knowing" is knowing something without knowing exactly *why* you know it. As I've said before, my father-in-law used to say, "I know, that I know, that I know." His "knowing" was claircognizance. He would have knowledge about something without any logical reason.

I think claircognizance is probably the most widely used of the four Cs because we don't often take time to figure out *why* we know what we know. Why are we able

"For awhile he [Edgar Cayce] could evidently see an astonishing array of facts with his psychic vision, he called on his talent only to train others to use their OWN talents; their hunches, their impressions, their promptings, and their dreams."
Harmon H. Bro,
Edgar Cayce on Dreams

to quickly remember a name from twenty years ago, find our way around a strange town without directions, or know the answer to some obscure or trivial question? Why do we remember just as we are walking out the door that we forgot to grab the theater tickets, a sweater, or a briefcase? How many of us reach for the phone instinctively knowing who's there? We never consider we might have received assistance from an internal guidance system helping us to know these things. We just presume it's from ourselves and brag about how smart we are. "Boy, I sure pulled that answer from out of no where." Or did we?

Just after I turned seven, my family moved to Ohio so we could be closer to my father's sales territory. Over the weeks leading up to our move, we made many trips there and back. As the trips grew more frequent, we made a game of crossing under the "Welcome to Ohio" sign. As soon as we would see the sign, the whole family let out a tremendous cheer as we knew this move would allow my father to spend more time at home. On one of these occasions, I followed the cheer by saying matter-of-factly, "Someday I'm coming back to Pennsylvania." My mother offered a maternal reply to the effect of, "That's nice, dear," which really meant "You're too young to know what you're saying." So I said, again, *"After I'm married, I'm coming back."* Still humoring me, my mother teased, "What if your husband doesn't want to live in Pennsylvania?" But I just replied, "He will." It irritated me that she didn't believe me because I *knew* it was true.

Some fourteen years passed. By that time, I'd lived most of my life in Ohio. Living in Pennsylvania was nothing more than a childhood memory. I don't think either my mother or I ever thought of the car incident again until the day my husband's company offered him a promotion and raise if he would relocate to their branch in Pennsylvania. At the time, I didn't even know his company *had* a branch in Pennsylvania.

How did I know this at age seven? Coincidence? I don't think so. What I spoke that day in the car came from a place of *clear knowing*. I had *no doubt whatsoever* that what I said was true. I don't know why I knew it. Nothing I can think of premeditated my saying it, I heard no voice telling me, felt no internal nudgings, saw no visions. I just spoke my mind from what I somehow knew.

CLAIRSENTIENCE

On more than one occasion, my father-in-law called the house and asked if my husband was sick. On every occasion, I reported that he was. Whether bronchitis or flu or some other ailment, his dad always knew. My father-in-law would say, "I've been sick for two days and didn't know why." He would actually *feel* whatever illness my husband had even though we lived ninety miles away. As soon as my father-in-law verified the cause, within a few hours he would feel fine.

Clairsentience is the ability to feel intuitively. While psychic healers may feel another person's pain or injury, we all experience clairsentience more frequently than you might expect. Surely you've felt that knot in your stomach when you tell a lie or try to do something you *know* you shouldn't do? Have you ever gotten a headache when you were in some place you felt uncomfortable? Have you ever felt nausea during a situation of fear or worry? These are all examples of clairsentience.

CLAIRVOYANCE

Shortly after we moved to Ohio, I discovered books of fairy tales in the school library. I fell in love with the magical stories where seemingly ordinary people found the power to overcome adversity and strife not only by using charmed objects such as magic beans or cloaks, but also by their good virtue. I longed to have the powers of these mythical people but knew they were only stories.

About a year later, while in the fourth grade, I had a clairvoyant *(clear seeing)* experience. Sitting in my class-room, bored, I covered my eyes with my hands, and even pressed on them a bit.[1] Within a few seconds, I could see a tunnel as if it were a long hallway lined with windows. As I traveled down this hall, I moved faster and faster until the windows and their ambient light became a blur. Then, just as quickly, the movement stopped. All I could see was a closed door with a small window. Peeking through the window, a bedroom with all white furniture, including a canopy bed, a dresser, and a dressing table came into view. My vision allowed me to see each item one at a time in clear detail. Then, perhaps brought to attention by the teacher, the vision ended.

"As a child I was always drawn to television shows featuring characters with amazing abilities and special otherworldly powers . . . I was obsessed with 'I Dream of Jeannie.' . . . I imagined I had those powers—blink and make things happen."

John Edward,
One Last Time

193

"Ask for clarification. . . . Notice patterns—for instance repeatedly hearing a song, seeing a bumpersticker, or having a friend unknowingly repeat the very same message word for word as you first received it."
Doreen Virtue,
Divine Prescriptions

I had never had anything like that happen before, nor had anyone ever told me such things could happen. I don't even know why I did what I did on that day. Sometime afterwards, my mother announced that my cousin would be coming to live with us. We drove to her home in Chicago arriving at a house I'd never been to before. Once there, we picked up my cousin's things, including her bedroom furniture. When I walked into her bedroom for the first time, I saw a white Provincial canopy bed, matching dresser, and dressing table all laid out in the same floorplan I'd seen weeks earlier in my vision. Even more amazing, I'd never seen white furniture before. I didn't know such a thing as "Provincial" existed.

Nothing like that had ever happened to me before, but I liked it. I wanted it to happen again. Seeing events in the future gave me a sense of power and control, something that I didn't have much of in my life. I continuously tried to duplicate what I had done that day to cause me to travel down the windowed hall, but I was unable to see anything more. Eventually I gave up, but I didn't stop trying to find some means of making that magic happen again.

Years later, when I met my father-in-law and watched him using what he referred to as the *gifts of the spirit*, particularly the *gift of sight* (clairvoyance), I was reminded again of my own experience years earlier. My father-in-law had a tremendous ability to see coming or hidden events; I wanted that ability too, so I prayed for the gift. More importantly, I believed I would receive the ability and immediately started trying to "see" things. I would wait until I was home alone, then sit quietly trying to see the future. Pictures and impressions would cross through my mind, but I didn't always know what they meant.

This was very much a trial and error process. In time, I could "see," but it took more time to be able to make sense of what I'd seen, longer still to use the gift wisely. As with prayer, I learned there were times to tell others what I saw and times to keep my mouth shut. I learned quickly that if I revealed something beneficial or what someone wanted to hear, they were glad to hear the information and wanted to know more. But if I said something against what they believed, they became angry.

After a while, I stopped focusing on this type of seeing because I realized that knowing the future didn't neces-

"I discovered that if I said all the ideas that 'came' to me when in conversation, the other person would think me strange at best and frightening at worst."
Laura Day,
Practical Intuition

sarily help me in the present. I learned that knowing the future didn't mean I could change it. I also learned that it was a tremendous responsibility.

I believe anyone who wants this ability can receive it because clairvoyance isn't a bestowed-upon gift. It is a part of the four-Cs intuitive package built into our bodies. In order to begin seeing, one must merely be open to viewing and interpreting the images and impressions that come to mind after asking a question or thinking about a particular situation. We already know how to "see" via our imaginations and our memories of past events. Seeing via clairvoyance works much the same way.

(I will explain more about interpreting our impressions later in the sections on Dreams and Visions.)

TRUSTING THE FOUR CS

The more we work on the outer part of connection and on creating a cohesive link between our conscious and unconscious minds, the more our intuition and other internal sensory perceptions are able to function as they were designed. Perhaps our biggest downfall when it comes to these built-in tools is our inability to trust them. Despite any guidance we might receive, more often than not, we simply ignore it. We fail to follow through on whatever our "gut" is telling us to do.

If you find yourself being wary of your intuitive guidance, begin by trying things that don't matter one way or the other. See how they turn out. Keep in mind that intuition operates more efficiently the more you rely on it and, the more you rely on it, the more important the information will become. In other words, your intuitive mind knows when you're taking its messages seriously and responds appropriately. Since your body will provide you with information in whatever way you're most responsive, the more you focus on one or another of the four Cs, the more it will illuminate its messages to you in that means.

Could this be why you suffer from ailments? Do you give more attention to *them* than to the intuitive four Cs? Do you find ailments have consumed your life? If so, begin to listen for the messages from your intuition, and see if the messages from your ailments gradually subside.

For more information on how to "trust your gut" be

"The automated mechanism is unconscious. We cannot see the wheels turning. We cannot know what is taking place beneath the surface. And because it works spontaneously in reacting to present and current needs, we can have no intimation or certified guarantee in advance that it will come up with an answer. We are forced into a position of trust. And only by trusting and acting do we receive signs and wonders."
Maxwell Maltz,
Psycho-Cybernetics

sure to read the rest of this chapter and the next for other tips. You'll also read how I learned to trust my internal guidance in Chapter 20.

HOW PAST MEMORIES ILLUMINATE THE FUTURE

MEMORY TAGS AND WHY THEY ARE IMPORTANT

If nothing is an accident, if there are no coincidences, then anything that is brought to your conscious attention, anything that seems to stand out to you, anything at all, is a part of the hidden, intuitive language I have been speaking about in this chapter. Let me explain.

Our memories consist of millions of tiny bits of information. For a single moment in time, we may have stored information containing everything from the color and texture of our clothing; smells in the air; sounds we heard; feelings we felt; pictures on the walls; programs on the television; even the time on the clock. We gather similar information about other people involved, including their words, actions, and expressions, and even minute details, such as the twitch of their nose, the slight upturn of their lip, or the glint in their eye. In order for our minds to deal with this overload of data, it takes the many countless bits of information and smashes them down into compressed chunks. It then gives each data "chunk" a *memory tag* that it uses as a trigger to bring the essence of that situation back to us. A memory tag may be a hint of fragrance in the air, the clink of a spoon against a pan, even a flash of light caught by the eye in just the right way. The scent of a man's cologne might trigger a memory of father, seeing a petunia might trigger thoughts of mother, feeling a soft blanket might recollect memories from childhood, because in each situation the trigger is one of the many bits stored in that chunk or memory tag.

Dr. Eugene T. Gendlin *(Focusing)* refers to our ability to compress our experiences and recall them from these tags as our *felt sense*. All we need to do after our memory tag is in place is to see, hear, smell, or experience that tag

"The sense of 'all about Helen'—including every one of those thousands of bits of data that you have seen, felt, lived, and stored over the years—comes to you all at once, as a single great aura sensed in your body."

Eugene T. Gendlin,
Focusing

again and all that the symbol represents is brought back to mind—regardless of whether we want to remember it or not.

Whenever one of these tags is triggered, a rush of sensory information floods our minds from that past event. Knowing this, we can use our felt sense to help us recognize some of the messages our intuitive mind is sending. We can utilize what we know about the past as a form of guidance in the present.

(MPMs) – MEMORABLE PHYSICAL MANIFESTATIONS

In the movie *Signs*, Reverend Graham Hess (Mel Gibson) has a recurring dream about his wife's death where she says, "Swing away, Merrill." The reverend rationalizes that as his wife died, her fleeting thoughts caused her to say whatever came to mind. "Swing away, Merrill" referred to a situation where Merrill Hess, the reverend's baseball playing brother, had too many strike-outs and became afraid to swing the bat. What Reverend Hess tries to understand throughout the movie is why he is having this dream and memory of his wife—now. His wife has been dead for nearly a year, yet the dream persists, almost haunting him. Why?

That is our job too. Why is something triggering our memory from the past—now?

My name for any situation that triggers such a reaction is a *memorable physical manifestation* or *MPM*. A memorable physical manifestation plays off of the memory tags we've stored away from the past. When a present happening triggers a memory from the past, it means something is connected about the two situations. It's by finding the connection that we are able to gain a valuable, maybe even vital, message about the present.

In the movie *Dragonfly*, Joe Darrow (Kevin Costner) associates his loving memories for his deceased wife with dragonflies. Emily Darrow (Susanna Thompson) had a dragonfly birthmark and often collected dragonfly objects, so now dragonflies are a memory tag for Joe. Just seeing one calls up Joe's felt sense memories connected to his wife, stirring his emotions, playing with his heart, and even driving him a little crazy. While for anyone else the bug might go totally unnoticed, Joe is drawn to them, even

"Every moment—past, present, and future—has a meaning. Every sign, every act, every deed, every thing we notice can be traced to the past and is being noticed in the present through the filter we're using in the moment."

Laura Day,
Practical Intuition

197

fixated on them. He can't help it. Each time he sees one, whether real or unreal, it triggers the memory tag associated with his feelings for his wife. His emotions flow through him almost out of control. No one else in the movie can understand why Joe goes a little off the wall about dragonflies, after all, to them a dragonfly is just another insect. To Joe, it represents everything; to Joe it is a symbol of his wife.

In the end, because of Joe's strong feelings associated with dragonflies, he is drawn to discover something about his wife that he might not have found otherwise—something vital.

That is why MPMs are so important to us. If we can only take them to the next level, figure out how a trigger from the past relates to the here and now, we have the opportunity to learn something life-enhancing, valuable, maybe even vital to our goals, our purpose, and our life.

So how do we do that?

WHERE AND HOW TO FIND MEMORABLE PHYSICAL MANIFESTATIONS

MPMs are found anywhere and everywhere. However, keep in mind they must also carry a personal, internal reaction. Without the reaction, there is no connection. It is the *reaction,* not the object, which is the signal that an MPM offers you a personal message or guidance.

A *memorable physical manifestation* is any occurrence or object that triggers an emotional reaction within you. It is the kind of situation where you might feel as if "the light went on," or think to yourself "I felt my heart flutter." Some refer to the associated feeling as an "aha moment." In these situations, words leap off the page, a friend's words stick in your mind, objects reach out and grab your attention. You can't help but notice. A stronger reaction feels as if the object (or situation) has grabbed you by the shirt, held you in its grasp, forced you to see whatever it is you are to see. You may even stop and stare in a momentary trance.

Let me share a personal example. Right before my hysterectomy, I read a novel about a character who almost died. At the last minute, he came back to life through the tears of a magical phoenix bird. This wasn't the MPM. The

"Out of the welter of information around us, your subconscious tells you what you should notice. It knows what is important for you, and it selects and coalesces information into a meaningful pattern."
Laura Day,
Practical Intuition

story, however, left a lasting impression, one of those things from which my mind compressed all the data into a memory tag to be recalled later. Not long after, my husband showed me a photograph of an antique plate he wanted to buy. Suddenly the image of the phoenix bird leapt from the photograph and grabbed my attention. I found it intriguing that I had never recognized the stylized image on the plate as a phoenix even though I'd seen the plates many times before. That was the first of my phoenix MPMs.

Afterwards, the bird began showing up in other areas of my life in almost surreal fashion. I felt as if someone pointed theater spotlights on these items. I also started noticing peacocks, which are often associated with the mythical phoenix.

The most startling of these MPMs happened at a local pet store just a few days before my surgery. Standing in the pet food aisle, I saw a women carrying a beautiful peacock pillow in her shopping cart. The colors of the pillow were so brilliant and beautiful I knew I must find which aisle they were sold in so I could buy one too.

As she rolled her cart closer and closer to mine, I suddenly realized she did not have a pillow in her cart at all, but a real and very live bird. I could hardly believe my eyes, the bird sat so calmly in the cart as if this were a perfectly normal experience, even when four or five people walked over to see and pet him.

I do not know what the odds were of my walking into a pet store and seeing a woman carrying a live peacock in her shopping cart. I do know that for me, it was a very memorable and physical manifestation with a definite internal reaction.

What did all those peacocks and phoenix birds mean to me? Each occurrence of the phoenix image reminded me of the original memory tag, the story of the character who had nearly died. While I wouldn't know for sure until afterward, I felt that somehow the phoenix MPMs were a warning of what might occur during my surgery, even though my doctors expected it to be a typical procedure.

Because of this warning, I told my husband as we walked out of the house for the hospital, "If anything happens to me during surgery, don't worry; I'll be okay." "Don't talk like that," he said, so I let it go.

"The intuitive mind [is] . . . able to tap into a deep storehouse of knowledge and wisdom, the universal mind. It also is able to sort out this information and supply us with exactly what we need, when we need it."
Shakti Gawain,
Living in the Light

After the operation, due to complications, I nearly died. My husband says that although the doctors doubted I would survive, he continually told them I would. For three days I lay in intensive care, unconscious. When I awoke, it was as if I'd been touched by some magical power. Within a week of my initial surgery, I returned home. Had I been cured by the touch of the phoenix bird? Probably not. But I had been given an indication of what was to come, allowing me to warn my husband—a warning that gave my husband hope and faith during a fearful and trying situation.

Remember, MPMs work off of your felt sense. While you may be taking part in a perfectly mundane situation, suddenly the memory tag from some past experience will come to mind, alerting you to its presence. You'll have that "ting" inside you notifying you of the significance of it. You won't need confirmation that you've "been tagged" because the memory will be there. However, you may need to force yourself to acknowledge the MPM has occurred because this kind of thing happens to us so frequently that we tend to ignore them.

"A felt sense doesn't come to you in the form of thoughts or words or other separate units, but as a single (though often puzzling and very complex) bodily feeling."

Eugene T. Gendlin,
Focusing

HOW TO INTERPRET AN MPM

In the movie *Paycheck*, Michael Jennings (Ben Affleck) is a reverse engineer, which means he takes things apart to see how they work. He usually applies this skill to software but, in his present situation, he now must apply his skill to nineteen seemingly unconnected objects he mailed to himself before losing his memory.

We can use the basic concept of reverse engineering on MPMs in order to better understand their meaning. It is by interpreting the MPMs present meaning that we can gain a clearer understanding of the message it has for us. An MPM can shed light on who we are meant to be, where we should be going, or how to proceed in doing so. An MPM might also offer a glimpse into our future.

According to a paper called *A Pattern Language of Reverse Engineering*,[2] the basic steps for reverse engineering are as follows:

1. First contact

2. Extract the architecture

200

3. Focus on hot areas

4. Prepare for reengineering

When I interpret an MPM, I utilize the steps above in a similar manner. Here's how.

Step one, *first contact*, is my first recognition that a memorable physical manifestation has occurred. One part of first contact, according to reverse engineering, is to "read all the code within an hour." For an MPM that means I make a quick assessment of the situation at the time it happens, saving the memory for later when I have more time to contemplate what it means. For example, when I saw the peacock in the shopping cart, I thought to myself, "Wow! That is a major MPM." I knew it connected to the story I had read, but I had to finish my shopping, so I set aside any further thought of it until later.

Step two is *extract the architecture*. Reverse engineers "check the database" and "guess objects." For me, it simply means I look back in my mind at the initial memory tag, the situation that pulled me to notice the MPM in the first place. I allow myself a few minutes of quiet time to attempt to tap into the memory as fully as possible. Then I look for ways to connect the two situations using known objects, feelings, situations, people, and any other connections that stand out in my mind. Next, I speculate as to what the connections mean ("guess objects"). I "guessed" that the phoenix bird connected to my upcoming hysterectomy since the surgery was the most likely connection but an MPM might connect to a coming, but unknown situation.

The third step in reverse engineering is to *focus on hot areas*. For an MPM, a "hot area" is any situation or problem taking up your thoughts at that time. This could be a situation that causes you worry, fear, anger, concern, or puzzlement. It even might be a situation that makes you happy. At any rate, a hot area is some emotional component that you have spent time thinking of or worrying about over the past days, weeks, or months. It will be something in your focus right now—as my coming surgery would have been to me at that time.

The fourth step in reverse engineering is to "prepare for reengineering." Reverse engineers take things apart when they don't know how they work so they can under-

"Omens are manifestations of Spirit, messages from the abyss of creation."
Ken Eagle Feather,
A Toltec Path

"You are where your attention takes you."
Kenneth X. Carey,
The Starseed Transmissions

201

stand how to rebuild them or build them better. In this step they, "refactor to understand." We are, in a sense, taking what we know about ourselves and using it as a guide to gain understanding about what we don't know. The more we practice with our mental and intuitive capabilities, the more we will learn about ourselves. The more we learn about ourselves, the better we will be able to use these abilities in beneficial ways to help ourselves be healthier, happier beings. Isn't that in a sense reengineering ourselves?

MORE TIPS FOR INTERPRETING A MEMORABLE PHYSICAL MANIFESTATION (MPM)

Remember that an MPM is a "memorable," "physical" "manifestation." It is something that will stand out to you—you'll remember it. It will be visible (something you can see) or physical (something you experience). You'll later understand how your having seen it or experienced it caused its creation (manifestation) to be symbolic guidance in your life.

Some of the messages are simple to interpret, such as my peacock just before my surgery. However, sometimes it might be difficult to see these occurrences in context with a present situation, which may be why we tend to ignore them. Trying to make sense of the less prominent ones can become tedious, even frustrating. For that reason, I recommend only focusing on those MPMs that offer a strong trigger, one that practically forces you to notice its presence (i.e., a peacock in a shopping cart). If you focus on those, you'll have a better chance of interpreting the messages correctly.

Here are some questions to ask yourself to help understand your MPMs' meaning:

- *What memory does the MPM recall?*

- *How might this memory apply to my present situation?*

- *Does the message offered somehow connect to my life's path, my heart's desires, or my present goals?*

- *Does the message and meaning come easily and quickly with hardly any thought? (It should. Never*

". . . heightened awareness brings dreamlike qualities to life. Inanimate objects possess vitality. Messages on billboards abruptly and magically change. Paintings hanging on walls spring to life as the features in them move about. Trees gesture, often showing which way to proceed. And rocks glow, illuminating narrow paths at night."
Ken Eagle Feather,
A Toltec Path

202

try to contrive or adapt a message into a more complex meaning. There should be no need to twist or turn it to make the meaning fit.)

• *Did the occurrence of the MPM happen when least expected? (Unexpected occurrences are of the greatest significance. In other words, looking for peacocks is not the same as stumbling upon one.)*

When all else fails, you'll probably learn the precise meaning of the MPM after the connected future event has taken place. They have a way of popping into your mind right at that moment. The more you practice interpreting them, the better you'll become at understanding them.

EXERCISE 15–DREAMS

A dream doesn't have to be sensible to be valuable. A dream can relay all sorts of information to us through its encoded pictures. Even better, since the images come from within, they are already intricately correlated with icons and familiar symbols. All we have to do is interpret those symbols and we will have a wealth of information at our fingertips. This exercise focuses on how to do that.

1. First, in order to better understand a dream, you need to understand that each and every object or person in your dream is in some way a reflection of yourself. Regardless of whether it's a house, a car, a tree, or a clock; your mother, a guide, the President of the United States, Brittany Spears, Bart Simpson, or Smokey the Bear. Such people or objects are a reflection of some aspect of your personality and motivations.

2. Numbers or duplicates of items often relate to time.

3. In order to interpret a dream, the first step is to list all the people and objects from that dream. The list might look something like this:

   • *A broken wristwatch*
   • *A ferocious tiger*

"The universal dreamer rises up above his earthly burden."
Jeff Lynne,
Eldorado

203

- *An empty dresser drawer*
- *A tree house*

4. Create a second list with all the *actions* of the dream. This list should include all actions carried out by you, by others, or by any objects in the dream. Here is an example list:

- *Climbing a tree*
- *Opening a drawer*
- *Breaking an arm*
- *Falling*

5. Next, make a list of the *feelings* and *impressions* you experienced during the dream in association with these items and people. Note how you felt or reacted, and also how the other people, situations, and objects felt or reacted.

- *I felt relief when I saw the broken wristwatch. I had the feeling that a painful time had somehow ended.*

- *As the cat climbed the tree, I felt incredibly sad, but did not really know why.*

6. Interpret each item in the list, looking for some way it correlates to yourself or your present situations. Look for word associations as described with interpreting ailments, and watch for "hits" or that intuitive knowing inside that you've chosen the right meaning.

7. Consider if any of the dream's messages should be taken literally or figuratively.

8. Don't worry about what you can't remember as it's not vital to the core message. As you begin interpreting the dream, other images will return to your mind if they're needed.

Here is an example taken from one of my dreams:

> My mother and stepfather are standing in the living room. Their appearance amazes me as both have been gone for more than a decade. I ask my mother if I can touch her and wonder if she is really

"We may give the dream a name . . . indicating also the primary image in it. As we do this, the identifying image becomes the title of the dream and gives us an easy means of referring to it if we have occasion to work with the material from that dream . . ."

Ira Progoff,
At a Journal Workshop

there. Is she solid . . . physical? She is.

My mother says, "We want to start our lives over so we thought we should try to be in an accident."

I think to myself, *That isn't right! If they are already dead, how can they be in an accident and die again?* Something about their statement leaves me feeling uneasy and confused.

Then we are standing in the back yard looking at a stone-lined pond that has dried up. As I peer into an opening in the rocks where water should flow through, I notice garbage has blocked the flow. The problem seems obvious and easy to fix.

Then my parents walk away. I notice my mother looks younger than when she died and has long hair even though I don't recall her ever having long hair during her lifetime.

I feel as though something about the pair is unnatural and I think of the movie, *Death Becomes Her* where the two main characters drink a magical fluid that prevents them from dying, yet they aren't really alive.

Here is the list I created of the main people and objects from my dream:

- *My mother*
- *My stepfather*
- *A dried up pond*
- *Garbage*
- *Rocks*
- *Mother's unusually long hair*

The actions in the dream were:

- *My mother's statement about death*
- *Wondering about her state of being*
- *Seeing the blocked pond (water)*
- *My parents walking away*

"Dreams from the subconscious levels of the mind . . . mostly concern the conditions of the body, symbolized by vehicles; the mind, represented by hair and clothing; and emotions, often indicated by water."
Wilda B. Tanner,
The Mystical, Magical, Marvelous World of Dream

"We can harness our dreams to help us overcome challenges in our lives, energize us and give us the wisdom we need to help us follow our own true path."
Kathy and Amy Eldon,
Soul Catcher Journal

My feelings in the dream included the following:

- *Confused by my mother's statement*
- *Disturbed by the garbage clogging the pond*
- *Noticing my mother's unnatural appearance*

Now that I have my lists, I work through one item at a time using word associations and symbolism to help me find any important connections. I also consider any recent life happenings, problems, or questions I may have been facing before the dream, along with any intuitive insights I may have recently received. I break the dream into "scenes" and interpret each separately knowing they somehow have to interconnect.

In this case, the part of the dream that seems the most logical to interpret is that of the blocked pond. I'd been eating a lot of garbage food lately and felt those foods affected not only the flow of my bodily systems but also the flow of my life. I recognized that when I ate them I felt sluggish and had less energy. I'd been receiving intuitive insights about eating healthier and about avoiding certain foods, so this is my first assessment of the dream. However, I don't feel the "hit" of that interpretation being right and also don't know how that interpretation ties together with the rest of the dream—as it should—so I keep going.

Next, I put myself in the role of each of the people and objects and think about why I might be doing what occurred in the dream. In other words, if I were my mother, why would I say what she said? It doesn't make sense to me at first. Then I decide that it's either because she doesn't realize she is already dead, or because she somehow feels trapped in her situation and is looking to break free of it. When I take this idea out of context—which is often an important step in interpreting a dream—it makes a lot more sense. I ask myself, "Do I feel trapped in some situation?" "Am I 'stuck' in a rut?" "Am I looking to 'break free' of something?"

I give myself some time to ponder this while looking at the other objects in the dream. What is my state of being if I am the pond? The stones? The garbage? My mother's long hair?

I think again about the pond being blocked. The pond

"Remember, your dreams are important coded messages to yourself, from yourself, for yourself."

Wilda B. Tanner,
The Mystical, Magical, Marvelous World of Dreams

being "blocked" in scene two and my mother being "stuck" in scene one, are similar situations. Perhaps I'm getting closer to the meaning of this dream.

I return to the image of my mother's hair. For most of my life, she wore it on top of her head in a bouffant hairdo, kept in place with countless bobby pins and hair clips. Maybe the message of her hair was to "let down your hair, relax, and *go with the flow*,'" which coincides with the message of being 'blocked' or 'stuck.'

I find I am stumped by one thing about the dream. It is the first time since my stepfather's death that he has appeared in one of my dreams. His special appearance must have some significance. Like with the other symbols of the dream, I consider several other options before deciding that my stepfather had been a unique teacher to me in other ways and must be serving as such in my dream as well.

Like my mother, my stepfather took a lot of pride in how he dressed. He insisted that when they went out, he and my mother were color coordinated. If she wore red, so did he, if she wore pink, he did too, if she wore shamrock green, he followed suit. After he retired, he typically wore golf pants and a matching shirt, but whenever he dressed up, he wore his signature bow tie. In fact, I don't think he owned a regular tie. The bow tie is what I see in my dream. The bow tie reminds me of how he didn't mind being himself and how he liked standing out in a crowd. I remember that in whatever I do it is okay to be comfortable with who I am and be myself.

I come away from the dream with a positive message reminding me to 'stop worrying about things that don't matter' (garbage), to 'let down my hair,' and 'go with the flow,' (the water). By doing so, I will be able to remove whatever obstacles (stones/garbage) that stand in my way (blocked)—all which coincide with situations I'd been struggling to work through prior to the dream.

Depending on how long I work with the dream, I'll come up with other subtle messages entwined within the symbols and layers. For example, the food message I came up with as my first interpretation can still serve as a reminder to me about how I should eat. For now, I am happy with the result and that I spent time working through the dream.

"By constructively using your dream time you always wake up to a world full of adventure, challenge, knowledge, and positive anticipation."
Ken Eagle Feather,
A Toltec Path

VISIONS

Visions are much like a dream, except they take place while when we are awake. I maintain that visions are far different from having psychic ability. Many people do not agree with me and put visions in the same category with clairvoyance. My feeling is that a person who is psychic sees a movie-like image *in exact detail* without having been in a position to have physically experienced it. For a psychic, it is as if they can freely step in and out of time to view events exactly as they happened or will happen.

On the other hand, a vision is an in-mind movie that typically consists of *symbolic* images and persons. Like a dream, a vision must first be properly interpreted before it is of any use. Most people who see visions on a regular basis have developed their gift to an extent that they know certain images correlate to specific meanings. John Edward *(Crossing Over)* often explained this during his television show while demonstrating his ability to communicate with those who have died.

Visions carry many of the pratfalls of the intuitive hunches I spoke of earlier in this section. If a vision can't be interpreted, or is interpreted incorrectly, it's useless. Case in point, in February 1985, I had an unusual and very vivid vision where I saw myself walking through a room of fire. Although the whole house seemed to be up in flames, I walked through and wasn't harmed. Once through, I walked outside into a beautiful green valley.

Try as I might, I could not figure out what this might mean other than I would face some trial and that I would come through unharmed. In my journal I actually wrote to my husband, though I laugh about it now, "something will happen concerning you." (It's very easy to be blind to self events.) I had no clue of the coming trial—which is probably a good thing since eight weeks later, doctors diagnosed me with Hodgkins Disease. Now I know that the "fire" referred to my radiation treatments and that I would come through the cancer experience fine. I also learned that "a valley" can be a trial as well, green or not so green.

Just over a year later, I had another vision. While pregnant with my second son, I saw an intricate maple-like leaf with five large tines, each tine with three smaller tines. Combined together, I came up with the number combination of 5-3-15. I knew this mathematical riddle had some connection to my unborn baby, but what? I tried working countless mathematical equations trying to figure out what it meant, but nothing made sense.

Five days later, my son was born. He weighed *three* pounds, *fifteen* ounces. The vision's puzzle (5-3-15) fit the situation exactly. However, he had arrived seven and a half weeks early. No wonder none of my earlier equations made sense!

Why are we sometimes given information that we cannot understand until *after* the fact? I believe this is God's way of showing us that we are connected, that we can receive answers to our many questions. But, in some instances, we are not to know of a coming situation as it would be too stressful, detrimental, or useless for us to know. I believe there are some things along our path that are simply meant to be, and in the case of something traumatic or life-changing, we are best left in the dark if there is nothing about the situation we can alter.

For example, I once foresaw myself in a horrible auto collision. I gained much understanding from that vision on how a person in such a situation sees their life flash before them, how in a split second, they must decide between life or death. For two weeks, I drove with extreme caution, always fearful for my life. Then we received a call that a cousin had been killed instantly by a drunk driver. Only then did I realized the vision had not been about me. The "who" had been hidden from me because the situation itself was out of my hands. Instead, I had been given a unique insight into what had taken place.

There have been just as many times when I could interpret a vision. In those times, the information served as a means for solving problems, as a guide to finding the right path, or as a warning to avoid hardships, mishaps, or danger.

Once, I had a vision of my husband driving a race car. Midway through the race, he drove into the pits and another driver took his place. I then saw him outside of another of his company's branches. I had the sense that he was in charge, but not the owner. I didn't know at the time that a racecar driver could be traded out and had asked my husband about it. He assured me that they could in some cases. I told him I thought he was going to change positions soon in his work. Not long after, another man

"The messages I received at this point early in my development were often very cryptic and disjointed. The language is very symbolic, rarely literal, and it would take years for me to understand it with any reliability or fluency."

John Edward,
One Last Time

took over my husband's position at his branch and he became the director of all of the branches.

In another example, before I had any children, I used to worry I'd never get pregnant. I'd had a miscarriage in our first year of marriage, and even though we tried again, nothing happened. Three years passed. One night as I lay in bed, I had a vision of a very special baby. However, this child lay in a hospital incubator surrounded by wires, machines, and other medical devices. I heard the doctors whispering that they didn't think the baby would live, but another voice coming from someone I couldn't see said the baby would live. As I looked at the child in my vision, I knew one day a baby would come, yet I also recognized this baby came with a price. I didn't know if I was ready to handle such a responsibility. I understood why there had been a delay in the baby's coming. Since I didn't feel ready for the baby shown, I prayed and asked God to send me another child first, a son to carry on my husband's family name, and he did.

When my second son was conceived just after my last radiation treatment, the doctors did whisper. And when my son arrived seven and a half weeks early, he spent thirty-one days in a hospital incubator. Like the vision had said, he did survive (and has definitely thrived).

The vision, the connection to the world beyond, had given me hope in a time when I feared I would never have children. More than that, the vision's message carried me through the difficult days of my cancer as I would often remember the baby vision and feel driven to survive for that God-given child destined to come.

HOW TO INTERPRET A VISION

Visions, like any of the four Cs are available to anyone. Only believe. It is in interpreting them that answers are given and connection is made.

To interpret a vision, utilize the skills I've shared in the section on dreams because the only difference between the two seems to be whether the images are seen while asleep or awake.

I've found dream books, such as Wilda B. Tanner's *Mystical, Magical, Marvelous World of Dreams* to be the most helpful in teaching me to understand how the

> *"We most often fail to think of those pictures which commonly come to our minds as visions because (1) our own minds seemed to be doing it, (2) it was so quick and easy, (3) we may not have been in prayer at all. . . . We who belong to the Lord should at least not exclude the possibility that God would speak to us by a vision. We need only ask by what source our imaginations are being stirred."*
> John and Paula Sandford,
> *The Elijah Task*

symbols relate to myself and my world. I particularly like Tanner's book since she recommends going beyond one-size-fits-all definitions for each symbol found in most dream books and she teaches the reader how to personalize the meaning of what is seen.

REFLECTIONS

Imagine that every day you go to work and, for some reason, your new boss, a fellow just transferred in from a branch upstate, is in your face—again. Your coworker calls it a "personality conflict," but no matter how hard you try to get along with him, you can't seem to make it through the day without some kind of confrontation.

At home, you switch on the television or hide behind the newspaper, trying to forget the frustration this guy is causing you. But you can't. This man's presence follows you home so that even if he is out of sight, he isn't out of mind. Arrrggg! Why won't that guy just leave you alone?

In the next exercise, we are going to take a look at people in your daily experience, people such as the in-your-face boss. We will also take a look at those who hold a strong influence over you whether they are present on a daily basis or not, persons such as your parents, siblings, coworkers, clients, neighbors, and friends. Of course, we won't leave out those most likely to be front and center in your life, your spouse (or lover), your children, and even the family pet.

EXERCISE 16–IMAGE BALLOONS

I'm about to share with you one of the most important exercises in this book. In order for it to be all it can be, I'm going to ask you not to work ahead. Stick with me on this because by doing so, you will have a tremendous opportunity to learn something fabulous about yourself and those around you. Are you ready to begin?

(Read all the directions, 1-9, before beginning.)

1. On page 209 is a sheet filled with blank balloons.

"We have an even greater responsibility to obey visions . . . in visions, since we are awake, we are fully responsible not to forget."
John and Paula Sandford,
The Elijah Task

"Every person, all the events in your life are there because you have drawn them there. What you choose to do with them is up to you."
Richard Bach,
Illusions

211

Make a photocopy of that page (you may want to do the exercise more than once) or hand draw a similar example on your own blank sheet of paper. The design does not have to be exact.

2. Write a name on each balloon, naming it after a person in your life and selecting from the variety of persons in the list that follows.

3. For the best results, you will need to include a minimum of five individuals that you know, but for even better results, choose at least ten, half from the 'family' list, half from the 'other' list, and no more than one from the 'pet' list. Feel free to substitute similar individuals for those listed here. For example, you may exchange "lover" for "spouse" or "partner" for "boss." Use persons who are most appropriate for your life and situations.

Family:	*Other:*
Mother	*Best Friend*
Father	*Coworker*
Spouse	*Boss*
Sibling	*Admired Celebrity*
Son	*Memorable Stranger*
Daughter	*Familiar Acquaintance*
Mother-in-law	*Classmate*
Father-in-law	*Neighbor*
Aunt	*Repairman*
Uncle	*Family Friend*
Cousin	*Doctor or Professional*

Pets:
Dog, Cat, Reptile, Fish, Rabbit, Hamster, Guinea Pig, Ferret, or other family pet

4. Write your descriptions using one word if possible, but no more than three. It's okay if more than one individual has the same trait(s).

5. You are to think of each person named in turn while considering their personality traits, those traits which most stand out about them and which come to mind quickly. *(See key words list for examples)*

6. For those individuals you know well, you should be able to easily write five or six character traits on

BALLOON EXERCISE

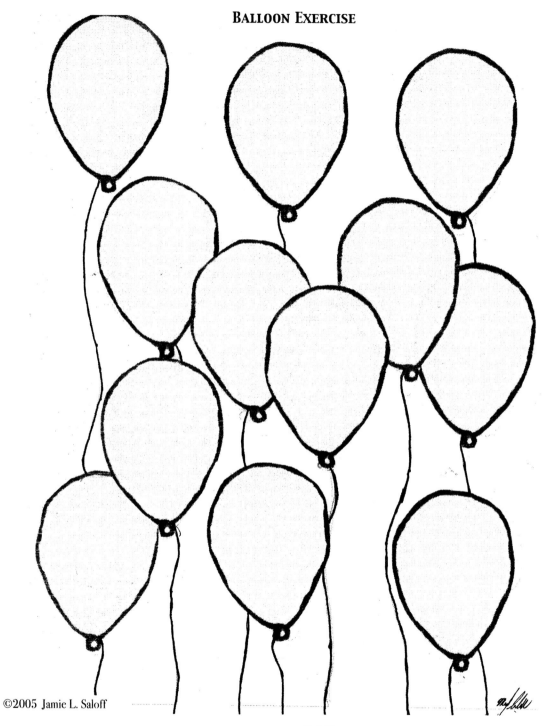

"Tell me what a person strives for and I'll tell you the kind of person he is."
unknown, as quoted by
Jack M. Bickham,
Writing Novels That Sell

each balloon. For those individuals you don't know well, write only the one or two traits that quickly come to mind.

7. Focus on *character* traits. A character trait is what motivates a person to act as they do or a common way they respond to situations in life. A few examples are listed below. **Avoid** using physical traits— tall, short, muscular, overweight, trim, blond, green-eyed, buxom, —as they **do not apply** to this exercise.

The following lists are for example only and just to get you started. Your options are limitless. Don't be afraid to think outside the box.

- *Character traits: sense of humor, hard working, stoic, humanitarian, workaholic, creative, happy-go-lucky, worrywart, space cadet, unfeeling, joyous, exuberant.*

- *Ethics: honest, trustworthy, chronic liar, loyal, two-faced, cheat, etc.*

- *How they predominantly treat others and themselves: generous, critical, abusive, disgruntled, kind, etc.*

8. Work through each person until you have filled in all the balloons that you chose.

9. If you get stuck, try thinking along these lines:

- *If I could offer this person some advice or direction, what would it be?*

- *I just wish he/she would . . .*

- *I always feel or sense he/she . . .*
    - *is mad at the world*
    - *is holding back anger*
    - *is troubled by something*
    - *is hiding a secret*
    - *really dislikes me*

Revise your thoughts so they are a single keyword or two-word phrase before writing on the balloon. Then return here when you have finished this part of the exercise. Do not read forward until you do.

After you have completed the exercise, compile a list in the following manner:

1. Make a list of each character trait listed.

2. It's okay if a trait shows up more than once. Checkmark the entry, don't add it twice. *(See the example on page 212.)*

3. If a trait shows up three, four, or more times, just continue to checkmark the already listed trait again, once for each time it appears on the balloons.

4. When you are done compiling the list, rewrite it, putting first those traits most often checkmarked, then those listed only once after. If you want to break a tie, the closer, more influential the person is to you and your life, the more powerful the trait.

Set all of this aside and we will come back to it later.

> *"In every recorded age there is the standard belief that 'no human being is either all good or all evil.'"*
>
> Leonard Bishop,
> *Dare to Be a Great Writer*

THE MAGIC MIRROR

As a kid growing up in the sixties, I would watch a kinder-show on TV every weekday morning called *Romper Room*. The host, Miss Sally,[3] would close each show by taking a "magic" mirror off the shelf so she could "see" the kids back home. Miss Sally used a hand mirror rigged so the center, or mirror portion, could be removed. This allowed her to "see" the kids at home, or so we believed. She would speak to the kids she could see saying, "I see Billy, and Wendy, Mary, and Martin," (the names changed after each show).

I am going to borrow from Miss Sally's magic mirror to explain how you can use this same "magic" to learn something about yourself. Imagine you have your own magic mirror. Hold it up in the air and imagine you can see some recently past event in your life. Through this magic mirror, see the argument you had yesterday morning with your spouse; see the manicurist at the beauty salon talking about her boyfriend; see the bank

215

BALLOON EXERCISE EXAMPLE

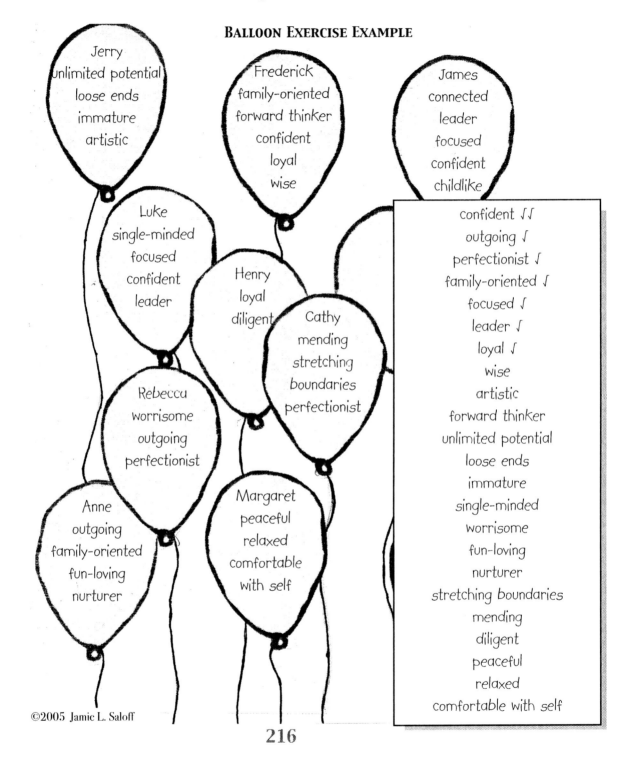

Jerry
unlimited potential
loose ends
immature
artistic

Frederick
family-oriented
forward thinker
confident
loyal
wise

James
connected
leader
focused
confident
childlike

Luke
single-minded
focused
confident
leader

Henry
loyal
diligent

Cathy
mending
stretching
boundaries
perfectionist

Rebecca
worrisome
outgoing
perfectionist

Anne
outgoing
family-oriented
fun-loving
nurturer

Margaret
peaceful
relaxed
comfortable
with self

confident √√
outgoing √
perfectionist √
family-oriented √
focused √
leader √
loyal √
wise
artistic
forward thinker
unlimited potential
loose ends
immature
single-minded
worrisome
fun-loving
nurturer
stretching boundaries
mending
diligent
peaceful
relaxed
comfortable with self

teller at your local bank complaining about the rain. Look at all these people and any others you can recently remember through the magic mirror you are envisioning in your hand.

Now, just like Miss Sally, we will work the magic of the mirror. Like Miss Sally, imagine you can take out the center of the mirror to magically see through it. But with this magic, the people we see through the looking glass become ourselves—ourselves acting as the people we see. Let me explain further.

Our outer life is a symbol and a metaphor for our inner thoughts and actions. Whatever lessons we're attempting to learn, we'll view on those around us and in our world. Seeing our reflected selves in this way is like looking into a mirror, except, instead of standing in front of a mirrored glass and seeing our own face, we see our reflection through the actions of other individuals or situations.

At first this idea might seem ridiculous. It's particularly difficult to accept that someone you adamantly dislike or who might act in some disgusting or immoral way might in any way be a reflection of you. Just as difficult might be to see yourself as the reflection of someone you truly admire, someone you look up to for their great courage or exceptional achievements.

Keep in mind that these individuals are not you, but they are somehow reflecting you, and probably not as a whole. In other words, seeing a drunk beggar on the street doesn't mean you are a drunk beggar. Rather, these persons are somehow reflecting a quality, trait, or motivation similar to an ability, desire, or trait you have. In some cases these might be traits you'd like to acquire; in other cases, you'll find traits you'd like to disown and aren't necessarily ready to admit. When you look for the truth, the latter will show themselves to you without a doubt. In such a case, you may not want to admit it to others, but you will know the reflection is there.

Regardless, you might have to think about it a little bit. Usually the "mirrors" who come into your life do so in an exaggerated way. By doing so, they tend to call your attention to themselves and force you to notice them. (Remember the in-your-face-boss I mentioned earlier?) Keep in mind too that, as stated previously, the closer and

"You can also learn to use Symbolic Sight, to intuitively interpret the power symbols in your life, to reveal where you have invested your personal energy, to uncover the greater meaning of your life's challenges apart from the literal events, and to discover how this all connects to your health."

Carolyn Myss,
Why People Don't Heal

more influential the person is over you, the stronger the reflected message tends to be for you.

Let me offer a reflection example. I once referred to our bedroom as "the land of chairs" because it had become a catchall for any furniture we didn't have a place to store, including some twenty different chairs. There were so many chairs, I practiced speeches in there, pretending my visualized audience filled the many available seats.

Exactly one day after I finished redecorating, and felt so excited at the prospect of having my bedroom back, my husband bought a weight bench and put it in the open space I had designated for yoga. The next morning, for no apparent reason, the dog woke up, walked over to the weight bench—where my husband happened to be doing sit-ups—and lifted his leg against the bench. The following morning, again without reason, the dog did the same thing. We were shocked because our dog had rarely had any accidents.

I asked myself if this could be a mirror. The first thing that came to mind was, "Am I *pissed off* about anything?" which seemed an appropriate question under the circumstances. Well, there was the obvious fact that my husband had put a weight bench in my newly decorated bedroom. I might as well have done the deed myself.

I have to admit that whenever I see these kinds of reflections, I am a little bit embarrassed. I rarely tell anyone, especially since I have usually made some not so complimentary remark before recognizing myself in them. I tend to slink away after seeing the mirror and quietly go work on myself. I can say, however, that the more I have recognized these self-reflecting mirrors, the less I have criticized others because I see that I am really criticizing myself. However, in the case of the weight bench—and I might add, the more appropriate way to handle such a reflection—I decided to talk to my husband about why he had put the bench in our bedroom. I felt better after talking to him. I even decided the weight bench could stay.

I had to speak up about my feelings toward the bench and clear the air before the reflected action would stop. Once I did, the dog never lifted his leg to it again, and a few weeks later, my son moved the bench into his bedroom.

"We're creating our lives as we go along; therefore, our experiences and needs give us an instant, ongoing reflection of ourselves."

Shakti Gawain,
Living in the Light

WELCOME TO ALICE'S WONDERLAND AND THE OTHER SIDE OF THE MIRROR

Now that you know how people and things can be a mirror and a means of sending you a message, you can go back to our discussion and exercise on balloons completed earlier. *(If you haven't yet done this exercise, do it before continuing to read further.)*

What you created with the traits on the balloons and the list of those traits was a mirror of yourself. The traits checkmarked the most, those near the top of your list, are the traits most predominant in your character, at least in some form. The items written toward the bottom of your list are traits or *tendencies* that you have.

Surprised? Doubtful?

If something shows up strongly on your list, something you feel is definitely not you, whether negative or positive, it simply means that the trait is a strong possibility open to you in the future, or that it's a trait which has heavily influenced you and how you make decisions.

For example, if you have never taken a drink in your life, but the word "alcoholic" shows up on the face of several balloons, it demonstrates how strongly this disease has affected your life and the decisions you make.

On the other hand, if you see positive traits which don't seem to reflect your present ability or skills, they are probably foretelling your potential.

Many years ago, I met a person for whom I would have chosen the balloon words "writer," "teacher," and "dynamic speaker." I had a great admiration for this person and never believed I had any of these qualities myself. However, over the course of the next few years, it quickly became apparent I *could* acquire those traits and, in fact, wanted to. I never realized in the beginning how this person had been reflecting my *own* possibilities.

The balloon exercise you completed earlier is important for two reasons.:

1. If you know what your character traits are, you can change them or enhance them accordingly.

2. If you know you are seeing yourself in others, you can change your reaction toward them because you're not reacting to something they have done

". . . always remember that the situation or person who has the ability to upset you the most, to pull you off-center, is your greatest teacher."

Lynn V. Andrews,
Love and Power

219

or said, but rather you're reacting to your own reflection.

To explain these points further here are a couple of examples:

On one of our many trips, we were riding in the car for quite a long distance. In this situation, I suffer a lot of stress because of my fear of having an accident, especially when my husband drives agressively in a heavy traffic. At first, I wanted to criticize his driving, but having tried that in the past, I knew it only made things worse. I've tried sleeping but being unconscious doesn't make for an interesting trip. So, on this particular occasion, I asked myself about the possibility of a mirror.

Here are the steps I used to work through this particular mirrored image:

1. I asked myself what feelings and motivations I saw my husband exerting as he drove in this manner (aggressive impatience). Doing so separates the actual act of driving from the connected and reflected emotions.

2. Separating the emotions from the act allowed me to put those same emotions on whatever it was I'd been dealing with in my life. I asked myself, "In what situations have I been 'aggressively impatient'?"

3. Next, I asked myself what advice or change I would like to see in my husband's actions. Easy! I wanted him to SLOW DOWN; take it easy; we weren't in that big of a rush.

4. Then, I applied this advice to my own situation. Did I need to be more patient with myself in some situation? Being so aggressive might not be the right answer. In this example, I had been pressing myself aggressively to finish my book. (Typically this is where the "you won the prize" bell goes off in my head.)

5. Lastly, I asked myself if I could now see reasons for my husband's actions. Having looked at the situation from a different perspective—and having argued with myself as to why it was okay for me but not for him—I had better insight into why he

"If there is a behavior which we detest in others, it is extremely likely that we do this ourselves, and have judged it to be wrong. It is on the wrong side of our imaginary line, and we hate ourselves every time we do it. And because we hate it so much, we pretend that we never behave like that."

Susanna Thorpe-Clark,
Changing the Thought

might be doing what he was doing. If I wanted to change his actions, then I first had to change mine. He would continue to mirror my actions until I had affected mine. In addition, having done this analysis, I found it was considerably more difficult to criticize his actions when, in essence, I would be criticizing my own. If his actions were inappropriate, than probably mine were as well, or why would God be trying to show it to me as such?

6. Later, I reevaluated. I discovered that on the trip home, I didn't feel quite so bothered by my husband's driving. I couldn't really tell if he had driven less aggressively, or if I just no longer reacted to it. In either case, I felt less stress on the return trip because I had recognized and acted against the mirrored reflection.

Here's another example:

1. My son has a room that is so messy we tease him that any strangers entering his room might become forever lost.

2. What are his motivations? In analyzing the situation, I realize there is more than one problem involved. I have to ask myself, is the problem the mess itself, or how he creates it? I decide that in order for him to clean up the mess in the long-term, he would first have to learn how to stop creating them. In other words, he needs to first work on the cause before the mess can be cured. So what is the cause? I decided to sidestep laziness and lack of concern because I've seen him in other situations where these traits are not typical of him. My assessment instead is that his problem is one of distraction. He has so many things he is interested in, working on, exploring, planning to fix, that he is easily distracted from finishing any one thing, whether it's finishing some art project, putting away his clothes, or returning dirty dishes to the kitchen.

3. Looking at these newly discovered motivations (again, based on my assessments, not his), and in separating the action from the motivation, I see an

"Judge not, that ye be not judged. For with what judgment ye judge, ye shall be judged: and with what measure ye mete, it shall be measured to you again. And why beholdest thou the mote that is in thy brother's eye, but considerest not the beam that is in thine own eye?"
Matthew 7:1-3,
King James Version

221

interesting pattern forming. Is there some area in my life where I have too many things going? (Oh, boy . . . I get one of those "ting" feelings inside myself. . . actually, it's more like a fanatic "ting, ting, ting, ting," but that's another story.)

4. What is my advice to him? To simplify, get rid of the amount of things in his room so that overall it's easier to keep clean. With less to distract him, he'll be less likely to leave something undone. Now the question is, will I apply this to my own life? Until I do, he will continue to have a messy room. I know this because he and I have gone through this reflection before with different motivations and meanings. I find that when I clear my own situations, he will stay up all night to clean his room —without being asked. If I don't clear my own situation, I can beg, plead, scold, holler, punish, or clean the room myself, but it will always return to the same state.

As a side note, I asked my husband why he drove so aggressively. He admitted what I'd already recognized, that he's impatient. However, when I asked my son what caused him to have his room in such a state, he offered a widely different answer. He doesn't want to deal with the mess, but on the other hand, he is too attached to some of his items. He wishes someone would steal them away in the night without him looking at any of it as he knows if he sees it, he will find some reason to hold on to it.

This is a reminder that the reflections belong to *ourselves*. What we perceive of others is not necessarily what others see about themselves. What they reflect to us is merely a perception we have placed on them. It is part of the life game we play with ourselves that I mentioned in Chapter 16.

It's important we don't trick ourselves into thinking the reflections we see are the Truth about those we love. By not forcing them to wear false reflections, we open ourselves to seeing other people in our lives as individuals who have come to help us. We might even see how, in certain situations, they have given their lives to helping us learn an important lesson in ours. When we criticize them, we are only tearing ourselves down. Learn to read the

"If you accept that every time a problem occurs the universe is showing you something, you will make rapid progress on your journey of self-discovery."
Shakti Gawain,
Living in the Light

importance of reflections and counteract them, then the people in your life will take on an expanded and joyous purpose. You will have more love for those in your life and find you are more forgiving. You will no longer feel as critical of them when you learn to see yourself in them.

SWANS—EVERYDAY PEOPLE WITH EXTRAORDINARY POWER TO INFLUENCE AND ENCOURAGE OUR LIVES

Earlier in this book, I wrote about the Ugly Duckling and the tremendous transformation that took place in his life. But one other important miracle occurred in his life that played a big role in his transformation.

Up until the day the Ugly Duckling left the old woman, cat, and hen, he had no reason to believe he might be anything other than what he'd been told because he had no knowledge that he could be otherwise. He had never even seen another swan. But as he left the trio's shack that day, an amazing thing happened. He heard a mysterious, yet stirring noise above him, and as he looked up, he spied a flock of swans flying overhead.

Even though he was about to enter into the most difficult period of his life, and although he could not yet accept that he might be one, for the first time he knew of their existence. That knowledge would later allow him to break free from his long-held mistaken perception. Without that glimpse, that Truth planted within him, he might never have discovered his real identity. His glimpse of those swans saved his life.

Swans are a special kind of mirror. They're the people and characters who teach us indirectly about who we are. They mirror our highest potential and ignite within us a desire and admiration of their ability. This admiration will one day be the spark we need to reach loftier goals.

Swans are often ordinary people who present themselves to us in our day-to-day living, but they might also show themselves from within books, movies, and dreams. They peek at us from the pages of history and appear to us symbolically through a variety of other means. Though like the Ugly Duckling we may not realize the power of their presence, we'll one day see the evidence materialize in our own lives.

". . . the ugly little Duckling had such a strange feeling as it watched them. It did not know the name of those birds, nor whither they were flying; but it loved them as it had never loved anyone before."

Hans Christian Andersen,
The Ugly Duckling

223

More Ways to View Reflections

Reflecting Backward

Looking backward at my major life situations, I have gained a new and different perspective on some of those events. For example, how can I ever forget the physical pain my father endured in his last days? But as a mirror, what would that mean to me?

If it had not been for his pain, I don't know if I would have questioned suffering. I don't know if I would have sought so diligently to find an answer for escaping pain, illness, and the other life-debilitating maladies that block our lives. However, today I see my father's pain as a reflection of what my mother, my cousin, and I felt inside as we watched him die. None of us openly complained or spoke of the horror we saw. We held it all inside. But he reflected our pain. He let it out when we couldn't.

I believe, too, that by releasing his pain he freed me from suffering a similar fate. I often look at the reflections I've passed to my children and at the heritage I've left for them *(See: Section III)*. My father met his challenge so I won't have to make it mine.

Our children have an uncanny way of reflecting ourselves back at us. Knowing this, I recalled some of my childhood situations and asked myself, "Could this have been a reflection of my parents?" Of course, like an ailment, a mirror is best interpreted by the individual themselves, but since my parents are no longer alive to do that for me, I took a few liberties on their behalf, knowing my assumptions were, at best, intuitive guesses.

At the age of seven, I fell against the coffee table and cut the corner of my mouth. The stitches left me barely able to talk and I could only eat through a straw. To interpret the reflection, I first tried to determine what the situation represented. The part that most stood out to me was how I couldn't open my mouth. Then I considered how my *closed mouth* might have been a reflection of my parents. I thought about all of their grief and how they no longer communicated with each other, or even with themselves. I thought about the many painful things that transpired with the loss of their first daughter. I specu-

"The greatest opportunity we have for growth is in our relationship with others. It is only as we see ourselves reflected in them that we get feedback on who we are. If you can see the issues your children bring up for you as opportunities for character development for both you and them, you will find the problems much less troublesome."
Melanie Melvin,
Respecting the Indigo Children
as told by Lee Carroll and
Jan Tober, *The Indigo Children*

lated that my closed mouth reflected their closed mouths, or their refusal to speak of my sister and their pain.

I learned many things about myself and them by interpreting these memorable situations. Seeing the reflections from this vantage point offered me the means of forgiving them for many things.

REFLECTING FORWARD

As mentioned before, some mirrors are reflections of actions we could be doing but aren't. I already mentioned the person who reflected the possibility of my becoming a writer, speaker, and teacher. Many other people in my life have reflected other important possibilities to me as well. I call these "forward reflections" since they are actions that could help in moving me forward toward my goals and purpose if I would act on them.

While I recuperated from my hysterectomy, my husband and sons took turns doing all my housework. Actually, most of the work fell to my husband and younger son due to my older son's work schedule. One night, my husband looked at my older son and said, "Tonight, it's your turn to do the dinner dishes." My older son said, "No, I'm not doing that." Then he went to his room.

My husband and I were so stunned by his blatant lack of consideration, we did nothing to reprimand him. Later, I asked myself if my son's actions might be a mirror of myself. What I discovered is a great example of a forward reflection.

For a long time, I had done a lot of things out of guilt or obligation, always being afraid to say no for fear of what would happen. Suddenly, here was a perfect example of what did happen . . . nothing! Lightning didn't crash from the sky, the earth didn't split open, no one even got mad. While I realized that if I started saying no to everyone, I likely would face some consequences, some hurt feelings, and some displays of anger, I could see from my son's reflected action that ultimately nothing disastrous happened. Even better, by saying "no," my son didn't have to do something he didn't want to do. Here was a reflection I could use! I gradually started trying it out on things that weren't quite so important, but eventually learned to be more honest and say no more often. Just as my son, I

"The world can give you only what you gave it, for being nothing but your own projection, it has no meaning apart from what you found in it and placed your faith in."
Foundation for Inner Peace,
A Course in Miracles

225

suffered no disastrous repercussions. At most, someone would grumble. My son's disobedience actually turned out to be a good thing.

MIRRORS IN OUR ENVIRONMENT

I believe we've been given the tool of reflection because it's easier for us to see and learn from others than it is for us to recognize certain traits in ourselves. While in the past we used these reflections as a means to criticize and ridicule those around us, now we can see how the actions of others, whether negative or positive, can actually be a means of guidance for ourselves.

Remember too how I explained in the beginning of this book that before we develop an ailment, the universe will first attempt to show us whatever message it's trying to convey through situations in our environment. Using the four Cs, MPMs, and reflections, we have the opportunity to learn the message before it reaches a crisis point.

The key to reflections is to use them as a reminder to change our own actions. The only way we can clear the reflection fully from our lives is by first clearing them from within. Unfortunately, that's not always easy to do because we become so caught up in the situation, we forget to look at the innermost cause . . . ourselves.

For example, my husband had been recuperating from major back surgery, and after five months in bed, he'd finally been released to drive, attend therapy, and begin the long process of recovery. In an attempt to revive myself from the tiring ordeal, I made plans to attend the writer's retreat I mentioned previously.

A dear friend who agreed to meet up with me along the way, called a few days before we were to leave to say she had suffered a back injury and didn't know if she could make the trip. I worried about going that far alone, so my friend decided to risk it. She suffered the entire trip with severe back spasms and spent each night lying on the floor of our hotel room moaning and groaning, without relief. I felt helpless to do anything for her and couldn't understand how this could happen. I had left one bad back at home only to find another.

I had gone to Arizona in hopes of finding relief not only from the situation at home, but from one of the worst

"Travel transforms us. . . . At the heart of that journey 'out,' we happen upon the deepest mysteries 'within.' There, the possibility of realizing the highest version of self lies waiting—waiting for us to recognize it, claim it, and begin on the path back home victorious."

Joseph Dispenza,
The Way of the Traveler

winters we'd experienced in many years. Of course, it snowed in Arizona the day after my arrival. The snowfall topped records going back more than thirty years.

To make matters worse, I felt as if I couldn't write a word. Everything seemed to be against me. I felt so angry and frustrated. Why was this happening to me?

There was a lot going on with me at that time. A lot of my "stuff" had come to a head. It would take hours to detail all of the reflections taking place at that time. However, I ultimately gained this message: I can't run away from myself.

I did receive a reprieve from caring for my husband on a daily basis and had a week to care for myself. However, the reflections from my interior situations went with me wherever I went. I could not run away from them. Not in Arizona, not anywhere in the world.

Take a moment to look around you. What happenings do you notice in your surrounding environment? As I write this, our next-door neighbor is significantly remodeling their home. Last year, the neighbor on the other side of our home did the same. To me, those are significant reflections of what is going on in my life as I write this book, but in fact, is also a significant reflection in the lives of everyone in this house, all who are showing major signs of change, growth, and improvement.

Our environment is only too happy to provide whatever reflections we need no matter where we might try to hide. I remember I had a friend who lived in a rough part of town. He worried about his family and the effect that crime, drugs, and poverty had on them. Eventually, he moved, only to find a similar situation shortly after his relocation—even though the environment hadn't been as such before. I pointed out to him how his environment merely reflected his inner self. He began to analyze all the reflections as he saw them. A year or so later, he moved again and found a quiet community with no crime, no poverty, no nightly drug busts. He had cleared the mirrored reflection from the inside.

". . . no matter where you go, there you are."

Confucius

"The reality you experience is a mirror image of your expectations. If you project the same images every day, your reality will be the same every day."
Deepak Chopra,
The Way of the Wizard

REFLECTED HISTORY

We have many different layers of experience in our lives. There are those events that affect us directly and personally, then those that affect us in our local community or sphere of influence. As we move away from the closer layers of our daily experience, we become a player in a wider realm of social and political events. These, too, are reflections of us, both personally and culturally.

The day Princess Diana died, I stared at the television in disbelief as scenes of the accident splashed across the screen, proving what we all hoped wasn't so. Princess Diana was dead. In my mind is the image of the millions of flowers lining the gates at the palace, a symbol of just how respected this woman was in all of our minds. Looking at her reflection on a personal and social level, she represented a person who fearlessly broke many long-held social and traditional boundaries. For too long, we (as a society) had been accepting of some situations without thought as to whether they were right or wrong. We accepted them simply because tradition demanded it be so. Diana stood up and said "no more." She made us look at ourselves and ask if our own lives had boundaries we needed to tear down.

How many women took a closer look at their marriages because of Princess Diana? How many paid closer attention to how they were being controlled by their in-laws? How many became more aware of their eating disorders or the importance of their own inner truth? Even our views of royalty changed. I saw all these things in a woman I've come to respect. The image she forged will forever be with me and the world she left behind.

There are times when the only way we can heal from the burdens placed on us by social traditions and expectations, is by living through a tragedy visible for all to see. Whether race riots, war, 9/11, or any other widely recognized event, by becoming a part of these larger images, the gears in our own minds begin to turn; we see ourselves in a new way. Because of them, we make dedicated changes in our laws and our lives to better ourselves, our cultures, and our societies. If we don't, the image lost would be for nothing.

In our town, we have the image of a teacher shot down in his prime. Due to his tragic death, many teachers in our area looked at students in a new way. Up until this time, they believed the "bad" kids came from a certain section of town, were poor, or wore a particular type of clothing. They

"What we think is what we create and if enough people are thinking the same thought, then we are definitely going to see it in operation around us."
Susanna Thorpe-Clark,
Changing the Thought

allowed their stereotypes to direct their feelings toward these kids. The murder of this teacher by one of the "good" kids showed our town that stereotypes didn't mean what they thought. After this horrific tragedy, quite a few of the local teachers changed jobs or left teaching altogether. Many of the town's residents, particularly the students who witnessed the murder, were profoundly changed after that night.

The fallen teacher's basic goal had been to inspire students to greatness. I have sometimes wondered if God had a larger plan for this man. Because of his tragic death, his image will not soon be forgotten. His death has inspired far more students than his life ever could. While there is not one person in this town who would not wish to bring him back, surely this vivid image will go far in fulfilling his original goal. For many years to come, he will be a sparkling icon, an image to uphold.

Many other events such as this have transpired all over the world. Some affecting a town, some a country, others, the world. To be a mirror, we must look at how it reflects on us personally, and to clear the mirror, we must work on ourselves.

There are countless events which have touched large numbers of people. These events show how many of us are like-minded. It takes a powerful and memorable event to show us such a collective need. What should we make of events such as the Black Plague, the Civil War, World War I and II, The Holocaust, The Great Depression, Vietnam, the fall of the Berlin Wall, and countless other events which have not only served to change our world but also remain in our minds unforgotten? Don't these and other events still serve us today as mirrors? Why would we continue to recall them unless their personal message to us had not been cleared? And what of those such as Marilyn Monroe, Dr. Martin Luther King, President John F. Kennedy, James Dean, and other iconic individuals who we continually hold up as memorable? They must be mirrors as well.

We can go as far back in history as we like, or look in the daily newspaper, to find events which can offer us personal meaning if we are only willing to uncover it. As I write this, the war in Iraq continues. In January of 2005, Iraq held its amazing elections where thousands of people

"What was happening globally in the present mirrored their own spiritual challenges. What the Earth as a whole was undergoing was exactly what they were experiencing personally."
Scott Mandelker,
From Elsewhere

"Most of us, when we first acknowledge that there is a problem in the world, want to do something about it. We spend all our moments trying to come up with ways to make the world a better place. Eventually this transforms into an obsession and becomes a beautiful way to completely ignore our own 'stuff'. We eventually see 'out there', all the problems that we tend not to want to look at, 'in here'"

Mark Vicente,
What the Bleep Do We Know?

"Notice the social, political, and environmental issues around you. Pay particular attention to those that trigger the most emotional reaction in you. Ask to see how they may reflect your personal issues, fears, beliefs, and patterns."
Shakti Gawain,
Living in the Light

literally risked their lives for the right and opportunity to have a democratic nation ruled by leadership of their choice. Still, the violence continues to rage. What I see in their situation is an exaggerated reflection of our own society here in the States. Our elections in 2004 were wrought with their own kind of violence, though not fought with guns and explosions, but with explosive words and negative attacks.

In this country, we have two divided factions who see only their way of doing things and, for whatever stubborn reason, refuse to compromise to find solutions beneficial to all. While I believe there are issues and beliefs worth fighting for, there are many more, such as education and health care where this country's people continue to suffer while the main factions hold out for their own agenda.

The book *A Course of Miracles* teaches that any answer of truth and love will not cause harm to one while lifting up another. Rather, an answer born of love will offer a solution that brings harmony to all. Before we can ever see peace throughout the world, we must first seek peace within our own borders and within our own hearts.

On a personal level, we need to look within ourselves to see where the conflict lies. Are you working at a job you know deep within is unsatisfying to you? Are you holding back from making some decision in your life, afraid of what those around you will say? Are you fighting against yourself, stubbornly waiting for an answer to come about in a particular way? Are you like the fly I spoke of earlier, continually banging your head against the closed window while a few yards away the door of opportunity is open?

Again, what is in your outer world is a reflection of your inner world. The more you are affected by events in the outer world, the stronger their reflections are on you. Look for your personal interpretation of these events to see what meaning you can extract from them. Then turn their message around and point it squarely at your life. Where is the parallel? Keep looking as, I assure you, it is there.

REACHING THE HIGHEST FORM OF CONNECTION

I read[4] of a man with epilepsy who as part of his treatment received split-brain surgery *(also called commissurotom)*. In this procedure, doctors severed his corpus callosum, preventing his right and left hemispheres from intercommunicating. According to the report, due to this man's unique situation, his doctors were able to interview each side of his brain independently. Unlike ourselves where our right and left fight between themselves for control, this man could offer each side's viewpoint without the other cutting in. One thing revealed by this unique interview was the man's career choices based on the thoughts of each brain's hemisphere. The man's right brain desired to be a racecar driver while the left longed to be a draftsman.

We all have this dualist battle going on inside of us. It's been referred to as everything from the angel and devil sitting on our shoulders, to our inner masculine and feminine, to yin and yang, and darkness versus light. Some teach us to listen to our feeling hearts over our logical minds. Others teach us to seek balance and right from wrong, but how does one find those answers in a world where the meaning of anything—right, wrong, love, hate, peace, war—is only what *we* make it?

When I read of this man's opposing inner ideals, I understood for the first time the inner battles we all face as we try to make decisions in our life. Forget trying to sift through the differing guidance we receive from our parents, spouses, siblings, and other loved ones; there's a battle raging inside our own heads. How do we find our way when even our own inner mind conflicts with itself?

There must be an easier way—and there is. We need to move our minds out of the left and right hemispheres of our brain, out of the contradictory information we receive that keeps us in a constant tug of war. We need to reach higher and tap into the connected plane.

While I am unable to explain this process technically, I can tell you how to get there through love. Love—which is much more than the human meaning we associate with relationships—is the answer. Love is the key.

But how do we find this thing called love? How do we

"'When I use a word,' Humpty Dumpty said, in rather a scornful tone, 'it means just what I choose it to mean—neither more nor less.'"

Lewis Carroll,
Through the Looking Glass

231

"The more I meditated, the more I understood how easily we all could get answers and information simply by asking."
Doreen Virtue,
The Lightworker's Way

"Jesus said, 'Seek and you will find. Yet, what you asked me about in former times and which I did not tell you then, now I do desire to tell, but you do not inquire after it.'"
The Gospel of Thomas,
The Nag Hammadi Library

find and tap into this invisible force we all know of, all seek, yet almost always find elusive?

Ask.

ASK-SEEK-KNOCK

Ask means to ask questions as you are moving into the appropriate state of mind. Ask for the fulfillment of your needs, your goals, your desires. Ask for assistance with those things which you don't understand or cannot manage to do alone. One bible verse says:

> . . . ask and it shall be given you; seek and
> ye shall find; knock, and it shall be
> opened unto you. (Luke 11:9 KJV)

Seek means that once you are in a higher state of consciousness, expect to find whatever it is you are looking for. Be open to suggestions and inspirations, even if they are unusual. Expect to find an answer if you've asked for one, but don't force the answer into being what you expect. Look around you to see what is open to you right now. There may be an open door that makes a way where there seemingly is no way.

Knock means that when you know what the answer is, you're watching for opportunities to put that information to use. You're keeping your eyes open for people who can help you or for situations that will lend to what you need. "Knock" is a call to action.

If all of this still seems a bit vague, don't worry. There is yet another way to reach the higher plane of connection.

Chapter Twenty:
The Still, Small Voice:
A Guide to Lead Us

20

It Began With a Dozen Eggs

My children were still very small and my time away from them short. A typical outing consisted of running to the grocery store and pharmacy before rushing home again. In those days, I ranked near professional as a coupon queen and would fill my cart with every bargain I could find to feed my two rapidly growing boys. Every dollar counted, and I made sure to get my penny's worth.

On one of those weekly trips to the store, I'd already filled my cart to the brim. I stood in the dairy department with the Saturday crowd and checked off the last few items on my list: milk, butter, orange juice. The thought suddenly crossed my mind that I needed eggs.

Now I have always taken great care in making sure any of the family's food needs were on my list, particularly in the days when, as a coupon queen, I needed to search out a deal for each and every item. Eggs were not there. That meant we had eggs in the fridge—period. Still, the thought persisted.

On any other day, I would have passed it off as nothing and continued to the checkout without a care. But something

"Beyond the reach of the Censor's babble we find our own quiet center, the place where we hear the still, small voice that is at once our creator's and our own."

Julia Cameron,
The Artist's Way

". . . tell them everyone has a direct dial to God. No one needs to go through an operator."
Julia Cameron,
The Artist's Way

about this need for eggs troubled me. For one thing, I don't eat eggs—ever, at least not the regular cooked varieties. I hadn't since I was three. So I didn't commonly think about eggs. In fact, I couldn't understand why I'd thought of eggs at all—that's what troubled me. So, I thought to myself— and don't ask me why I even took the time—did I just *coincidentally* think of eggs (which seemed unlikely) or did something or someone other than me offer this thought since, for some good reason, I really did need eggs?

I pondered this amid a bustle of other ladies' carts in a heavily congested dairy aisle where every few seconds another cart wanted to get by or accidentally bumped into mine. I needed to make a decision and get out of the way.

All this silliness about *eggs*. . . I needed to get home! At last, I decided they were neither on the list nor in the budget; I left them behind and headed for the checkout.

Once I'd reached the front of the store and its long lines, my thoughts turned again to the eggs and the oddity of thinking of them. I wondered to myself, could these thoughts—whoever or whatever they were—help me with other things in my life, such as getting me through the checkout quickly and on my way home again? I immediately got the impression—I can't say it was anything more than a hunch—to choose one of the longest lines. Well, that settled it right there. I knew I'd just gone loony, too much thought about coupons and pennies and who had the best deals. So I totally ignored this "valuable" bit of advice and stepped into the shortest line.

The gal ringing the register for this line was apparently having a bad day. I heard her cabitzing with the woman checking out ahead of me but paid little attention. I still had my mind on those darn eggs and the possibility that not all our thoughts are our own. I also did not yet see how quickly the longer line shortened, while mine, for some reason, had come to a standstill.

At last, my turn came. I had an overflowing cart, a coupon for every item, and a checker who apparently had no love for the fine art of saving over fifty percent off one's grocery bill. She seemed to question every coupon I handed her. My patience waned. I quickly found myself in a loud argument with her over the matter of twenty cents off some cans of cat food. We were so loud that the store manager stepped over to the register to see what the

"My specialty is being right when other people are wrong."
George Bernard Shaw

234

commotion could be. By the time the argument had been settled—the checker won the dispute—the other line had long since cleared.

When I got home, hot under the collar and bothered by all that had transpired, I opened the fridge to put away the milk and other cold items. I immediately noticed there were no eggs. I didn't think it really mattered at that point. It was just one of those oddities in life, a coincidence. It wasn't until later, when my husband asked if I had any brownies I could mix up, that I realized the ingredients required . . . *eggs.*

Who knew? Someone did and had tried to warn me, but I hadn't listened, which in itself was a more memorable lesson than if I had purchased the eggs and never given it another thought. From then on, I started listening more closely to those hunches. *(Well, for the most part.)* It also got me thinking. What was this "voice" that told me to buy eggs?

THE VOICE WITHIN

Hearing the voice within isn't a special ability. The voice within is merely one more of the connection tools available to us all—should we choose to use it. In order to do so, we need to become aware of it, listen for it, and trust it.

After the situation with the eggs, I started listening a lot more and noted the following:

1. In the beginning, in two out of three incidents, my listening to the voice (or hunch) didn't make any difference one way or the other. (That also meant in one out of three incidents, it did.)

2. In some cases, the information coming through didn't make much sense until after, when it was too late to make any use of it.

3. At times, I was too caught up in myself to pay attention to any suggestion or hunch. I can only say I must have heard it because I'd realize later that I had. I just didn't consciously acknowledge I'd heard it at the time it initially spoke.

"You have this guide by your side all the time, It never stops whispering in your ear. . . . You may not see a burning bush, or have a life-transforming, mystical experience. . . . But it is there, in its quietly insistent way, no matter how many times you turn it off."
Lindsay C. Gibson,
Who You Were Meant to Be

"Receiving is just letting in what's already been there for you."
Michael Lee,
Phoenix Rising Yoga Therapy

"Even if your guides suggest areas of improvements or changes they would like to see you make, they will not fault you later if you decide not to take the advice. . . . Their suggestions are not orders but reflect views from where they are looking."

Iris Belhayes,
Spirit Guides

4. In some instances, I couldn't bring myself to do what the hunch suggested. It's not that the suggestion had been bad, rather I simply didn't have the guts or courage to act on it. For example, one evening as I sat in a church listening to a very inspiring missionary speak, I felt nudged to contribute something to his cause. Unfortunately, I had another engagement and had to leave before his talk would conclude and the offering plate would be passed. The idea occurred to me that I should stand up and enthusiastically say, "I'd like to contribute to your cause!" But I couldn't bring myself to do it. I felt it would be too disruptive to his talk—though it might have also inspired the rest of the audience to contribute wholeheartedly. I'll never know. Instead, I left some money with the usher at the door.

5. In some incidents, I did follow the advice given to me and found it helpful in a variety of ways to my health, my well-being, and my happiness.

I eventually came to the conclusion that I would at the very least *acknowledge* all of these suggestions either by:

> *a) Writing them down,*
> *b) Speaking them out loud, or*
> *c) Acting on them.*

After I had acknowledged them, I could then decide if I wanted to use the information or not. I felt by simply acknowledging them, I would at least be honoring whatever or whomever had given the suggestion to me. This turned out to be an important aspect.

One thing I noticed about these suggestions, though—and this is something that helped me accept them as real and not just of myself—if I *did not* follow them, at the very moment the suggestion would have come into play, I immediately remembered having ignored it—*"Aw, I knew I should have brought an umbrella. Would you look at this rain?"*

I noticed one other thing about paying attention to these subtle suggestions. The more often I listened, the more were given, and not only that, but the *more valuable* the suggestions and the more clearly I understood them.

236

So, while I still might be reminded to *buy eggs*, I also might be advised as to what job to take (or not) or what plane to get on (or not) and so on. But I'm getting ahead of myself because, after all, I'm still talking about mere hunches and subtle hints. Connection is more than that alone—*much more.*

HEARING VOICES

I don't "hear" voices. I *sense* them. In the same way visions don't involve the physical eye—they are seen in the mind—the voice within is not heard with the ear. It too is in the mind.

What I sense is a voice without sound, a language unlike my own, a guidance that feels more evolved than I could ever be. What I "hear" is the *voice within*—the bible writer's *still small voice*—to some, the Holy Spirit, to others, God, to others still, an angel, the higher self, superconscious, or guide.

How do I explain a voice without sound, a language without words, reception without wires?

"What does is sound like?" asked one friend.

"It sounds like . . . me . . . well, sort of."

It is me, but it isn't. It can't be me—can it? If it tells me things I don't know, how can it be me? It's really quite confusing, and yet, it's also absolutely amazing.

I spent a considerable amount of time trying to figure out the voice within. I don't mean a couple of hours, I mean years. From that study, I learned there is more than one kind of voice. I've differentiated them into three types of voices by how they are used so I can explain each a little better.

I've also spent a lot time worrying about the idea of hearing voices. It's a very difficult thing to tell someone. "Oh, yeah, and by the way, I hear voices." That's not the kind of thing I wanted to put in a book for everyone to read. The only reason I'm doing so is because I think we all hear them, we just don't recognize them.

However, just to be on the safe side, I asked a psychiatric nurse about them. I was very concerned about the hearing them because not long before I sat down to write an entire chapter on voices, a young boy in our town

"I have much more to say to you, more than you can now bear. But when he, the Spirit of truth, comes, he will guide you into all truth. He will not speak on his own; he will speak only what he hears and he will bring glory to me by taking from what is mine and making it known to you . . ."

John 16:12-15
New International Version

237

stabbed his father to death after being directed to do so by "voices" he heard. I wanted to be sure I wasn't suffering from some type of disease or disorder, even though I was fairly certain I wasn't. The nurse assured me the voice within was not dysfunctional, and that hearing it was a normal, natural thing we all experience. If you still have your doubts, that's okay with me, but you might want to continue reading because you're about to learn you hear voices too. Honest.

THE THREE VOICES

As I mentioned above, after considerable study, I separated the voices into three types. The three types are as follows:

- *The angelic voice—an audible whisper in the ear, typically in situations affecting life or death.*

- *The teacher voice—a playful voice that offers us instruction, guidance, and a means to walk through life situations before they happen, or in order to relive them afterwards.*

- *The prophetic voice—the still, small guiding voice within, an empowered voice that most often speaks of future happenings.*

THE ANGELIC VOICE

I've already explained the *angelic voice* a couple of times earlier in the book. I admit, they are not commonly noticed by most individuals, so you may not remember ever having heard one. Unlike the teacher voice and the prophetic voice, the angelic voice is perceived as audible and seemingly heard by me as if someone whispered near my right ear. Unlike a human's voice, there is no breath of wind, no sound of breathing, just the voice itself.

There is another, very important aspect about this voice, at least as far as my experience has been concerned. All three times I heard this audiblel-like voice, the words concerned life or death or the preservation thereof. That leads me to believe this type of voice is typically used only

"When we finally accept that some of our loved ones are not the best ones to be relied upon for good advice aobut our future, we are free to turn to our own inner guide."
Lindsay C. Gibson,
Who You Were Meant to Be

"Whether or not you believe in angels and guardians, I believe each of us can contact higher consciousness and see that form as we choose. . ."
Lynn V. Andrews,
Love and Power

as a last resort or when the message being given is so important the sender wants to be sure the message is received without any doubt or confusion. (There are some individuals who hear them in other kinds of situations.)

I've already shared the experience of hearing the angel's voice in the basement and how I'd been warned about one day having cancer. During the early days of my cancer testing, I heard another voice.

Two doctors had just finished giving me a CT Scan covering the upper regions of my body. I'd been left by myself in a long L-shaped hallway to wait for my next test. As I sat there, I began to hear the Twenty-third Psalm:

> *The LORD is my shepherd; I shall not want. He maketh me to lie down in green pastures: he leadeth me beside the still waters. He restoreth my soul: he leadeth me in the paths of righteousness for his name's sake. Yea, though I walk through the valley of the shadow of death, I will fear no evil: for thou art with me; thy rod and thy staff they comfort me. Thou preparest a table before me in the presence of mine enemies: thou anointest my head with oil; my cup runneth over. Surely goodness and mercy shall follow me all the days of my life: and I will dwell in the house of the LORD for ever. (KJV)*

Now, I'd been a bible reader for quite a few years by then, but I can tell you, I didn't have the Twenty-third Psalm memorized. In fact, to add it here, I had to look it up in order to remember all the lines. So to hear it spoken to me word-for-word, flowing, not just through my mind, but through my heart, I knew it wasn't just me entertaining myself. Moreover, when the angel finished reciting the psalm, he said, "Do not fear. I will never leave you or forsake you."

Then something else unusual happened. Way down at the other end of the hall, two men in doctors' white coats exited a room on the right and were quietly talking to themselves and headed toward the CT room from where I'd just come. They were only in sight for a moment as they crossed to the left and disappeared from view. Looking at

"For the next few years, each time I questioned or doubted myself and the work I had begun to do, I would hear those voices, those angels singing, and always the same hymn. The Twenty-third Psalm."
Rosemary Altea,
The Eagle and the Rose

"In each person there resides 'a personal guide,' a sort of internal mentor, which each of us is given to show us our own wisdom."
Spencer Johnson,
Yes or No

239

a hospital chart as he walked, the one said, ". . . with my luck, she won't have anymore . . ."

The two men were unusually far away for me to have understood their conversation, but I did. And even if that weren't odd, why were they discussing patients in the hall, and why did I *just happen* to hear that particular part?

Looking around the area, the only other patients nearby were an elderly man and a newborn baby boy. Neither of them was a "she," so the two doctors had very likely been talking about me.

Within minutes of this happening, a nurse came to get me. She explained I would be having a second, unscheduled CT Scan to cover the lower extremities of my body. Which I did. The results of that second scan showed I had cancer throughout my body.

Something about the doctors' conversation had immediately made me feel uneasy. I didn't know why, but didn't think my fear had to do with my concerns of having the test. Rather, my concerns focused on the idea that these doctors were under pressure not to do any unnecessary testing. If this second test were clear, that would be the case.

Something happens to a person when they go through a life-threatening experience such as cancer. In my case, I became very vocal. I asked my doctors a lot of questions about everything. I asked to see the results of the second CT Scan. My doctor refused to show it to me. He said I wouldn't understand the results. Then he changed the subject in an attempt to prevent me from asking any further questions about it. I decided that if my doctor ever lost his job, he'd make a great used car salesman. He could talk for ten minutes about a question without ever answering it.

Two months went by. I still had not received any treatment. The problem seemed to be that even though the test results showed I had cancer throughout my body, my symptoms didn't match the diagnosis. In fact, I didn't have *any* cancer symptoms in the beginning. During those two months, I underwent every test known at the time to prove or disprove the results of the CT. When none proved the results, my doctors scheduled a laparotomy.

The funny thing is that it all came down to my not wanting the laparotomy. This is a surgery where an inci-

"If you don't receive an immediate answer, let go and go about your life. The answer will come later, either from inside of you in the form of a feeling or idea, or from outside through a person, a book, an event, or whatever."

Shakti Gawain,
Living in the Light

240

sion is made across the belly from one side to the other so the doctors can look around at everything. I'd endured all those other tests because my doctors said they couldn't see any reason to open me up. I didn't have a tumor or something they could just cut out. Having a laparotomy wouldn't really accomplish anything. I couldn't understand why after having done everything to avoid it, they now had decided to do one anyway.

I should also mention that throughout the ordeal, I kept remembering a silly statement my Aunt Neenie made years before. She used to say that if you opened someone who had cancer, the air would hit the disease and make it worse, killing the person within a very short time. As far as I know, that's nothing but an old wives' tale, but I still worried about it, nonetheless.

As I said, I became very vocal. I had put up with a lot, and the laparotomy became the last straw. I told my husband to take me to a bigger hospital. I'd realized by then that no one had a larger stake in saving my life than I did. I had to do what I had to do if I wanted to live. I didn't care who got mad anymore. This was about saving my life not someone's feelings.

Unfortunately, the doctors at the Cleveland Clinic told me I did have to have a laparotomy. In fact, the Clinic doctors said that had I come there first, I wouldn't have had any of the other tests. They felt they were outmoded. I had endured two months of painful testing for nothing.

After the laparotomy, I learned why the angel wanted me to hear the words of those two doctors in the hall. The laparotomy proved the only cancer in my body was located in my upper chest in the initial spot discovered by a standard chest x-ray. When I asked about the CT Scan showing I had cancer throughout my body, the Cleveland doctors told me something to the effect of, "That was only gas," and they weren't in the least bit concerned about it.

Now, you can believe one of two things happened. Either I'd experienced a tremendous and wonderful miracle between the time I had that CT Scan and I went to Cleveland, or I had been terribly misdiagnosed.

I actually prefer the latter. However, I believe that had it not been for the angel who allowed me to hear the discussion of the two doctors in the hall, I would never have questioned the test results. And if I hadn't stood up

"A strong body/personality structure is not created by eating certain foods, doing certain exercises, or following anybody's rules or good ideas. It is created by trusting your intuition and learning to follow its direction."
Shakti Gwain,
Living in the Light

for myself, and forced my husband and my doctor to allow me to go to Cleveland, I might never have learned the truth. Because of my doubts, my fears, my prayers, and the knowledge given to me by the angel, my diagnosis changed for the better. To me, that was a miracle.

A few years ago, I had an occasion to return to the hospital and to the area where I'd heard the angel's voice. Over the many years I'd allowed myself to shorten the length of the hall and diminish the miracle of having heard the two doctors' conversation. I have to say, the hallway was two or three times *longer* than I'd remembered.

THE TEACHER VOICE

The *teacher voice* is perhaps the most disregarded of the three voices. This is the one voice I know we all hear. The real question is how many of us appreciate its scope and ability?

One morning while taking a shower, I found myself rehashing an argument I'd had with a friend. I began imagining what I'd say the next time we talked. I could see the whole conversation in my mind—me talking to her, her replying back, and on and on until it hit me—the whole discussion didn't mean a thing because I had no idea what she would *really* say if I were to call her that minute.

Yet, in my mind, I could see her likeness. I could hear her voice. I could feel the intensity of the conversation. Her image responded to my questions and accusations with the same feelings, emotions, and gestures she would have had if she'd been standing there at that moment. Even if I went over the same part of the conversation ten different times in ten different ways, I could still see and hear her perfectly in my mind.

So, I wondered to myself, if this is only my imagination, if I'm not talking to *her*, who *am* I talking to? Who is playing her role? The obvious answer was me, yet I couldn't help but acknowledge the presence of a higher reasoning involved. By having these periods of imaginary role-playing in my mind, I learned to look at situations in different ways, something I could do without actually calling my friend on the phone and yelling at her. I could work through problems without making a situation worse. I could come to an understanding of why my friend acted

"The universe has both personal and impersonal aspects: as I surrender and trust more, I find my relationship with this higher power becoming more personal. I can literally feel a presence within me, guiding me, loving me, teaching me, encouraging me. In this personal aspect the universe can be teacher, guide, friend, mother, father, lover, creative genius, fairy godmother, even Santa Claus. In other words, whatever I feel I need or want can be fulfilled through this inner connection."

Shakti Gawain,
Living in the Light

in a particular way. I could even get really mad and throw things without breaking anything or causing any harm. In the meantime, I had a chance to calm down and to think more clearly before I actually talked to her again. My imaginary conversations had a purpose. They had a learning opportunity attached to them.

After my initial recognition in the shower, I took a closer look at the imaginary role-playing going on in my mind. Through the conversations in my head, I frequently spoke to family members, coworkers, and friends, but also to celebrities, dignitaries, persons who were deceased, even characters from books and movies. I not only had conversations with people I knew regarding things that had happened in the past, I had conversations with people I didn't know regarding things of the future. I started noticing that in some of my internal conversations, I gained information about subjects I previously knew nothing about. If I wanted to know something about the theory of relativity, I didn't have an imaginary conversation with my husband. What did he know about it? I discussed it with Albert Einstein.

In addition, I realized the voice had incredible spontaneity. I didn't have to think "Hey, I'd like to speak to Albert Einstein." It just happened. I might even go as far to say I didn't have any control, though I could stop at any time if interrupted or simply bored by it all.

You can probably think of an occasion earlier today where you had just such a conversation (though women are more prone to this than men). Whether with your spouse or lover or sister or mother, they magically appeared in your head, ready and willing to play out the role you imagined for them. (If you can't think of such an example, you're probably arguing with me in your head right now . . . and that counts.)

The leap here is not in recognizing the conversations exist or that they have a learning value. The leap comes in recognizing these other people are being role-played by something alive, interactive, and intelligent—the teacher. I like to think of it as having a twenty-four/seven, in-house playmate because isn't that how we refer to our imaginations? As a child's plaything?

The important thing is that it doesn't matter how you perceive the teacher, real or imagined. What matters is

"Consciousness is so broad, so abstract, and so diffuse that we can only study its manifestations. While these manifestations may be considered by some to be nothing but a veil of illusion, it is certainly a most well-ordered illusion!"
Anodea Judith,
Wheels of Life

243

that you have the ability to access this teacher at any given moment to walk through presentations or to discuss micro-fusion, or to simply talk to yourself about the content of the latest article you've read.

All my life I've had imaginary discussions in my head without ever realizing they had such an important impact on my life. They were a teaching device. They were a way to learn, to dream, to figure things out.

THE PROPHETIC VOICE

Let's return to the story of the eggs and the voice one more time. The voice I heard on that day I refer to as the *prophetic voice*. Why prophetic? Because it's the voice that tells of coming events. I'm sure eggs aren't high on your list of prophetic revelation, but weren't they? Wasn't the fact that I should buy eggs actually foretelling that I would soon need them? Of course it was.

Like the teacher voice, the prophetic voice is available all the time. Since it is a part of the body's intuitive reasoning package, it responds independently—as needed in its opinion. In other words, it's not open to our whims. Like the angel voice, its messages are typically of a guiding, helpful nature, but above all, of love, the latter being its most important aspect.

The prophetic voice is innately personal, knowing what makes you laugh, what gets your attention, what you know, and what you don't. It knows what you need, what you want, and probably, what you're going to get. I suppose we could refer to it as the "Santa" voice since it knows if you've been 'naughty or nice,' one moment offering a humbling reprimand, the next, uplifting encouragement. If the teacher voice teaches, then the prophetic voice is like a father who mentors and guides.

There are many things in our lives we wish to know more about. Why is life the way it is? What decision should I make about my job? My boyfriend? The money I spend? What is good? What is evil? What is love? We look for answers in a variety of places, but how many of us think to look within ourselves?

Perhaps we are waiting for an image of God to appear in the clouds and speak to us with a booming, audible voice. Now that would be a voice! But don't expect some-

"I then heard a calm, fatherly Voice speaking to me out of the surrounding atmosphere. . . . it was a different Voice whose commentary was not vague or general. It was very direct and specific. And above all, It was suffused with an all-encompassing, sublime love that is nonexistent on Earth."

Saint Germain (Spirit), Channeled by Philip Burley, *To Master Self Is to Master Life*

thing like that to happen. Think of how disruptive it would be if God talked to all of us in that way. It's very impractical. Instead, God has given us this very personal, private, intimate means of receiving information. All we need to do is listen to ourselves think. Inside ourselves we have access to perhaps the most powerful of all divination.

HOW TO RECOGNIZE THE PROPHETIC VOICE WITHIN

I can say almost for sure that you 'hear' the prophetic voice all the time. It is the voice that reminds you to grab your umbrella on the way out of the house, it's the voice that gives you your hunches and sometimes your doubts. It's the voice that reminds you the tickets are on the counter when you're halfway to the show. It says a lot more too, more than you've recognized up to this point because you have yet to fully differentiate between it and you. Once you do, it will tell you much, much more.

I don't know any easy way to teach someone how to recognize the prophetic voice. There are a lot of finer points, which I'll explain in a moment, but there aren't any easy steps or simple exercises other than just learning how to listen. The reason for this is because the voice is telepathic. It intermingles in and amid your internal dialogue so that unless you know how to tell the difference, you might not hear it at all, or you might otherwise determine the information came from yourself.

A few years ago, my husband and I took the boys to the Ontario Science Centre in Toronto, Canada. They had a display showing what happens when the brain hears multiple conversations at once. I walked into a semi-enclosed cubical where speakers on all the walls and ceiling each were playing different conversations. It's amazing how the brain seems to listen everywhere, but the conscious mind can follow only one conversation at a time. I could only pick up a few bits of the conversation before being distracted by another. After a while, my mind became tired of trying to listen, and all the conversations blurred into one of indistinct noise.

A friend of mine gave me some self-improvement tapes that work from the same premise. The tapes play two messages at the same time, one in each ear. The conscious mind can only comprehend one, so it begins

"Most, if not all, communication. . . is telepathic, or directly apprehended in some other way . . . . Communication from another entity often sounds and feels as thought the entity is right inside your head."
Ken Eagle Feather,
The Toltec Path

"A healed mind does not plan. It carries out the plans that it receives through listening to wisdom that is not its own. It waits until it has been taught what should be done, and then proceeds to do it. It does not depend upon itself for anything except its adequacy to fulfill the plans assigned to it."
Foundation for Inner Peace,
A Course in Miracles

combining the two benign stories into a powerful subconscious message for self-change, whether it be quitting smoking, losing weight, or being more creative. The conscious mind can't outsmart the trick, thus allowing a new, positive message to form.

Remember, the prophetic voice has no sound, and so what is spoken blends into our own chattering inner dialogue. While the subconscious mind receives its message, the conscious mind doesn't differentiate between the two unless we teach it how, and I can help you do that.

I had a friend who swore she heard no voices whatsoever, didn't plan to. She felt certain I couldn't help her. Part of her denial had to do with fear, part with a lack of confidence. But after some time and practice, she let me know that she did hear . . . *something*. While she couldn't say for sure she heard a voice, she knew beyond a doubt the messages coming through were alerting her to many possibilities in her life. Over the next few years, her life dramatically changed in many positive ways.

"The voice of the Inner Self . . . can only speak through your own quiet, calmed, alert personality because emotional static drowns out its call."
Scott Mandelker,
From Elsewhere

EXERCISE 17—LISTEN

This is a very simple assignment. *Begin to listen.*

First acknowledge that you are *willing* to listen to any suggestion that would enhance and benefit your life and the lives of those around you. It certainly doesn't hurt to add that you are interested in finding direction towards your higher purpose. You might want to add as well that you'd like to be alerted to these messages in a gentle way. If you've been ignoring them for many years (and I assure you we all get them), this extra notation will help ensure you will be made aware of them.

Remember, too, the technique of making sure to always *acknowledge* them *even if you're not totally sure you really received one.* Use one of the ways previously described: *write it down, speak it out,* or *act on it.* While you may choose not to follow the advice, acknowledging receipt of it is vital.

Next, sit back over the next few days and see what happens. There is so much waiting for you when you fully plug in and make this strong connection.

"Listening is not passive; God does not write on us like chalk on a board. Listening is active work, although the key to it is restful abiding in trust."
John and Paula Sandford,
The Elijah Task

THE FINER POINTS

THE VOICE KNOWS IF YOU ARE LISTENING

Let me restate what I said earlier: Intuitive hunches and other means of deep intercommunication provide information based on the recipient's trust and receptivity. It knows how seriously you take this information. It knows your learning curve. If it has an important message to offer and you're not listening through this channel, the message will be sent through some other means—the one you're most likely to hear. The message might come from one of the reflections we spoke of earlier, or from something you see or read, or it might come from an ailment whose debilitation forces you to turn in another direction than the one you've been going.

If, on the other hand, you're open to hearing the intuitive nudges and the voices your body gave you at birth, the message can come from one of those directions. If you think about it, our bodies are pretty flexible. They are changeable and adaptable to whatever boundaries we have placed on them.

"My thoughts flow into your consciousness in each moment, with each breath. On the current of your awareness they enter."
Kenneth X. Carey,
The Third Millennium

YOU CAN FEEL THE VOICE

Hearing the voice for me begins with a feeling. Knowing the voice has spoken starts with my feeling a sensation within my body. What does it feel like?

Imagine standing at the edge of a large pond. You find a pebble in the grass. It's not a very large pebble, not compared to the vastness of the pond, but you toss it into the water. The pebble disappears into the water with hardly a sound. Then, as you watch, tiny ripples make their way from where the pebble entered the water to where you are standing on the shore. Those ripples represent what I feel. Although by the time I feel the so-called ripple, the "pebble" has long since entered and disappeared.

I can't explain how the ripples feel. They just are. I think it's possibly a type of electrical impulse. Maybe a disturbance of my body's electro-magnetism. I can't say. I just know when I hear the voice, I feel the ripple, and then I know the voice is there. In fact, it might even work back-

"Why does time go forward? It turns out that the forward motion of time is an illusion rooted deeply in the Western psyche, founded in one single concept—that time is linear."
Fred Alan Wolf,
The Yoga of Time Travel

247

wards so that when I feel the ripple, I recognize a message has been given. Then to retreive the message, it's almost as if I go back in time to where the voice entered so I can hear what it said, then I leap forward in time to the present so I am back in sync with time.

While you're learning to hear the voice, also take time to note any feelings or sensations you may notice in association with the messages you receive. At first, you may not notice anything at all. The sensation is very subtle. Keep trying and soon you'll learn to hear and feel the voice.

You Do Not Have to Hear Distinct Words

Especially in the beginning, you may not recognize the prophetic voice as offering direct statements with words. It may remain blended within your inner dialogue so that you do not recognize it.

Many years ago, before I understood any of what the voice was about, before I understood we all hear the voice by some means, I remember hearing a pastor explain how he heard the Holy Spirit.

Pastor Fisher was leaving our congregation as assistant pastor to direct another church. In his farewell sermon, he talked about the different ways to hear from God. He said, "God speaks to each of you in many ways," and he went on to describe how we have thoughts about things. He said, those thoughts could be God's thoughts.

Pastor Fisher asked, "If you happen to be driving your car and out of the blue you think, 'I wonder when I last checked the oil?' Then you check the oil, and it's low. Is that a coincidence?" According to Pastor Fisher, there are no coincidences; rather, these subtle thoughts are God's way of gently speaking to us.

By allowing myself to be aware of thoughts such as these, I showed trust in the power of intuition and trust in God. My awareness and trust became the stepping stones for my later hearing the voice.

I will always be grateful for Pastor Fisher's talk because he gave me an open door to experiment with what I heard even before the incident with the eggs. Long before I worried about hearing voices, I had been gaining trust in the inner voice not through its words, but by examining coincidence and opportunity.

"The answers may come in words or in feelings or images. The answers are usually very simple, they relate to the present moment (not the past or future), and they 'feel right.'"

Shakti Gawain,
Living in the Light

248

THE VOICE SPEAKS A FOREIGN LANGUAGE

There's another unusual thing about the prophetic voice. When I hear it, the words, feelings, expressions, and explanations, make perfect sense. I feel as if I've understood it perfectly. But afterwards, if I attempt to write the message down word for word, I discover that I can't. There is a gap between what I heard and its written translation. Even when I think I've heard a specific direction, when I try to write it down, I find I need a multitude of explanations in between the lines or it doesn't make sense. You might think this would make it harder to understand the voice, but it actually makes it easier.

Although a breakdown in communication may occur when trying to translate the inner prophetic voice to the written word, the problem isn't so much one of not understanding as it is simply having a lack of words that can convey the truest meaning. The reason for this is because the voice uses a higher form of language, one that goes beyond words.

As the saying goes, a picture is worth a thousand words. The language of this voice works along similar lines. Utilizing all that I have known, felt, seen, heard, and experienced—even if it has no interconnection otherwise—I'm somehow able to translate those many bits of essence into something I interpret as words. From that essence, I am able to gain a concept. From the concept, I then determine a means to explain the concept in a way more easily understandable, like Jesus using parables. What I write down then, such as the concepts in this book, are my means of understanding the higher direction I've received.

THE VOICE REMEMBERS WHAT IT TOLD YOU

The prophetic voice almost always offers an "I told you so" at the moment the projected event occurs. For example, while you're standing in the rain without your umbrella, you'll remember the earlier moment when you could have grabbed your umbrella, and didn't go back for it. You'll know you had the opportunity to avoid this moment, and ignored the message you received.

The prophetic voice seems to take great pleasure in the "I told you so." I suspect this is how the voice gains our

"Thoughts do not come in any verbal formulation. I rarely think in words at all. A thought comes, and I try to express it in words afterwards."

Albert Einstein

attention so it can remind us of the importance of listening to its suggestions in the first place. With the "I told you so," you are more likely to listen the next time around.

TRUST, ACKNOWLEDGE, AND OFFER GRATITUDE TO THE VOICE

Earlier, I mentioned how the voice knows our abilities and beliefs. It knows if we are taking the idea of listening seriously. One way to build trust is by acknowledging anything you believe you might have heard, even if you think it might only be your imagination. By acknowledging any helpful information that comes to mind, you are offering recognition to the source of that wisdom. You are letting it know that you're listening and open to guidance.

The best way to acknowledge a message is to either write it down, speak it out loud, or act on the knowledge received. Start by doing this with little hunches and gradually the knowledge received will come more frequently and be of greater value. Simply say something like, "Oh, I wonder if I should take a sweater?" or "I'm thinking I might need my class notebook." If, after acknowledging the information, you decide not to follow through with it, "I know the professor said we didn't need our notebooks today"—that's okay. Later, when you get the "I told you so," at the very least, you'll have your confirmation that the information came from the voice.

Note, you may not be able to rationalize why the information is important. For example, with the notebook example above, you may think, "I know I don't need my notebook for class." But realize later when you get the "I told you so" that you had written a client's phone number on one of the pages. When you thought of the notebook initially, your mind tried to think of its use logically. The prophetic voice knew it had another purpose. You only realize this at the moment you need the phone number. Had you listened to the reminder earlier, and not concerned yourself with the logic of its request, you would have had the phone number when you needed it.

Gratitude is another part of the acknowledgment process. When you receive knowledge, whether or not you acted on the knowledge, offer thanks for having had the opportunity. Thank God, Jesus, your angel, guide, "the

"When your heart is filled with gratitude, it is grateful for everything and cannot focus on what is missing. When your attention is on your scarcity, you are telling the universal spirit that you need more and are not grateful for all that you have."
Wayne W. Dyer,
Manifest Your Destiny

250

voice," or whatever entity is in keeping with your beliefs. By offering gratitude, you affirm you recognized your opportunity to receive the information. You're continuing to build trust, and you're proving your intention to receive information by this means.

YOU CAN ASK THE VOICE QUESTIONS

I have asked many questions and received many answers. The catch seems to be that the answers don't necessarily come when I want them to come. Rather, they seem to show up in their good old time. Some answers arrive within minutes of my asking, some within days, some within months, others take years.

In some cases, I blame myself because I know the prophetic voice must wait until my understanding or lifestyle can comprehend the answer. This may mean waiting until I've had some parallel experience that can be compared to whatever it is I want to know. In the same way Jesus spoke in parables to explain spiritual matters to his followers, the prophetic voice (and also the teacher voice) often uses comparisons to things I know to explain things I don't. But understanding isn't always the problem.

Sometimes I ask and receive the answer too late. Does some unseen force block the answer from coming? In the bible, Daniel wrote of waiting twenty-one days for an answer.

> . . . Fear not, Daniel: for from the first day that thou didst set thine heart to understand, and to chasten thyself before thy God, thy words were heard, and I am come for thy words. But the prince of the kingdom of Persia withstood me one and twenty days: but, lo, Michael, one of the chief princes, came to help me; and I remained there with the kings of Persia. Now I am come to make thee understand what shall befall thy people . . . (Daniel 10:12-14)

Or maybe the voice is like a parent who, when their child can't spell a word says, "go look it up." In other

"I ask myself, 'Am I making my decision with fear or enthusiasm?' and I remember that the word 'enthusiasm' comes from the Greek 'entheos,' which means 'The God within.'"
Spencer Johnson,
Yes or No

"Our guides don't try to answer all our questions for us or try to solve all our problems as much as they help us contact our own inner selves. In other words, they validate our own abilities to find answers for ourselves. They guide us to our own beingness. That is what is meant by 'guiding.'"
Iris Belhayes,
Spirit Guides

251

"As a practicing intuitive, I am frequently asked, 'If you're so intuitive, why don't you have all the answers?' I don't have all the answers because I don't have all the questions."

Laura Day
Practical Intuition

words, maybe there's a line drawn between learning a lesson and using the voice as a crutch. We don't know where the line is so we never if the answer will be forthcoming. It might be that the search for the answer is in itself part of our path. Knowing the answer without the search might prevent us from obtaining skills, meeting people, or completing roles needed to fulfill our purpose.

Perhaps our rush-and-hurry lifestyle blocks the answers. If we haven't taken time to make a strong connection and aren't fully "plugged in," we might miss hearing an answer due to the other distractions in our lives.

There are many things that remain closed to our full understanding, but in all things, we can be guided if we ask and are open for the answer.

THE VOICE HAS ITS OWN AGENDA AND REMAINS FOCUSED ON THE ULTIMATE GOAL AT ALL TIMES

Picture this scene. I'm listening to my husband as he describes his day when suddenly, something he has just said triggers the prophetic voice into action. I now have two dialogues going at once, one between my husband and me, and another with the voice inside my head.

I remember my father-in-law doing this. Sometimes while sitting with us, we'd all be talking, and I'd notice how during the conversations his eyes would glaze over. I knew he was no longer with us. His mind was somewhere else. He would be there physically, he'd have his eyes open, but he'd be looking blindly into space. I knew he was listening to the prophetic voice.

"I banished all my doubts and began listening to the inner voices that kept telling me I would receive the guidance I needed . . ."

Wayne W. Dyer,
Manifest Your Destiny

We're only human and we aren't very good at listening to two conversations at once. We tend to zone out the background noise, even if that "noise" is our spouse, our parent, a friend, or our boss. But why would the voice interrupt a conversation? Doesn't it have any manners? How could something so loving and helpful be so rude?

The phophetic voice is at all times in direct communion with God and in full recognition of everything we are meant to learn and accomplish. Our highest purpose is always at the forefront of anything we do and, thus, takes precedence over everything—and I do mean everything—else. That means that no matter what we might be doing at any given moment—even if someone is dying—if the opportunity arises for us to gain important information that we need to further our purpose, that knowledge or lesson is offered right then and there.

Much of what we learn is based on what we already know. We might gain understanding about the softness of a pillow by comparing it to the hardness of a tabletop. We might gain understanding about the brightness of light by comparing it to the darkness of night. Babies learn by experimenting with objects. They lick them, throw them, pick them up and squeeze them. They learn that when dropped, a ball falls to the floor and rolls or bounces, but mother's favorite vase breaks when it hits the floor.

Thus, in order for us to learn whatever lessons we might need, we are taught by comparing what we know to what we don't know. However, as adults, we have billions upon billions of known bits of information all stored in our amazing brains. Some of this information might be harder to access since it might not be as vital to our daily lives.

In our minds, we have pockets of thoughts. Associated thoughts are connected by an electrical strand. Write the word "rabbit" on a blank sheet of paper and your mind will immediately begin to tell you countless associations you have for "rabbit." However, if the prophetic voice wants to tell you something about rabbits, and wants you to remember a piece of knowledge you have about rabbits so as to compare it to something you don't know, it first needs some happening to occur to cause you to remember rabbits.

The voice will wait patiently for as long as it takes for that trigger to occur. Then, the moment one of the connected mind pockets is triggered, say by the conversation mentioned earlier with my husband, BAM! I'm rushed via a series of associated thoughts to that remote pocket. Once there, the parallel thought explains something I didn't know by means of something I did.

Unfortunately, this could happen smack dab in the middle of someone else's conversation. The voice's agenda of offering necessary information will supercede everything else. This presesnts a few minor problems. For example, there is nothing more embarrassing than having the voice say something funny while I'm talking to someone about something serious.

The voice's instruction will likely be something

"Once you do have a memory, it remains persistently fixed in the mind—even if you think you can't remember it. It lurks there in your unconscious, ready to jump out at you the first chance it gets."

Fred Alan Wolf,
The Yoga of Time Travel

253

personal, maybe even intimate. The voice probably will have pointed out something about me that I need to fix, some trait I've just recognized or some flaw that suddenly jumped out like a second left foot. It's not going to be something I want to share with the person I've just laughed at, so I may have some explaining to do.

There's more. Nobody likes to be zoned out, and nine times out of ten, they will know I've left them behind because the voice's dialogue will have distracted me from whatever the person might have been saying. I'll pick up their conversation mid-sentence and hear something like, ". . . so I didn't know why it turned out red. What do you think?" I won't have the slightest clue as to what they are talking about. Did I lose one sentence? Two? A whole story? I won't know.

Fortunately, these minor annoyances aren't fatal and they carry with them the bonus of whatever valuable lesson might have just been learned.

THE VOICE REPRESENTS ONLY TRUTH AND LOVE

What I receive from the voice represents only Truth and Love. Nothing it's ever told me has been negative, hurtful, degrading, or inaccurate. There have been times when I misinterpreted what I heard or when I didn't understand its meaning. There have been times when I felt humbled or scolded. In contrast, the voice displays a great sense of humor and knows how to make me laugh.

I remember years ago hearing of a man who attempted to bomb a church because "a voice told him to." I know this inner voice would never instruct anyone to do something violent, murderous, or destructive. Such acts are not of its nature nor in keeping with the lessons of love it teaches. I can only believe this man suffered from some psychotic disorder, as did the boy I mentioned previously who stabbed his father.

When in doubt, weigh any message alongside Truth and Love to determine if it's truly the prophetic voice within. Lindsay Gibson *(Who You Were Meant to Be)* writes of the voice that it:

- *Is supportive*

- *Tells it like it is*

"Your spiritual helpers will never ask you to do anything that would hurt you or your loved ones. They help you so that you can help the world."
Doreen Virtue,
The Lightworker's Way

"Another guideline by which we can test what we hear is God's love. He speaks in love. . . . God will never speak in hate, bitter condemnation, or malice."
John and Paula Sandford,
The Elijah Task

254

- *Tends to make us feel relieved and at peace*

- *Offers a quiet realization of one fact at a time*

- *Is not emotional*

If the statements we hear are not in keeping with the above qualities and are not of Truth and Love, they are ego-based or a part of our ongoing inner dialogue. Gibson reminds us of the tactics the ego uses to pull us off track, saying the ego is *wordy, anxious, emotional, conflicted, fearful,* and *resistant to change.* She warns that the ego will set up *contradictory goals.* But we are all familiar with these things for they are revealed in our daily lives when we are avoiding connection and not listening to our *Body's Songs.* The ensuing chaos might even have been the conditions that brought you to this book. But now you have a series of strategies to overcome the ego's chaos. Now you have the keys to connection and well-being: *relief, commitment, goals, connection,* and *synchronicity.*

THE VOICE KNOWS LOVE AND PAIN

As you enter into deeper and deeper levels of connection, you will learn what I have, that there is no human relationship that can compare to the immense love given through this voice and its connection.

Saint Teresa of Avila compared the intensity of this love to pain. She saw a vision of an illuminated angel stabbing her heart with a flaming arrow. She wrote:

> . . . *so excessive was the sweetness caused me by this intense pain that one can never wish to lose it, nor will one's soul be content with anything less than God. It is not bodily pain, but spiritual, though the body has a share in it—indeed a great share.*[1]

If there is a fine line between love and hate then, too, perhaps the line between pain and love is also minute. Is it possible that we overindulge in alcohol, sex, drugs, and the power of affliction because we are seeking our lost connection and substituting that missing love for the next best thing?

"The ego is the hit man of the psyche."

Lindsay C. Gibson,
Who You Were Meant to Be

Chapter Twenty-One: Taking Your Connection to the Next Level

21

Pain and Connection—for the Greater Good

Between 1990 and 1991, my faith faced many trials. During those two years, my best friend moved away, my mother died, my family more or less disowned me, my step-father and I lost contact as he began dating, then married his third wife. Late in 1990, I joined a writer's group. Its few members became my support and surrogate family through many of my difficult days. Within eight months, I lost them as well.

Around that same time, my older son lost his first tooth. Unlike most children who can't wait to put the tooth beneath their pillow, my son refused to give his up. I found him a while later sitting by the sandbox, tears streaming down his face. When I asked him why he was crying, he said he didn't want his tooth to fall out. I assured him it was part of growing up, something to be excited about, heralded, even cheered. He would have none of it. "I don't want to grow up," he said.

We talked some more. I got him a popsicle; he dried his

"Now we are entering another dimension, widening our vision, exploring facets of ourselves we may have never explored before. Our goal is to encounter other realities, to take off the blinders, which can take us to a higher level of understanding we never before dreamed possible."

Rosemary Altea,
You Own the Power

eyes, and returned to play. All was right in the world, except he never did give his tooth to the tooth fairy.

Looking back on it now, I see how his refusal to accept the inevitably of growth mirrored my own feelings. While I reassured him about the loss of his tooth, something I viewed as a small stepping stone along his life's journey, I couldn't see my own resistance and lack of acceptance of the stepping stones along my own. I didn't want to "grow up" because it hurt too much. I couldn't see my way past the pain to the good things to come.

The changes in my life were symptoms of something greater. They foretold of a coming change where the old fell away and the new, higher understanding entered into my life.

WHEN LIFE CHANGES

Change is the pattern of growth. A seed becomes a fledgling plant, a plant sprouts a bud that blooms, a flower gives way to seed, withers, and dies. Change, no matter how fortunate or unfortunate, is inevitable.

Just when we think we have our lives figured out, something happens to challenge all that we know. Change steps in to make sure we continue on the prescribed path. Change is the kick in the pants that reminds us what we came here to do. Change prevents us from staying at a standstill, even if we want to.

For some, this is the point where their spouse has a heart attack and dies or, without warning, their longtime employment comes to an end. Change could be a tornado destroying a home. Maybe a business fails, leaving the owner bankrupt. Change might be a divorce, moving to a new state, or a legal summons for a crime. Change could be learning of a cancerous tumor, or the moment an automobile accident takes a limb.

I tried to resist change. Like my son and his tooth, I tried to prevent growth. I didn't see growth as something exciting, invigorating, and challenging. I only knew that change hurt. I knew I couldn't replace the loved ones I'd lost, so instead of looking forward to the new beginnings in my life, I clung to the past in fear of what was to come.

It had been five years since my cancer experience. My life had once again become routine and bordered on the

"We begin to sense our real potential and the wide range of possibilities open to us. That scares us. So we all reach for blocks to slow our growth. If we are honest with ourselves, we all know which blocks are toxic ones for us. Clue: this is the block we defend as our right."

Julia Cameron,
The Artist's Way

mundane. I'd become comfortable. I felt safe. Change tested my boundaries and pulled me away from safety. I didn't want change.

YOU CAN'T STOP GROWTH

While losing my mother, my best friend, and the support of my family pained my heart, through it all, my faith never waivered. I had a strong trust and belief in God to encourage me through those dark days. Then something happened that threatened even my belief in God. Change had come.

Earlier in the book, I discussed how we can easily find plenty of evidence to prove a belief, but it only takes the tiniest of contradictions to change our perception of that belief. You may recall my telling the story where I struggled to remove the white lid from the blue thermos only to realize the lid wasn't the lid at all, but the secured bottom. In a sense, this is what happened to my beliefs about God.

After having believed a particular way for many years, suddenly my beliefs were turned upside down. From then on, my beliefs of God took on a new perspective. It began subtly, snuck up on me, then hit me from behind.

Beginning in mid-1989, I found myself writing nearly every day, filling notebook after notebook as if driven by an unseen mandate. I'd always been a writer, but at this time in my life, writing seemed to consume me. It was almost as if I *had* to write.

Then, late in 1990, I joined a small writer's group. It was then I first began writing a book about healing. The book focused on my cancer experience and mentioned the voices within. To my surprise, publisher after publisher rejected the book, not because of the quality of writing, but because of its message.

I received many notes from editors telling me their publisher's doctrines didn't accept the voices as I'd depicted them. This was my first hint that anything about my beliefs might be different than what I'd been taught in church. I'd been an evangelical for nearly sixteen years. I'd devoted my life to God and followed what I believed to be a good and God-fearing life. In writing the book, I'd merely

"No amount of experimentation can ever prove me right; a single experiment can prove me wrong."

Albert Einstein

"I believe that catalysts are presented to us in various stages throughout our lives. They force us to either go forward, change our rhythm, or retreat. I believe that fear sometimes forces us to make our most monumental decisions."

Willie Stargell,
as told to Tom Bird,
Releasing Your Artist Within

followed the internal guidance I'd received after hours of prayer, so this bit of information came as quite a shock.

Around the same time, another change occurred. One afternoon, I received a phone call from the head of the writer's group telling me not to come back. While most of the closeknit members were like family, one woman did not like me. There had been some words. For a moment, things had gotten ugly. The argument, too, centered around my beliefs. I felt more humiliated than angry; nevertheless, for the sake of all parties involved, I'd been expelled.

This is what growth change is like. While I clung to safety with one hand, change pulled at the grip of my fingers. Anything keeping me from moving toward growth was, one by one, falling away.

The writer's group and the friends I'd made there had been my buffer from all the pain and heartache I'd endured over the past year. Without them as my safety net, I quickly plummeted into a downward spiral. The loss of my friends, my mother, my stepfather, all came to a head at once. I fell in to a deep, dark depression as all my repressed grief now rose to the surface.

For the next forty five days, I did not write, not even a grocery list. Except for necessary errands, I did not leave the house. I spent every day sitting in the living room reading, listening to music, and praying.

What happened to me during those days sounds awfully melodramatic now—even to me. Only those who've faced a depression will truly understand that it doesn't matter how good or bad life is because it's not just a mental problem. There's a physical heaviness that goes with it. On some days it's like walking through thick, wet sand on a foggy day. Nothing matters. Not even life itself.

I survived by doing meaningless, benign things, as they offered the easiest means of existence. I'd go through the motions of living, following my routine, avoiding anything too strenuous or social, doing as little as possible to escape having to feel because feeling anything simply hurt too much.

Then, just when I thought I could go no further, when I had done all I thought possible to suppress the pain, without success, I gave up. I stopped fighting. I quit resisting the pain and let it hit me full force.

What happened next was both incredible and scary.

"Because of the commitment to trust yourself, everything in your life changes rapidly. At first, when you make the choice to let go of your old patterns, it may appear that things in your life are falling apart. If you decide to go all the way in this process, you will eventually let go of everything you've been attached to. But this will be a joyful experience, because your true happiness comes from your connection with the universe."
Shakti Gawain,
Living in the Light

260

Incredible, because of how it changed my life and lifted me up to a place where I not only felt better about myself but also became inspired to help others. Scary, because it led me through paths I would not have chosen on my own. Scary, because it caused me to believe things I could not have believed possible. Scary, because in order to go forward, I had to let go of what I'd believed in the past.

In the book *Eagle and the Rose*, Rosemary Altea tells of her life's journey. Like me, she faced many days of worry and stress wondering what all the happenings in her life could mean. Those events were not typical, not expected, not normally to be believed. Yet, because she lived them, she did believe, and they changed her life for good. What happened to me changed mine. Ultimately, that is what growth change is about.

A MIRACLE IN MY LIVING ROOM

Earlier in the book I explained how, without a miracle, I would never have come out of my depression or survived it. I've not yet told what that miracle was. I decided to share it here since it shows how growth change pushes us toward the next level of life experience, and because it explains the next plateau for the three voices.

At the height of my depression, I came to the point where I felt I could not make it even one more day. I prayed and begged God to let me die. I said, "Give me a heart attack, strike me down, anything, just release me from my miserable existence." I didn't even think of how my death might affect my husband, my sons, or other friends and family. I just wanted freedom from my burden of pain. Like the biblical Job, I'd faced illness, I'd faced the loss of my loved ones, and now I'd been chastised by my friends. With the exception of my immediate family and home, I felt as though everything of meaning had been taken from me. Fortunately, my beliefs prevented me from committing suicide.

I remember putting on my headphones and standing in the living room listening to music. I had my eyes closed and gently swayed in time to the rhythm, listening for the voice to comfort me, just like I always did. Then the music paused, so I opened my eyes.

"Pain is resistance to growth. If you are in pain, which can manifest in anything from frustration to anger to depression, it is because you are resisting the life-enhancing growth that we have all worked so long to be a part of."

Tom Bird,
Rollercoasters

"All miracles mean life, and God is the giver of life. His Voice will direct you very specifically. You will be told all you need to know."

Foundation for Inner Truth,
A Course in Miracles

261

"Although the Lord gives you the bread of adversity and the water of affliction, your teachers will be hidden no more; with your own eyes you will see them. Whether you turn to the right or to the left, your ears will hear a voice behind you, saying, 'This is the way; walk in it.'"

Isaiah 30:20-21,
New International Version

"They answered my questions with questions and pointed me into the night. The power that bore me had left me alone to figure out which way was right."

Manfred Mann,
Questions

When I opened my eyes, a being—a man—was standing there.

He had on brown loafers.

I noticed his shoes first because I'd had my head bowed and, when I opened my eyes, his shoes were the first things I saw.

Next, looking farther up, I noticed light-colored slacks and a white fisherman's knit sweater. Then white-blond, shoulder-length hair that framed a clean-shaven, fair-skinned, benevolent face.

Looking into his eyes, I became mesmerized by them. They were blue, the bluest blue I'd ever seen. They weren't sky blue or Caribbean blue, or any earthly blue. They were the blue that all other blues have ever been made of—effervescent, alive, illuminated. Looking into his eyes, I became engulfed by blue until he had drawn me out of reality and away from my distress. We were not in another place. He had merely separated me from my damaging, conscious thoughts. I felt safe, protected, loved, healed, revived. Then, I felt nothing. For a moment it was as if I didn't exist at all. When I opened my eyes again, he was gone.

THE QUESTIONS I ASKED

The first thing I did was to sit down and ask myself, "What just happened?" I needed time to think it through. I found my thinking had somehow been altered. I now knew I had a purpose. I knew I would succeed in that purpose, and that I had been healed from the depression and pain I'd suffered. I also knew I'd been given other knowledge as well, but understood I wouldn't be aware of what it was until such time as I needed it. I didn't know how I knew these things other than they had been given to me while wrapped within the blue.

Then my mind filled with a million questions, too many to list here, though you probably would have asked the same questions yourself. Who was he? Where did he come from? Did he stand for good? Why did he appear to me? What did this mean? Did I even see him at all? Was I crazy?

I can't say 'veI received answers to all of them. In fact, there are many things I've never fully understood and probably never will.

262

As soon as I started thinking and began to analyze what had transpired, the three voices, particularly that of the teacher voice, offered their help as well. I discovered that through the voices and their roll-playing I could communicate with the being I'd just seen and ask him questions. From these conversations, I learned several important things.

More than anything else, I wanted to know who he was and why he had come. He said that he himself was of little importance. His answers focused on my well-being and my fulfilling my purpose. As with the voices, his messages centered on the immense and unconditional love of God.

I pressed him further, asking, "Do you have a name?" I half expected him to say something like "Michael" or "Gabriel" or some other angel-like name. Those are the kinds of names I would have chosen for him. Instead, he said that his name would be too difficult for me to pronounce. As an example, he showed me names akin to Aztec or Mayan civilizations where lots of consonants like X and L ran together. He suggested a nickname and called himself "Jesse." Jesse, according to one of the books on my shelf at the time, meant "God exists," so I accepted "Jesse" as his name.

I wanted to understand *how* he had appeared to me. Jesse's presence had been holographic. He was there, yet he was not there.

My father-in-law used to describe angels he saw coming and going. He'd explain how the angels appeared from nowhere as if an elevator door had slid open and they stepped into the room from another dimension.[1] During one of my hospital stays when I had cancer, I'd seen an image of Jesus at the foot of my bed. As my father-in-law had described, Jesus appeared to be standing in an elevator-like box. I thought of it more as a doorway to a parallel dimension or the seam between our two worlds. Since I had not seen Jesse either come or go, I did not know if he used this means or not. I do know he did not use the front door.

Paul writes, "For now we are looking in a mirror that gives only a dim reflection of reality, but when perfection comes we shall see reality, and face to face!" (*Paraphrased from 1 Corinthians 13:12, Amplified Bible*)[2]

". . . these very solid-looking people had apparently materialized out of nowhere. . . . They didn't look anything like I might have imagined that angels, or ascended masters, or any other kind of divine beings might look."

Gary R. Renard,
The Disappearance of the Universe

263

"When angels visit us, we do not hear the rustle of wings, nor feel the feathery touch of the breast of a dove; but we know their presence by the love they create in our hearts. Oh, may you feel this touch. . ."
Mary Baker Eddy,
Miscellaneous Writings

"And I will pray the Father, and he shall give you another Comforter, that he may abide with you for ever; Even the Spirit of truth; whom the world cannot receive, because it seeth him not, neither knoweth him: but ye know him; for he dwelleth with you, and shall be in you."
John 14:16-17,
King James Version

Omm Sety, an Egyptologist who attempted to explain the first visits of her own otherworld contact said, "Every time I tried to touch him, or he tried to touch me, it was as if there were a thick pane of glass between us."

I knew Jesse had been there. I couldn't have simply made it up. The changes that took place both immediately and over time were evidence that I'd been touched in some miraculous way by a healing and loving source. Almost immediately after having seen him, I began writing again and, most importantly, started living again. However, despite these marvelous changes, there were several things I continued to struggle with in my mind.

For one thing, I had a difficult time referring to Jesse as an angel. He didn't fit the stereotype image that I had of angels. Where was his white robe, harp, and wings? In an attempt to understand, I wrote about what happened. Then, in the company of several close writing friends, I shared the story with them, testing the idea that Jesse might be an alien. I reasoned that all angels were technically aliens anyway since they were neither human nor of our world. My friends rejected the idea. Apparently, they had no difficulty believing that an angel could appear in my living room, but could not stretch their imaginations far enough to accept that angels might be alien. They more or less insisted that I refer to Jesse as an angel. To me, we were simply disagreeing over semantics. To them, the idea of aliens appearing in our living rooms simply sounded too frightening.

There was another problem. Through subsequent conversations, I realized that Jesse had been with me as a kind of guardian and guide throughout my life. This was problematic since the doctrine I'd been following prohibited me from having a guide of this sort. Although I hadn't followed any particular denomination until after I turned sixteen, for the fifteen years following, I had. I well knew, according to their teachings, I had no choice, there was no other way, there was only one way.

Now my heart pulled me in another direction. I didn't know what to do. How could I turn away from all that had guided me, protected me, loved me through every trial I'd ever faced until that time? How could I give up on the guidance I'd received and refuse to listen to it again? This guidance had been with me through my cancer, through

The ground shook,
The air filled with smoke,
Fire rained down from the sky.
When the walls around me had finished crumbling,
When the air cleared,
I was still standing.

From amid the rubble,
I found one brick,
One brick which I could use to start again.
Then I searched and found another,
The second, charred, to be sure,
But still strong.

Thus I began rebuilding,
Blessed that though I had faced destruction,
Destruction had not destroyed me.

Jamie L. Saloff
8-21-91

(One of the first things I wrote after the occurrence of the visitation.)

the premature birth of my son, through the death of my mother, and even in my most darkest moments. From the time I'd clasped my hands together with God in vacation bible school at age seven, I'd sought only to serve God to the best of my ability. This visitation in my living room proved to me that God did watch over me, did care about me, did send help in my time of need. I couldn't see how something that had been such a positive force in my life could in any way be wrong.

So I decided to use a test. The prophetic voice had recently given me three prophecies that were soon to unfold. I would wait and see if they came true. If they did, and I could verify once and for all the guidance I received spoke only of truth, then I would continue to listen. If it didn't, then I would listen only to what I heard in church.

"Do not conform any longer to the pattern of this world, but be transformed by the renewing of your mind. Then you will be able to test and approve what God's will is—his good, pleasing and perfect will."

Romans 12:2,
New International Version

THE THREE PROPHECIES

The first of the three prophecies had to do with a friend's mother who had been very ill for quite some time. I knew it wouldn't be long before the mother died. The second prophecy said I would sell a book. I had recently sent out four proposals on a book I wanted to write. The third prophecy had to do with snow.

As I saw it, the prediction of an extremely ill, elderly person dying wasn't all that amazing. None of us escapes death. Selling a book, well, I didn't know what to think about that as I'd received sixty-three rejections on my first proposal and no sale. But, as it turned out, I did sell the book, coauthored by my husband. Looking back at the proposal many years later, a miracle must have occurred since we sent in a six-page proposal filled with typos, distorted color photocopies, and a two-paragraph bio that basically said we had absolutely no experience whatsoever. In addition, another individual with more experience and expertise had proposed a similar book; ours had won out. But honestly, selling a book didn't prove anything by itself.

The snow . . . now that was a different story.

THE PROPHECY OF SNOW

When my sister-in-law learned her baby's due date fell near the birth date of her sister's second son, October

8, she grumbled about it because her daughter had ironically been born on the same day as her sister's first son. She wanted her child to have his own special day and worried about it throughout her pregnancy.

As her delivery date neared, she asked me if I could tell her when the baby would be born. I explained that I didn't have the ability to predict dates. In fact, whenever I tried to find out a date for myself, they were rarely correct. As I said, the voice has its own agenda and didn't intend on being a sideshow for material profit or gain. But as we were speaking, I saw a vision of snow, and so told her I couldn't give her a date, but that it would snow.

If anything, I think my prediction made her feel worse instead of better. Unlike my sister-in-law, I live in the snowbelt where snow before Halloween is typical, but in mid-Ohio, having snow in early October would be more of a long shot. Had I just predicted she would go over her due date?

I remember her asking me many more questions, none of which I could answer. The only answer I could offer was that it would snow, and I didn't even know if that was accurate, especially with all the doubt I'd been feeling of late.

As my sister-in-law's delivery date neared, I found myself looking out the window first thing every morning. Any snow? No, just very green grass, colorful leaves, and bright sunny days. We had a gorgeous fall that year.

On the morning of September 29, the voice woke me just after dawn. The prophetic voice within told me to get up and look out the window for snow. I didn't. I know I should have, but I didn't. I hadn't had the opportunity to sleep in for many days, and the bed felt cozy. I soon fell back to sleep.

A couple of hours later, my brother-in-law called to say their son had been born. While on the phone, I reached for the curtains covering the glass sliding door and looked outside. I saw a beautiful sunny morning, green grass, fall leaves . . . no snow.

Now I had a decision to make. No snow meant the voice hadn't spoken the truth. What should I do now? I knew what I had promised, but suddenly I had second thoughts. Then scriptures poured through my mind, and I felt loved. I can't explain this in terms of human under-

"Listening to God is fun. God has not one but trillions of ways to speak to us. Even when we hear wrongly He turns it to glory, for we learn anew His grace."

John and Paula Sandford,
The Elijah Task

267

"Now faith is the substance of things hoped for, the evidence of things not seen."

Hebrews 11:1,
King James Version

standing. I just felt loved. I knew it didn't matter about the snow. I knew I would keep trusting the voice. I didn't know why it hadn't snowed, I just knew that right or wrong, I couldn't turn my back on the guidance. In all honesty, I didn't know if it were even possible, particularly since I believe hearing the voices within is a natural part of our human experience. Perhaps, at best, the only thing I could have done was to ignore the voices, which we have a tendency to do anyway, but having learned to trust them, I doubt I could have done even that.

Within minutes of having come to that conclusion, the phone rang. By now, the afternoon had set in, and my sister-in-law called to tell me about the baby. The first words out of her mouth were, "You were right! We were sitting here watching the news and it snowed today in Colorado." Her enthusiasm surprised me. She didn't seem to care in the least that the snowfall had occurred over a thousand miles away. But then, I never had said *where* it would snow. I don't know why, I'd just assumed it would be here. Still, I think she had more faith than I did about the snow.

The following morning, a friend called. Before I could get the word, "hello," out of my mouth, she asked, "Did you see the snow yesterday?"

"What snow?"

"It snowed here yesterday morning," she said. "Not a lot, just a dusting. It melted off quickly." I swear the next words out of her mouth were something like, "If you didn't get up early, you would have missed it."

There had been snow? Had I missed it by staying in bed? I'll never know for sure. I do know throughout the rest of the week, friends from all over called and told me about sightings of snow. In time, all three prophecies had come to pass.

WHY AN ANGEL IN MY LIVING ROOM IS IMPORTANT TO YOU

Jesse appearing in my living room is important because it's an illustration of the next step forward in making a connection to your higher mind. To make the

268

leap from feeling a knot in your stomach to a place where you can receive personalized, concrete answers, you need to utilize the imaging capabilities of your brain. In simple terms this means we relate better to principles we can see than to those we can't.

For example, understanding the nonmaterial concept of "love" is difficult for us to fully grasp because love can't be put in a box and given as a birthday gift. In order to understand love, we relate it to physical concepts we do understand, such as a hug, a kiss, or a loving relationship. We do the same thing with the Holy Trinity. God the father, God the son, and God the Holy Spirit are visual ways for us to personify nonmaterial concepts of faith, hope, and love.

When I spoke of the "teacher voice," I explained how we use the power of our mind to revisit an argument or other past event in a visual way by examining our memories. In doing so, we move past what we've stored in our memory banks to our imaginations where we allow ourselves to visualize whatever situation we are trying to figure out.

What I want to make clear is that the visual aspects of our mind are the human brain's strength. It's by bringing the three voices and external guidance into a visual sense, in whatever context we are led, that we can make the leap to the next plateau in connection.

At the end of Chapter 19, I wrote about the next level of connection. I explained how we need to rise to a higher mind in order to tap into our greatest potential, and that to do so we need to seek love. In order to obtain this higher level of love, this nearly indescribable form of unconditional love, we need a guide to show us the way. That guidance begins with our putting our trust in the voices within, but expands when we can personify the voices into a trusted being or entity. To some, this guide might be a visual concept of God, Jesus, or the Holy Spirit. To others, it might be an angelic being, a high priestess, goddess, or Tibetan wise man because there is no limitation on what this perceived guide might be.

When I initially worked with Tom Bird in his Intensive Writer's Program, he never spoke of guides. However, both his directed visual meditations and mentored writing exercises often directed me to visualize

"Things become clearer when we give them visual form, for it communicates something tangible. From the visual form comes the verbal expression."
Anodea Judith,
Wheels of Life

269

> *"One of the most important things to keep in mind, though, is that your Transformational Archetype usually appears in the form of someone or something with which you are familiar or trust, so as to be able to reach way deep down inside you and to deliver a message. That message is always one of love: love for yourself."*
>
> Tom Bird,
> *Releasing Your Artist Within*

> *"I come now to knock upon the door of your heart. There are those here with me of the angelic realms who, though they cannot open the door for you—you alone must do that—will illuminate the doorway and encourage you in spirit."*
>
> Kenneth X. Carey,
> *The Third Millennium*

individuals he led me to meet. Later in his book, ~~Write~~ *Right From God*, he wrote extensively about the use of what he called archetypes and how these characters could lead a writer to not only write a bestseller but also fulfill the purpose of their life.

However, the exciting thing is that you do not have to wait until "an angel" appears in your living room. You can play a role in bringing this being into your mind's forefront through writing, guided visual meditation, or prayer.

ONE LAST NOTE

Some of what we have discussed in this chapter has been mind-boggling. I have challenged you to stretch your boundaries of belief. By doing so, you have explored concepts that might seem ridiculous. If you don't want to explore them or even consider them, that's okay. Think of these concepts as the advanced manual, the part to explore when everything else has come together and you are ready to go to the next level.

In the meantime, concentrate on making a solid connection to God every day and in doing whatever is necessary in your life to find your own personal definition of total well-being. If you do that, the other parts of your life will come together and be in sync.

CHAPTER TWENTY-TWO: TROUBLESHOOTING CONNECTION: WHEN THINGS GO WRONG

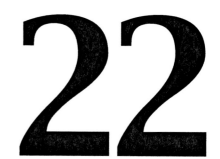

BREAKDOWNS AND WHAT TO DO ABOUT THEM

It was July. I was finalizing preparations for a party we were throwing the next day to celebrate the Fourth, a huge event in our community. The phone rang.

Though it had been some time since I had worked with Tom Bird in a student/mentor relationship, he immediately picked up on my stress. He asked me how things were going, not just with my writing but with life in general.

I sounded like so many other people we all know, complaining about not having enough hours in the day, feeling frustrated, tired, overstressed. My nerves were on edge. I kept snapping at the kids and my husband for insignificant things. No matter what I tried to do, something broke down or someone interrupted me. I couldn't accomplish anything. In everything I did, Murphy's Law applied—what could go wrong, did.

Tom said very simply and matter-of-factly, "You're not connected." And perhaps for the first time, I listened. Maybe I

"Oftentimes, like with any trip, routes and eventual destinations change. Your tension is a friend, a sign that you may have taken a wrong turn or that you may need to go in another direction."

Tom Bird,
Riding the Wave

had finally reached my limit in dealing with all of life's nonsense, or maybe I had finally gathered all the little pieces of necessary knowledge to fully understand the importance of being connected. Whatever the case, I not only listened to what Tom had to say, I did it.

Tom offered a little piece of advice which turned out to be the most valuable of any he'd ever given me. He said I needed to *connect every day.* Just like my dowsing friend had taught me before, Tom recommended I connect each morning, first thing, before I did anything else, and then to do so again mid-afternoon before continuing the balance of my day.

For two weeks I made a dedicated effort to connect on a daily basis. During that time much of the chaos in my life disappeared. In almost miraculous fashion, my workload became manageable, the kids started being more helpful, my husband became more attentive, and my time to be productive and work on my own projects increased tenfold. How could that be when just days before I had seen no end in sight?

The reason my life settled down was simple. Many of the distractions that had been plaguing me were symptoms of not being connected. They were environmental reflections and annoyances determined to grab my attention in hopes of delivering messages, since the normal lines of communication were down. Without making a connection to my higher mind on a daily basis, my body and the environment around me had teamed up to make sure the awaiting messages got through. And since it had been a long time since I had connected on any regular basis, the amount of messages waiting for me had backlogged—creating the chaos that ensued in my life.

Once my higher mind knew it could connect with me through the most direct means—subconscious to the conscious—the other message bearers were no longer needed, and they quickly subsided.

Does this mean I never have a chaotic day where nothing seems to go right or where I can't seem to move one step forward without first taking two steps back? I still have those occasionally, we all do. But by being connected, I have more productive days and more time to follow my desires. I am more adept at handling whatever life wants to throw at me.

"If you don't heed your inner voice, it will patiently repeat the advice until you are ready to hear it."

Doreen Virtue,
The Lightworker's Way

If you find you are facing way too many chaotic days, read through the following tips :

1. **Connect Every Day:** Without a commitment to do so, you may find it difficult to find time to connect on a daily basis. If you skip even one day that can quickly lead to two days, three days, or more. However, as soon as the chaos begins, remind yourself of the importance of connection and get back to it right away. The more you live in a connected space, the more you'll know the value of keeping that connection strong.

2. **Seek Out Relief:** If you're in pain, it's difficult to make a quality connection because your mind is focused on the pain—whether it be physical or emotional. Refer to the first section in this book on Relief to reaffirm how your connection can return to full power.

3. **Make a Commitment to Change:** Resisting growth can act as a connection block. If you are unwilling to move forward, like my son with his tooth, then you may be unable to recognize the messages and guidance coming your way. Review the second section of this book which focuses on Commitment and break through those barriers.

4. **Act on Your Purpose:** Each of us faces innate challenges that we must work through. Some of those stem from our heritage. You may not have recognized how your heritage plays a role in your ability to understand and clear away those issues. Return to the section on Goals for advice on how to use your heritage, skills, and heart's desires as a map to fulfilling your purpose. As you begin to clear away innate challenges and walk toward your higher purpose, you will find making a connection easier.

5. **Be Open to Opportunities:** Once you've set your goals in place, begin looking for doors of opportunity. Remember that you must take the action steps toward your desires, but by doing so, all of the universe will come together with guidance and direction to pull your life into sync.

"I know you have your doubts. You've been through something that no one should ever go through. You're going to be okay."

Dr. Daniel Jackson
to Col. O'Neill,
Stargate SG1, The Abyss

273

WHEN LIFE GRABS THE HELM

THE RAGING RAPIDS

At times, our lives feel as though we are a tiny boat tossed about by raging rapids. The rush of water looms around us, and we can do nothing except stay afloat, steer, if we can, and hold on for dear life.

Sometimes chaos is necessary to get us through precarious periods in our lives. This rush of life is designed to prevent us from making an error in our underlying life plan. There are times when life snags us by the collar and drags us through days or months (sometimes even a period of years) at such a fast pace, we feel we barely have time to take a breath. During those times, it seems we don't have the opportunity to make well-thought-out decisions, relax, or sit back and enjoy life. We are pulled quickly through each day with little opportunity for thought or reflection.

Those times are a means of protection and guidance, helping us through a part of life we would probably avoid, if we could, or where we would worry too much over the finer details. These might be periods where:

- *A loved one is ill and we spend hours at their bedside.*

- *Our employment takes a turn and our days are filled with travel, meetings, negotiations, or intense work.*

- *A severe ailment or injury pulls us away from our typical daily life, entwining us in a series of tests, treatments, or rehabilitation.*

- *A change of residence or heavy remodeling changes the landscape of our normal days.*

All of these things and more cause the days to speed by so quickly we simply don't have time to think or worry. When we look back in retrospect, we see how our lives were on autopilot as we had little or no control over the events that shaped that part of our life. Decisions we made at that time were possibly not well thought out—there simply wasn't time, so decisions were made on the fly and out of necessity rather than comfort.

In these periods of life, do not worry or fret. Just do

"Realize that by trying to push the river you're clogging vital energy. At all levels you'll accomplish less, not more."
Judith Orloff,
Dr. Judith Orloff's Guide to Intuitive Healing

274

the best you can to get through it. Once you reach the other side, you'll have time to regain your perspective, insight, and peace. Trust that you did the best you could during the turmoil and that the decisions you made were right for you at that moment, even if in retrospect you feel you might have made a better choice. Know, too, that overall those periods were probably for your own good and were intended to guarantee you would later have what you need to succeed.

NO WIND FOR OUR SAILS

In other times, our lives are like a small sailboat on an immense ocean without a breath of breeze to fill our sails. We long to move forward, to do anything to get moving again, but life is stuck at a standstill.

Some call this a void, others, the dark night of the soul. It is the space just before a major life event. These periods also serve an important purpose in our life.

I have faced voids several times in my life and can tell you without a doubt that if you can wade through them (wading is about all you can muster), on the other side you will find tremendous, positive change. Looking back over my life, after every void there occurred some beneficial event which changed my life dramatically.

During the void, I could see no way out and had no energy to fight it. At times, I longed to die. Yet, each time I pressed through one day (or sometimes, one hour) at a time, doing whatever I could to get to the other side.

Our lives are not a straight-line graph, always predictable, mundane, void of color. What kind of existence would that be? Instead, they are like that of the heartbeat on an EKG. They are a series of ups and downs, admittedly more severely so for some than others, but these life changes keep our lives fresh, new, revived, and moving forward.

When suffering from a void, I spend hours and hours listening to music, praying, and talking to God. I sleep a lot and take countless showers. I often read voraciously. The first book I will pull from my shelf is Carol Adrienne's *The Purpose of Your Life*. I turn directly to Chapter Ten where she writes about the void, what it might mean, and ways to attempt to overcome it.

"Rather than coming down hard on yourself as a failure, it might be more productive in the long run to think of the void as a rite of passage, an initiation to the next level of your life. It is a time of germinating the seeds of your new self, and a time-out while your inner processes sort, clear, and present you with new insights."

Carol Adrienne,
The Purpose of Your Life

275

In addition, you may also want to consult with a physician to see if you are suffering from a hormonal imbalance or vitamin deficiency, as both of those things have afflicted me at different times.

Sometimes a void is caused by our inability or even resistance to move forward toward our purpose. This may be caused by not fully understanding what our purpose is or, conversely, that we do know but are unsure how to begin. This may be because:

- *You think you lack the money, time, health, or education necessary and have not seen there is an alternate path.*

- *You are not sure what to do next, or how.*

- *You are faced with choosing between your purpose and something else you fear losing.*

To remedy any of the above, return to Section III and work through the exercises there.

In addition, you may find that consulting a numerologist may be of help, because through a numbers report a qualified professional can show the beginning and end of such a cycle. I once examined the chart of a cousin who'd committed suicide. I could see the downward spiral of the entrapping void and the coming trend of reprieve just weeks in the future from the day she died.

If you are in a void, take heart in knowing the end of your void is just around the corner. Like the song that says "the darkest hour is just before dawn" so, too, is a void. So many times I have seen friends and loved ones go through a "dark night of the soul" only to emerge into a wondrous new time in their lives.

After the loss of her husband, my mother-in-law emerged from her void to find a new love in her life. A friend's wife emerged from her void to discover she was pregnant. My son emerged from a void after landing a job he'd dreamed of having since he was a small child.

A void often occurs after a traumatic event or loss of a loved one. If you find yourself in such a void, think of it as a wound that must heal. Study again the section on Relief and understand that as long as you work toward healing and total well-being this, too, shall pass.

"Where you're going has nothing to do with where you are now. Nothing! You've got to remember that. This condition you see yourself in doesn't mean anything."

Lynn Grabhorn,
Excuse Me, Your Life Is Waiting

Section Five: Synchronicity

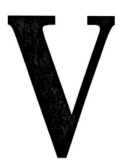

"Unless you believe we live in a random universe devoid of meaning, where chance and accidents are the norm, you probably see your life as a series of meaningful occurrences that happen for a reason."

Robert M. Williams,
The Missing ~~Piece~~ Peace in Your Life

CHAPTER TWENTY-THREE: LIVING YOUR LIFE 'IN SYNC'

23

In the fall of 2004, my son registered for Dale Carnegie Training, and since I'd previously taken the course, I decided to go along as a mentor. On the first night, we drove into town, a twenty-five mile drive, first taking the highway, then maneuvering through the five o'clock, rush hour traffic downtown. As we pulled into the parking garage, I stepped on my brake pedal and felt my foot go all the way to the floor.

I pumped the brake a few times, managed to get through the parking garage gate, then parked in the first available slot. Nothing appeared to be leaking, but it was obvious we weren't going to be able to drive the vehicle home.

As the dinner hour neared, I needed to call for help before the repair center closed. I worried about not attending the class and didn't want my son to miss any of the exciting lessons I remembered from my own participation.

I told my son I'd go with him to class, thinking I'd just let the instructor know I wouldn't be staying. My son immediately balked, saying he intended to stay with me so I didn't have to deal with the vehicle problem alone. We disagreed with each other all the way to the classroom, him saying he wasn't going to class, me saying he was, until we turned the corner and saw

"The more your life intuitively flows, the more it will be studded with synchronicities. You want this. It can spare you a chaotic day-to-day existence—a truth I keep relearning."

Judith Orloff,
Dr. Judith Orloff's Guide to Intuitive Healing

a large sign on the classroom door. The sign read: Due to a change in plans, we will begin the course next week.

We were both stunned. What an odd coincidence.

Soon a tow truck came and took my car for repairs.

I kept thinking about all the places I could have been when my brakes went out—on the busy highway, in congested traffic, traveling a long distance from home, all places I'd been with my car, or planned to be the next day. But instead, I'd pulled into a parking garage as if it were any other day, parked the car as if nothing were wrong, then walked safely away.

That is what synchronicity is to me. Synchronicity didn't prevent my car from having brake trouble, it permitted me to have brake trouble at a time when I could avoid disaster and not miss an important class.

> *"When we are clear about who we are and what we are doing, the energy flows freely and we experience no strain. When we resist what that energy might show us or where it might take us, we often experience a shaky, out-of-control feeling. We want to shut down the flow and regain our sense of control. We slam on the psychic brakes."*
>
> Julia Cameron,
> *The Artist's Way*

WE ALL FACE CHALLENGES

We all face challenges and struggles. The bible says that "the rain falls on the just and the unjust." What that means is we all find ourselves in difficult and trying situations from time to time. It's up to us to make the most of those challenges.

Look at it this way. A "good" game for a football team means they had the highest score at the end of the match. In order to win, they had to face the challenges of blocks, sacks, interceptions, and injured players. If they didn't have challenges, the game itself wouldn't have any purpose it wouldn't be any fun to play, and certainly wouldn't be any fun to watch. It's not whether or not they faced any challenges that makes a good team great, it's *how* they faced those challenges that defines the better players, coaches, and teams.

When you make a connection every day, you will find that your life usually flows with synchronistic ease. When it doesn't, and when you find yourself up against challenges, the difference between being connected and not, will affect how well you are able to meet those challenges.

When you are connected:

- *You have more patience for life's little annoyances*

280

- *You have more rescources to call on for answers to troubling situations*

- *You have access to people who can lend a hand when one is needed*

- *You have inner gifts that allow you to find solutions to previously unsolvable problems*

- *You have an inner calm amid chaos*

- *Your life will be "in sync"*

This section is written to assist you in creating synchronicity in your life by using the tools discussed so far, along with a few others described on the following pages. Together they'll lead to creating a life in sync with your purpose and goals. In addition, I've included a few more of the finer details designed to:

- *Clear out the last of your fears*

- *Break through your life blocks*

- *Expand your mind*

- *Reach your highest level of total well-being*

"There's always something to learn, something to know. Patience is being at peace with the process of life, knowing that everything happens in the perfect time/space sequence. If I'm not having completion now, then there's something more for me to know. Being impatient doesn't speed up the process; it only wastes time."

Louise Hay,
Present Moments

CHAPTER TWENTY-FOUR: THE LAST STAGES

LETTING GO, MOVING ON, BEING THE BEST YOU CAN BE

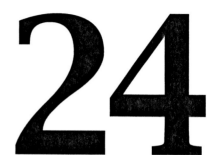

WHAT'S MINE IS MINE—TAKING BACK YOUR POWER

It was May of 1997. I had volunteered to coordinate a statewide writers' convention. Never mind that I already held the title of PTO president for our local elementary school and ran a busy, all-volunteer writing and publishing center for the school. Not only that, I'd organized two other major events for the students, and spent a week out of the country with my husband. I barely had time to scratch.

After a long day of preconference set up, a few nail-biting moments, and a tense meeting before the organization's board of directors, I was ready to call it a day. A friend and I sat on the hotel room floor eating carryout chicken dinners from plastic containers and rehashing the details of the next day.

We then talked about our many obligations. Although my volunteer contributions took up a large amount of my time, her list had to be at least double mine. We discussed our passions and the few personal projects we each had a desire to complete. I'd learned the hard way and the conference was to be my

> *"Quit trying to find yourself. Begin, instead, to allow yourself."*
> Lynn Grabhorn,
> *Excuse Me, Your Life Is Waiting*

volunteerism swan song. Come June and the end of the school year, all my major obligations would be fulfilled.

I'd come to an important realization during that year. Being a volunteer gave me a sense of being needed, of giving a vital contribution to the world, and a feeling of importance. When I realized why I volunteered so much, I decided I could get that same emotional payoff in other ways, including spending more time with my family who hadn't seen me much of late.

For my friend, many of the duties she'd taken on were just beginning. I sensed that she wished she could also call it quits. Her kind heart and moral sense of obligation had kept her from saying "no" too many times.

I suggested she opt out of a few things, because she obviously had more on her plate than she could handle. As I pointed out to her, in order to do so much, she had sacrificed herself and her own desires. In the long term, without her inner passions fueling her giving, everything she did eventually suffered from her half-hearted attempts.

She smiled and said, "How do you decide which ones to give up? They are all worthy causes."

I could answer this easily because I'd already been through it myself. I said, "Of course, they're all worthy. That is not the question. What you need to decide is which ones are also in keeping with your own path, goals, and purpose. If they are not furthering you along your desired path, then they are ultimately hindering you from being all you want and believe you can be."

She didn't say much after that. We still had a lot of preparations to finish for the coming day's events. But a few months later, she resigned from our group and several others as well. While the organization lost a dedicated volunteer, she regained her peace of mind and self-worth. She later joined a different organization that was more in keeping with her goals.

DON'T FEEL GUILTY

One of the main points of this chapter is: *Stop giving your life away*—and don't feel guilty about it. A *Course in Miracles* teaches that "guilt" is the opposite of love. When we abuse ourselves and the life we were given, we are not acting in love towards ourselves.

"The ability to say no to what doesn't support us is an essential part of our inner guidance system. It is never too late to start saying no to those things that drain you and yes to those that replenish you."
Christiane Northrup,
Women's Bodies, Women's Wisdom

284

Most of the people I know are good people. They want to help and give to others. They often go out of their way to be kindhearted. But for some, that help goes way beyond the call of duty. Like my friend, they have forgotten how to say "no." In the process, they have lost control of their lives and the ability to pursue their goals. They are so busy helping others, they no longer have time to help themselves—and that is eventually detrimental not just to themselves, but to those they want to help.

Giving too much of yourself only serves to drain you of your personal power. Though not something measurable by a standard blood test or chest x-ray, it still weighs heavy on your immune system and levels of stress. Giving too much of yourself takes a toll on your level of enthusiasm and passion for life. When you no longer have time for your own identity, ideas, pursuit of purpose, or (in the most dramatic of cases) personal care of yourself, you are draining your soul energy. While I believe wholeheartedly in giving—we can't outgive God nor ever run out of love, love is available in an unending supply—nevertheless, there are other subtle energies necessary to our body's wholeness that can be depleted. It's our pursuit of purpose and the fulfilling of our life's passions that refuels these energies and keeps them strong. It's our passions that call to love and brings love into our life in such great measure.

Since our purpose is so strongly tied to our physical being, it doesn't take long before our bodies begin sending ailment messages in an attempt to turn us around and get us back on our directed path.

How can you offer others love, joy, peace, hope, and kindheartedness, if you don't first offer these things to yourself? The more you love and take care of yourself, the more you'll respect yourself. The more you offer yourself unconditional love, the happier you'll be. When you are happy and filled with love, you'll be more able to give the same to others. And when you do give of yourself to others from this state of mind, you're giving comes from the purest, deepest part of your soul. You're actually giving more because you're giving from your fully charged, inner passions.

How do you stop? Many of the previous exercises in this book will give you the foundation you need. However, here are a few more tips.

"Guilt is an anchor that keeps us chained to time. Guilt is always associated with something we believe we did in the past. It makes the past seem real. Because we believe that what we 'did' happened in the past, it appears unchangeable. But through guilt we continue to feel affected by that past 'wrong doing.' Since guilt expects punishment, we expect our future will in some way punish us for our wrongdoing in the past. It doesn't seem to be even a matter of if, but when."

Pathways of Light,
Pathwaysoflight.org

285

"If you want to be in the flow of life, you can't struggle against it at the same time."

Deepak Chopra,
The Way of the Wizard

"We are all like tubes. Things flow into our lives, and we must let them flow out of our lives or we will become plugged up."

Doreen Virtue,
as told to her by her dad,
The Lightworker's Way

BALANCE AND FLOW

Part of being "in sync" is having a balance and flow to your life. As the saying goes, "All work and no play makes Jack a very dull boy." On the other hand, the fairy tale of the grasshopper and the ants tells what happens when the grasshopper doesn't work at all. (Luckily, the ants take him in come winter and he learns his lesson.)

If there are areas in your life where one thing or another occupies too much of your time, then your lifestyle might be out of balance. This disproportionate area that is consuming all your time is stealing energy away from other important areas of your life.

The energies in our life work much like the flow of electricity through a wire. In order for the electricity to work, energy flows in through one half of the wire, but then it must flow out the other half to complete the circuit. Without this cyclical flow, the power is blocked from illuminating a light, toasting a slice of bread, or spinning a compact disc.

In our lives, if all our power is going into our job, our household duties, the care of a loved one, or any other one thing, then we're robbing from the supply of energy we might use for other life-reviving activities. My husband is always reminding me, "All things in moderation," which if followed, does, indeed, create balance.

My mother used to spend as many as sixteen hours a day at her worktable where she made dolls to sell through her home business. When my father became ill, she divided her time between her work and his care. She had no time for anything else. She aged quickly during those years and lost much of her enthusiasm for life.

After my father died, my mother looked into the mirror and decided she wanted her life back. She did something none of us could ever have expected, but I admire her for having the ambition and courage to do it. By chance, she saw a plastic surgeon on a woman's talk show, who performed face-lifts. In those days, cosmetic surgery was typically reserved for celebrities or the rich and had not yet reached the popularity of today. After the show, my mother called the doctor's office and made an appointment. In order to have the procedure done, she had to fly halfway across the country, stay in a strange city and hosptial all alone, then fly home on a plane, looking like a battered wife. That took a lot of courage, but she did it.

Once healed from the surgery, she bought new clothes and a new car. She joined several women's groups, started going out occasionally with friends, and learned how to play golf. Eventually, she met and married my stepfather, who was a prominent attorney at the time. She had succeeded in revitalizing her life. She had restored the balance and flow and regained the creative energy she needed to take back a piece of what she had lost.

Note, it was not the face-lift that gave her back her power, rather it was when she took action toward loving herself and giving to herself that she regained her self-worth and personal power.

REGAINING YOUR LIFE'S BALANCE

In my own life, I've struggled with balance. I love to dive into whatever I'm doing and give it 110%. I love software gadgets, so I purchased a utility called *Life Balance[1],* and installed it on my computer and PDA.

The software works by first helping me to create a balance wheel based on the activities I wanted to track. I included everything from personal hygiene, work, household chores, and hobbies I never had time for in the past. Then the software asked me to create an outline of tasks that needed to be done in each area. A task might be "inline skate," "water the plants," "make phone calls for work," or "feed the dog." Each task belongs in its particular category. There are other settings as well that allow me to show what needs to be done in order of importance, based on the time of day and where I am located. It can even show me which stops are in the same locale so I can make my shopping trips more efficient.

Every week or so, I pull up the balance wheel. It shows my desired wheel in comparison to my actual wheel. This helps to alert me to what areas of my life I am neglecting and by how much, based on my own preferred balance settings. While I've yet to get the two wheels to match—my husband teases me about that—it has helped me to take control of the balance and flow in my life. Being able to see where I am putting my efforts, helps me adjust my life appropriately, even if I have to do so gradually.

". . . I was beginning to think of disease-related stress in terms of an information overload, a condition in which the mind-body network is so taxed by unprocessed sensory input in the form of suppressed trauma or undigested emotions that it has become bogged down and cannot flow freely . . ."

Judith Orloff,
Dr. Judith Orloff's Guide to Intuitive Healing

"Despite the fact that your ego hates unpredictability, the truth is that you have benefited from it again and again."
Deepak Chopra,
The Way of the Wizard

"Work isn't life, it's what we do to fund life."
Sue Christensen,
Making a Six-Figure Income on Your Terms

While the software has been immensely helpful to me, you don't need a computer program to do this. Simply draw a circle on paper, then divide it into "pie" slices based on how much preference you want each desired category to have. Next, make another wheel showing where those categories stand at present. Once a week or so, redraw your wheel to see how you are matching up to your desired balance wheel. Look at the areas that consume the largest pie pieces of your time and actively work at thinning down those areas while gradually adding to those so desperate for your attention. Think of those large slices as some fattening food you need to cut back on while adding some of the more enjoyable, "nutritious" slices of life to those areas you've cut too thin. If you're serious about making a change, this chart can help you to see where you need to make adjustments.

SIMPLIFY YOUR LIFE

In 2004, my husband came home from a men's golf weekend and announced he had purchased a small cottage. I thought he had lost his mind. While I knew some of the people from the tiny community, the cottage needed work and was situated more than two hours away from our home. I couldn't see how we would ever find time to go there when we barely had time to use the boat parked in our backyard. Like it or not, I soon began to learn the ins and outs of cottage life.

The most-heard saying in the community is "It's just a cottage," which is supposed to mean that "roughing it" is the first call to duty. But what it really means is that life at the cottage is slower, simpler, and more satisfying. I say satisfying because after we'd spent only a few visits there, we learned a lot about the simple life and just how good it could be.

To illustrate, imagine setting up a home in a two-car garage, including a shower, a bedroom, a kitchen, and all the living space. It doesn't take long to realize that a lot of the conveniences we think we need to live from day to day, we don't. While we opted for cable TV (it's a guy thing) and the Internet (so I could work on my writing) we have very few other conveniences—and we love it.

We never realized until we spent more and more time

at the cottage just how complicated our lives had become and how cluttered. Suddenly "housecleaning" took less than thirty minutes for a thorough scrub down, including running a small, hand-held vacuum and wiping down the shower. Clothing? It's no decision when I have two pairs of pants, four shirts, and three pairs of shoes to choose from.

At first, I thought I would miss all my things, but I quickly began to see how I didn't. In fact, we found the more we went to the cottage, the less we wanted to go back home to all our "stuff"—and I don't just mean our things. We found we also tended to leave behind many of our worries, stresses, and frustrations. My husband and I spent New Year's Eve at the cottage with some of the other residents there. What made this event so amazing was that we spent those hours in freezing temperatures, without running water. The inner peace that accompanies the simplier life is so powerful that when it came time to leave, we both paused at the front door, wishing we didn't have to go home.

I recently read a quote—I can't remember where—that said something to the effect of, "Have you ever noticed how many conveniences have been invented with the intention of simplifying our lives? Yet if you really want to experiece the simple life, go somewhere away from these conveniences." At our cottage this proved to be true.

Not everyone can do what we did; yet, by having both a home and a cottage, I had the ability to be without my things in a safe way since I still had what I thought was important back at home. However, having now lived for days on end in this way, I can easily part with much of what I have as I'm no longer attached to those items.

Several years ago, my husband and I read the widely popular book *Your Money or Your Life: Transforming Your Relationship With Money and Achieving Financial Independence*, by Joe Dominguez and Vicki Robin. The book talked a lot about simplifying our lives and becoming financially independent. It sounded like a nice dream when we read it, but even though we worked through the exercises and changed some of our buying habits, we really didn't take the "simplifying" part to heart. Yes, we wanted to be financially independent, but we also wanted a new car, new carpeting, and a big screen TV, not to

"By sorting through our possessions we literally bring up memories and thoughts which allow us to free ourselves of unwanted emotional clutter. In this way, we choose transformation."

Nell M. Rodgers,
Puppet or Puppeteer

"At the peak of the Fulfillment Curve we have enough. . . . Enough is a fearless place. A trusting place. . . . It's appreciating and fully enjoying what money brings into your life and yet never purchasing anything that isn't needed and wanted."
Joe Dominguez & Vicki Robin,
Your Money or Your Life

mention the day-to-day expenses of having two teenage boys at home.

After spending more time at the cottage, having so many "things" no longer seemed important. And while we don't necessarily prescribe *Your Money or Your Life*[2] as a financial planner, the exercises in the book are invaluable, particularly for individuals who have never looked at their financial situation with that kind of scrutiny.

There are two important points I want to make sure are clear. First, simplifying your life can make living a lot more comfortable, peaceful, and even financially stable. Secondly, and maybe more importantly, simplifying your life will teach you a lot about the attachments you have made in your life.

ATTACHMENTS

Letting go of the things you no longer need helps to promote flow in your life. As you let go of the old, you make room for the new. This applies not only to physical objects, but also to nonmaterial beliefs and obsessions too.

I always thought of an "attachment" as being in association with people. I'd lost so many loved ones, I knew all too well the sting of losing someone I'd been attached to. Such attachments come in many sizes, shapes, and forms.

A wise friend of mine caught me off guard one day by suggesting I take off my many rings. Most of the ten rings on my hands at the time hadn't been off since the day I'd received them, except to be cleaned or resized. I wore them proudly and loved the way they felt on my hands. The idea that I take them off actually made me angry. After I calmed down, I realized that something about them must really have pushed my emotional buttons, since I obviously had an attachment to them. Later, I found I didn't mind having them off as much as I believed I would. I put most of them away for a while.

Attachments can come in the form of an addiction to food, drugs, alcohol, cigarettes, or other vices. We also have attachments to the beliefs that we've formed. These attachments are perhaps the most damaging because, unlike an addiction where we have our underlying conscious reminding us it's wrong, a belief can block our visibility from seeing the Truth.

"It is when the material comforts become who we are and the focus of our lives that we lose our way. Life is to be lived from the inside out (from within your soul), not on the surface (the ego-dominated material life)."

Mary McGovern,
The Reason We Are Here

290

Our most strongly held beliefs center around religion, politics, education, medicine, law, and government. Once we form a belief in these areas, we often hold to it despite hearing contradicting information from the opposition. We become so firmly engrained in one way of thinking, we often can't see how another way might be equally as right. Even if we have the facts fully presented to us in black and white, we can not let the belief go. Instead, we make up false allegations and excuses as to why the information can't be so when, in the end, the only person we are lying to is ourselves.

When we hold too tightly to a worn-out belief, it is no different than wearing ragged clothes or driving a rusted, old car. Our stubbornness and refusal to let go of these beliefs creates a barrier blocking the flow in our life. Our refusal to rethink these beliefs may drive away those people in our lives who could offer us help, or who could show us a new path to take. Instead, we remain stuck in an old situation that is wearing us down, even making us ill. Sometimes we have to be willing to let go of what we have in order to obtain something better.

Here's one example of how a belief blocked my life. For years, I've been a very picky eater. As a child, my parents told everyone how bad my eating habits were. As a married woman, my husband joined their crusade. Later, my boys felt the need to chime in as well. Their feelings about my eating caused me to always feel guilty about the way I ate and to look for excuses or apologies for why I ate the way I did.

One day I sat down and made a list of all the foods I enjoyed and discovered I'd made a very long list, much longer than I'd expected. It included many foods from all the food groups . . . more delicious, healthy, good-for-you foods than even I realized. I liked more foods than anyone gave me credit for liking. My beliefs about food had been formed not by how I ate, but by my family beliefs and their imposition of their opinions on me about them.

Another breakthrough in my thinking occurred when, during a discussion about this with a friend, she pointed out how my way of eating had become a belief. She explained that the way I ate was not out of need, but a choice I made every time I picked up my fork. What changed after our conversation wasn't how I ate. What

"When you are attached, you become caught up in the emotions and the effects . . . Detachment is a way of creating an environment to allow the choices based on the values of the Truth, rather than the emotions of your ego."
Mary McGovern,
The Reason We Are Here

"Remember: Beliefs are taught to us by those who wish to control our thinking and actions. It is up to you to create those beliefs which are supportive and nurturing to your present life."
Nell M. Rodgers,
Puppet or Puppeteer

changed was how I *felt* about what I ate. I stopped offering apologies. I stopped offering explanations. I stopped feeling guilty about how I ate. Moreover, I started standing up for myself and asked my husband and kids to stop telling everyone about my eating habits. I didn't tell them how to eat, they had no right to tell me how to eat.

Recognizing how much food had become entwined in my beliefs about myself and my habits, and then allowing myself to let go of that belief and exchange it for a new, more beneficial one, made a big difference in how I felt about food. Having been told for more than forty years that I didn't eat right, I'd taken on the belief that I was in some way dysfunctional. Realizing I ate plenty of good foods, even if they weren't the same foods my family ate, allowed me to begin beleiving I ate well. This small change in beliefs created a large change in my well-being.

Remember in your own path that sometimes a belief is an attachment that must be broken in order that you might fulfill your higher purpose. Remember, too, that some of our beliefs are merely our perception and, like my beliefs about food, simply need restated in order that they properly reflect the Truth.

FORGET ABOUT THE NUMBERS

Our lives are entangled in numbers. We put numbers on everything even though they mean little. We assign numbers to time, size, weight, even to the portions of food we eat. We earn our livelihood providing numbers. We drive our cars by numbers. We live in homes listed by numbers; collect paychecks with numbers; even die with numbers. We create reams of statistics for our greatest athletes remarking on when, where, who, how high, how far, how deep, they achieved their greatness.

Unfortunately, we live in a society of numbers and, in some cases, we can't live in harmony with those around us without conforming to the unwritten laws of numbers. If we showed up at work at whatever time we pleased or walked into a doctor's office without a scheduled appointment, our actions would only make our lives more difficult due to the patterns set up by the status quo. However, there are many areas in our lives where we can turn off or release ourselves from numbers.

"Modern life is so full of pressures pushing this way and that that most of us react by trying to impose order upon it."
Deepak Chopra,
The Way of the Wizard

292

Begin by removing unnecessary clocks from your home, take the calendar off the fridge, hide the bathroom scale, carry your wristwatch in your purse or pocket so you don't look at it every five minutes. Don't eat because it's "lunchtime." Eat when your body says it's hungry. On days when you are not restricted by a time or particular date, allow your body to tell you what time to get up or what time to go to bed. Don't choose clothing because it is a certain size. Put on what feels good. Who cares if the size says it's two sizes too small or six sizes too big? As long as it fits correctly and comfortably, size doesn't matter.

What does the number on the bathroom scale mean? Does our weight in pounds or height in inches mean we are any less or better of a person? Our body's size and shape is a reflection of what we want it to be rather than what it is. Standing on the scale doesn't make us have any less or more worth. If we are overweight or underweight, it is only because we are comparing ourselves to someone else's numbers. For years I weigh 120 pounds and wore a size seven. My sister-in-law now weighs 120 and wears a size zero, so the numbers on the scale don't really mean anything.

When you begin to pull away from numbers that judge you, your life will be able to flow in true harmony with itself. I have several friends who live alone and who have jobs that do not depend on the clock. Yes, they still have occasional appointments and calendar dates they must keep, but when they are not under those restrictions, they allow their bodies to dictate their internal natural harmony. One friend rises at three or four a.m. to start her day and retires early, sometimes by eight p.m. She loves the quiet of the night and doesn't live her life according to the heartbeat of the city. Another friend doesn't have a second thought if he feels like staying in bed all day, maybe for several days in a row—and he is one of the most vitalized people I know.

A few years back, my husband stopped wearing a watch to work. He said it freed him from always wondering what time it was and allowed him to get work done more efficiently. While it may seem impossible, he found his internal guidance system always alerted him to look at the clock just before he needed to leave for an appointment.

When we live by the numbers, we place boundaries on our lives which we weren't intended to have. Escaping the numbers in our lives is just one more way we can move into a place of trust, harmony, and flow.

ATTITUDE ADJUSTMENT

In Section II, Commitment, I wrote about mouth confession and how what we say affects our daily lives. Our attitude about life also dictates much of how we see the world.

There have been people in my life that I literally stopped calling because I couldn't stand how negative they were about *everything*. No matter what happened to them, even if it might appear good, those people would find something wrong with it. It amazed me at how these people could twist something and make it sound so horrible.

An old Chinese tale teaches how any happening in our lives could be good or could be bad depending on what perspective we view it from. In the story, a boy falls into a well, which could be bad, but ends up being good when the soldiers arrive to take all young boys to war. Since the boy in the well can't be found, he can't go to war. The story continues with many threads from the boy falling into the well that are both good and bad.

If no matter what happens could be viewed from either a good or a bad viewpoint, then why focus on the bad when the good viewpoint:

- *Provides another opportunity to create positive energy around us*

- *Keeps us smiling and creates an environment everyone enjoys being around*

- *Can lead us to finding solutions instead of feeling stuck in problems*

- *Creates joy, which relieves stress and helps prevent ailments*

- *Offers peace, which softens pain*

- *Promotes unconditional love*

Tom Bird taught me years ago that negative people are "miserable and want to stay that way." He knew that

"Our thoughts, a major source of power and energy within our powerhouse, our physical body, need to be, to some extent, controlled. If we want our power to be creative, and if we want to advance our spiritual journey, then we must use our energy in the right way."
Rosemary Altea,
You Own the Power

294

for them, no matter what anyone did or said, it would never be good enough, and he taught us to stay away from individuals such as that, as they would bring us down too.

Guard your thoughts and spoken words. When you allow your thoughts and words to drift negatively, you are, in a sense, asking for these negative things to come into your life. Remember instead the bible writer's words to always think on good things.

> *Finally, brethren, whatsoever things are true, whatsoever things are honest, whatsoever things are just, whatsoever things are pure, whatsoever things are lovely, whatsoever things are of good report; if there be any virtue, and if there be any praise, think on these things. (Philippians 4:8) KJV*

EXERCISE 18–LETTING GO OF YOUR DEEPEST SECRETS

One afternoon, in an attempt to release my mind from all the many fears and problems that were cluttering it, I sat down with a deck of index cards and wrote down, one to a card, my worst, most horrible, darkest secrets. While I haven't committed any crimes and have done my best to live a good life, there were still many issues which I did not feel comfortable telling anyone about. They were plaguing my mind and stealing away my focus from the things I wanted to accomplish.

By using the exercise that follows, I released those items from my mind and made room so new information could pass through. I cleared my conscious of things that no longer mattered, but that I'd never released. In addition, I discovered that many of those old issues were not as terrible as I'd initially thought. Once I wrote them down, I found rational and logical reasons why I might have done them—reasons why anyone in my situation would have done them.

This exercise is very simple.

"Although the experience of memory sharing can be strongly emotional, it carries the possibility of external confirmation and the opportunity to rework our memories—to find new emphases and understandings."
Lenore Terr,
Unchained Memories

"When we have allowed ourselves a full emotional release, the body, mind, and spirit feel cleansed and free. Insights come up and long-buried self-understanding returns. I've watched people forgive themselves and others after deep process work because they are finally at peace with painful events in their past."

Christiane Northrup,
Women's Bodies,
Women's Wisdom

1. Using a stack of index cards, make a list of your deepest, darkest secrets and fears, one thought per card. Here are some questions you can ask to get you started:

- *I am afraid _____ because . . .*

- *I don't want anyone to know that ____ because . . .*

- *Secretely I wish that ____ because . . .*

- *I feel guilty or ashamed of myself when I ____ because . . .*

2. As you write each one on a card, consider why you did this particular thing. Decide if:

- *There was some rational and logical reason for doing it*

- *You were mature enough to understand why it was right or wrong*

- *It was something you could ask forgiveness for or make amends for*

3. When you are done writing, take the cards and burn them in a fireplace or other safe place. This last step is the most important because if you hold on to the cards, you could be tempted to go back and read through them from time to time. That would only cause you further pain and continue to dredge up these hurtful thoughts. Release them by burning the cards or by destroying the cards in such a way that they can never be read again. Do not save the ashes or scraps. Save nothing in order to release those thoughts from your life.

After you have done this, put these past deeds out of your mind. You might think of these things later on, but if you released them effectively, they will no longer plague your mind.

You may find this an effective exercise to do on an annual or semi-annual basis, such as on New Year's Eve, so that you can begin each new year fresh.

MENTORS

I will never forget the Christmas my cousins came from Southern Illinois to visit. Gifts stretched from the Christmas tree in the living room, around the corner, and into the dining room. Sweet treats and goodies galore. Later in the day, we had a huge family dinner with turkey and all the fixings. Yet, none of those things are what made this particular Christmas so special.

My favorite cousin and I had a special bond, so he always paid a lot of attention to me whenever he and his wife came to town. Later that evening, after all the festivities had ended, he and I settled in to play a board game I'd received as a gift.

I heard his stomach growl. He said, "Hey, squirt, how about making me a turkey sandwich?" I think I may have been ten years old at the time. I said, "I would, but I don't know how." He immediately stood up without giving it another thought, and said with a smile, "Let's go teach you how!"

I followed him into the kitchen where he helped me get everything we needed out of the refrigerator. Then he showed me how to make a sandwich. Making a sandwich with him didn't seem like a chore because the whole time he talked and laughed and was having a good time.

He was so encouraging about whatever we did, I never felt foolish or afraid to try something new. If I got stuck or had a hard time, he'd give me any help I needed. Once he helped me build a stobe light and something went wrong. When I came home from school the next day, I discovered he'd totally rebuilt it from scratch in order to find the problem. Another time, after I'd learned how to drive, he pulled his Corvette off the road, put me in the driver's seat, set me off down the road, all the while teaching me how to use a clutch and shift gears. (What a thrill that was!)

To me, he was the perfect example of what a mentor should be, but in reality, a mentor doesn't have to be any particular sort of person or personality.

In the movie *Karate Kid*, Daniel (Ralph Macchio) had to convince his mentor, Mr. Kesuke Miyagi (Noriyuki 'Pat' Morita), to help him learn martial arts. The methods taught by Mr. Miyagi were unusual to say the least. Daniel had a difficult time understanding how they would

"Do not underestimate the need for support, encouragement, and community with like-minded people."

Lindsay C. Gibson,
Who You Were Meant to Be

"Choose role models who are winners in all areas of their lives. . . . make an effort to get your hands on everything they've ever written or said. Really become a student of their work and of their lives. Don't just admire them, learn from them."

Denis Waitley,
Timing Is Everything

297

"Some of my greatest teachers were not formal teachers at all. They were everyday folks just like you and me."

Rhonda Jones,
Teaching Common Sense

help, but in the end, Daniel succeeded in winning a martial arts tournament.

In *Star Wars* lore, all the Jedi knights were mentored by other Jedis. Who can forget Yoda riding on the back of young Luke while he tried to learn his Jedi lessons? Dorothy had the good witch to guide her. Cinderella had her fairy godmother. Alice seemed to learn from all of the characters in Wonderland, but perhaps the strange Mad Hatter offered her the most. Fair-faced Snow White had the dwarfs to look out for her. Sleeping Beauty had her fairies. Even wooden Pinocchio had someone to help him along, little Jiminy Cricket.

Mentors are the people in our lives who see us for who we are and for all we can be. They inspire us or lead us in the direction we most need to go despite how unconventional their methods might be. Often it's with their help that we receive knowledge we need to move forward in our lives, or to break the spell of a mistaken perception that's long held us in its grip.

A mentor doesn't necessarily have to be a defined relationship. Mentors might simply be an ordinary person in your life who just happened to be at the right place at the right time to guide you and offer you the right advice—advice that later proves pivotal in an important life decision that you make. In fact, you might not even realize you're being mentored at the time—it just happens.

I never realized how many mentors I had in my life until I took time to write them down. I made a long list of people who taught me a vital skill, offered me sage advice, or guided me in doing something I now do well. Later, I thought about how amazing it was that these people came into my life at the time they did, and how perfectly they had fit into my life at the time, while the lessons learned might not be needed for years to come.

It occurred to me as well that we often think of these people later, just at the moment when we have to make an important life decision. Even their memory serves to show us the lighted way. Could this all be coincidence?

Lindsay Gibson says of mentors in her book *Who You Were Meant to Be*, "You need some people in your life who will hold the dream for you, remind you of it, and push as needed when you get scared and discouraged." But, unfortunately, for some of us no mentor appears. We have great ambitions, but no coach to lead us. What do we do until then?

While at any turn the cavalry might show up to knock down the fighting hoards, it is the hero of any great story who must stand up against the villian. No matter how much we wish to rely on a mentor, in order for us to truly transform our lives, we must rely on ourselves in the end. There are, however, a few things you can do to keep yourself going when all else fails.

For one, rely on your guide or angel. Do not be too proud to pray for help. When your source of support comes from within or from the higher heavenly realms, you have an open-ended supply for all the support you need.

Look for the book *Supplies* by Julia Cameron. Her cartoon style can't help but make you laugh while encouraging you at the same time. There are countless other motivational books, videos, and audios as well. Many can be rented for free from the library.

There is a story I love to tell about "shirt sleeves." My younger son had never been that great of a sport's fan, but dutifully went with us to countless hockey games because we had season tickets. He would quietly sit in his seat and play with a toy while waiting for his favorite part of the game—the intermissions. During the intermissions, 'Mac,' the zamboni driver, would appear to clean the ice. As Mac passed by the crowd he would throw shirts and hats to the cheering kids.

On one of those nights, my son rushed to win a prize. We saw him disappear under a pile of frantic kids, all vying for a T-shirt. My son came back wildly waving one sleeve.

"Why didn't you let go?" I asked. It embarassed me that he would rather have a sleeve that no one could use than to have let go so someone else could have worn the shirt. Every few mintues, he would wave the sleeve excitedly in the air, while I slunk farther down in my seat. We left the game early that night, but the incident did not end there.

A few days later, I thought of the incident again and burst into tears. I just couldn't understand why my son would have wanted that sleeve. Yet etched in my memory was him passionately waving it. That image bothered me for days. Then, one afternoon, it finally dawned on me as

". . . your mentor is suddenly gone, vanished, just when you needed him the most, or thought you did. . . . 'What am I supposed to do now?' you howl. You discover that when you ask, you do hear your mentor's voice— 'in here.'"

Julia Cameron,
Supplies

299

to why that sleeve was so important to him. I was admiring the clutter of signs, trinkets, and memorabilia I'd scattered around my office. Each fragment represented tiny crumbs of encouragement to me. While the bits of paper, colorful note cards, photographs, and poems would mean nothing to anyone else, to me they were vital. They inspired me and kept me going when everyone else didn't have time for me. They were my "shirt sleeves."

"Each winding marks a containment and a completed cycle in the development of the whole; but, as each is a part of the whole, the completion is also a beginning, so that the spiral shows the enclosure and 'rounded' quality we experience, and the equivalent points reached at every new winding."
Jill Purce,
The Mystic Spiral

SPIRALS

One of the concepts I've had a difficult time explaining to others are *life spirals*. You may have often heard the phrase "circle of life" and been told how history repeats itself. Life is not so much a circle as it is a spiral, a curve that spins back around to where you stood before, but from a new, higher, more knowledgeable perspective.

Imagine the spiral figure, not flat and one dimensional like a drawing, but rather like a spiral staircase that you must climb. Each time you go around the support post a full turn, and reach the spot where you once stood, you have completed a cycle. Only now, you stand a little bit higher, you can see a little bit farther, you can understand a little bit better than when you stood on that spot before.

It's much like returning to your hometown twenty years after you left. Many of the same buildings and people are there, but the way you view them has changed. You're older now. What might have been important then, isn't now. Maturity, life experience, and time itself offer you new points of view for looking at once familiar surroundings.

Such is true with life spirals. They are a kind of check system. Like *deja'vu*, you suddenly find yourself at a point in time where you're either viewing, working with, studying, or applying something as you did before. It may have been several months, several years, maybe decades, but there is that situation in some form again. No one will have to point it out to you. You will recognize the similarity from within.

This spiral viewpoint is a point in time to reassess your life in that area. How have you grown? How has your life changed? What has improved? What has gotten worse?

When you recognize a spiral in your life, this is a good

time to reevaluate your goals and purpose. Take a moment and reflect on how far you've come. Seeing the spiral may provide a wake-up call as you think, "Here I go again." It may be a kind of spiritual graduation where you recognize you've made it past some block or challenge.

Perhaps you'll notice that someone who once pushed your buttons, doesn't anymore. Maybe you no longer feel attached to an old vice. Maybe it's nothing more than realizing you have forgotten the name of that boy or girl you once thought as a youngster you couldn't live without. It's funny how things like that change as our lives spin through the spiral of life.

"You're always free to change your mind and choose a different future, or a different past."

Richard Bach,
Illusions

Chapter Twenty-Five: Who Am I—Really?

Alternative Realities and Why They Are Important

Do you know who you are—really?

A Hindu legend says that in order to know God we must first know ourselves. The more I learn about me, the closer I feel to God. The closer I feel to God, the more I feel I know God. Knowing God has molded me into a better person, allowing me to offer more compassion, love, and patience to my fellow human beings. More than anything else, knowing God has brought me an understanding of unconditional love, not only as a force for good, but also as a life-changing power.

So I am asking you, do you know who you are—really?

"With guidance, you will learn to release your definitions of who you think you are, open your self up to the experience of a much greater reality than you presently believe possible, and return to a level of consciousness where you will be able to communicate with us, not through cumbersome words and concepts, but directly, through communion with all that is."

Kenneth X. Carey,
The Starseed Transmissions

Trying on Different Aspects of Self

My journey to know who I am began not with me but with my mother (who probably carried it forward from her mother). After my sister's death, she sought for meaning from the tragedy and loss she felt. She filled an entire wall with books she'd read on a variety of religions in her search to find understanding. Near the end of her life she became a Catholic, not because that particular religion offered any different or better answers than any other, but rather, she had come to believe that no matter what religion she chose, God by any name, was the only solace she could find for her pain. There were other questions she had yet to resolve. Those ambiguous riddles were passed to me.

I began my search believing I wanted to find love. That eventually led me to a search for God. My mother had already explored religion in her journey, so my own search began where hers left off, going beyond the prescribed bounds of religion and into my heart and mind.

My search for who I am—really, took a giant leap when someone asked me, if I knew who I was. I had never been asked that question before so I had never thought about it. I just thought Jamie was Jamie. How could I be anything else? But the more I explored the question, the more I came up not only with an answer, but with different *ways* in which to answer. In other words, I found more than one way to define who I am.

Eileen Roe authored a children's picture book called, *All I Am*. Each page depicts a different title a person could use to refer to themselves. Following her examples, I could say of myself, "I am a mother, a daughter, a sister, a wife. I am a writer, a teacher, and an artist." I am also "an American, a Caucasian, a woman, a human." Each of these titles is one of many definitions I can give myself. Titles are only one of a multitude of ways to define who I am.

While each title or label placed boundaries on who I am, I learned I could alter those boundaries simply by using different labels or names.

The more I looked at the different ways to define myself, the more I learned about me. The search became a kind of game where I tried on many different costumes. Whenever I left the house, I wore my 'Jamie' costume. But in the back alleys of my mind, I played with a variety of costumes, labels, and distinctions. Each definition took me one step further in defining who I am—really—and altered the boundaries preventing me from obtaining my goals. Each definition offered me a better view of who I *could* be while allowing me to better understand who I really *wanted* to be.

The best way to explain the meaning of these definitions of self is to briefly share with you the different areas

"Find out who you are, and do it on purpose."

Dolly Parton

"We should take time out to really love, we should find out who we really are."

Lenny Kravitz

I searched and different answers I developed. What follows are *my* answers and involve *my* understandings of them. Your understandings may be different. In searching for who you are, you might disagree with my answers. That's fine because there isn't any one answer, but don't discount your own answers because each definition of self leads you to know and understand to a fuller extent who you are.

CHILDHOOD PERCEPTIONS

As a child, I didn't know about the many masks we wear. I just existed. The only boundaries I knew were those I'd given myself and those impressed on me by my parents from the day of my birth. As adults we forget we have multiple definitions of self or that we can alter who we are simply by taking on the role of a new identity[1]. As children, we thrive on new identities, role-playing wherever and whenever our imaginations allow.

For example, while still quite small, I received a set of books containing photos of exotic animals and faraway places. I didn't know how to read, so I just gazed at the pictures. More than any other, I most often turned to a photo of a jaguar perched in a low-lying tree. From the photo I gained an impression of its size, ability, and overall presence. I seemed to know instinctively of its search for food, water, and shelter. Since I couldn't see it, touch it, or feel it in person, I *became* it. I crawled around the floor on my hands and knees pretending to be a jaguar. My pretending allowed me to experience the animal more fully and to make it a part of my being.

A very different type of incident happened to me around six years of age. I often spent warm afternoons on my backyard swing set and, as many children do, I would sing songs and make up stories as I played on the swings, glider, and slide. One story in particular I've never forgotten.

The story told of a close-knit brother and sister traveling alone to a new world from a distant place. They had been spirited away in the night through some secretive mission of which the sister didn't fully understand even though she knew she had been training for it all of her life. Most of all, she worried about being separated from her

"Conventional thinking holds that masks conceal. Dionysius teaches that masks also reveal."
Keith Thompson,
Angels and Aliens

305

brother, who'd been charged with watching over her. He, having a fuller understanding of the journey and its purpose, assured her that all would be as it should and ominously told her not to worry if they should become separated, as they would find each other again.

The accompanying song I sang concerned the journey itself that took place first by horse, then by flight in a mystical vehicle, then on foot as the pair traveled a great distance to their new destination. Suddenly, they were blinded by a white light, and she lost her brother in its brilliance.

At that same moment, something startled me from the surreality of the story and, in doing so, burned the tale forever in my mind.

Looking across the landscape, I saw a man clearing brush in the woods on the edge of our property not far from where I played. Though only the next-door neighbor going about his Saturday afternoon yard work, I hadn't realized anyone had been watching or listening to me sing. Apologetic and recognizing he had startled me, he said, "Don't let me stop you. Keep singing," but the spell had been broken. Once again, I returned to being a six year old standing atop her sliding board—the magical mountain and loving brother were gone.

For a moment I'd been a dignitary, a being of another world. I did not have to ask myself if it were possible or even probable. As a child, I could tell myself any story I liked and live it to its fullest for as long as I pleased. No one questioned a child for doing so, though some might call it silly or make-believe.

A few years ago, I had the occasion to meet author Leonard Bishop who taught that in order to promote themselves successfully, all authors needed a story for themselves, a story to tell when explaining why as an author they were different or special. This is the story that makes them stand out as a writer or celebrity. Leonard claimed that he'd been a hobo before deciding to write a book. His story added character to the fictional tales he wrote as they caused his readers to wonder what parts of his novels might be taken from his true-life adventures.

The value and importance of this ability is often lost on us as adults. We don't realize that even today we are living out our stories. I hear stories being told all the time,

"How could it be that this went back into my childhood? How could it be? And if that wasn't true, and my mind had chosen to do this to itself, then what was it doing, and why?"

Whitley Strieber,
Communion

stories called "How ill I am," or "How poor I am," stories called, "Why I can never be a success," or "Why I can't change." Some stories are tragic, others sorrowful. Some are joyous too.

What is your story? What is the life you have created for yourself? What would happen if you stopped telling your particular story and changed it in some way? What could you become if you no longer focused on the story of "how I'm trapped in my job" or "How I am the only one who can care for my ill mother (father, sister, brother...)"?

When you meet someone for the first time and they ask you questions about who you are, how do you answer? I recently had an opportunity to speak with an acquaintance I hadn't seen for five or six years. Surprised to see him now in a wheelchair, I said, "How are you?" He said, "I have accepted the fact that I must stay in this chair." Yet he went on to explain how his being in the wheelchair had been a *choice* he'd made since he still had the ability to walk. He now chose to stay in the chair and made his repertoire from telling others the story of his chair. When the story no longer interests those he tells, will his story have to worsen? Will he need to become more ill to make his story valid and interesting again?

My mother used to complain that my father would exaggerate the stories he told. She didn't mind the exaggerations except, she said, after he told the story a few times, he began to believe them as fact. The more we tell the stories of who we are the more we believe them, the more our actions coincide with what we've said, the more our lives become our stories.

Rosemary Altea has an exercise in her book *You Own the Power* that asks the user to tell the same story of their life from three different perspectives: sad, happy, and inspirational. This shows how each of our stories can be remolded and redesigned from whatever perspective we wish. I wonder what would happen to my friend in the wheelchair if he began to say he would soon be getting out of the chair?

When I was a little girl and my family moved to Ohio, I wanted to be a new person. I wanted to rewrite the story of "Who I am." When I met the next-door neighbors and their kids, I told them my name was Lynn. I remained Lynn for several weeks, never giving it a second thought.

"The Way of Self-Reliance starts with recognizing who we are, what we've got to work with, and what works best for us."
Benjamin Hoff,
The Tao of Pooh

307

Then one afternoon the neighbor's father knocked on our door asking if he could take "Lynn" to get some ice cream. I had some explaining to do then, but I had learned an important lesson. I can be creative with myself. If I am dull and boring, mired in predictability, it is only because that's how I have created myself to be, that's how I've told my story. If, however, I write in my hopes of success, my ambitions toward my dreams, suddenly my stories begin to create for themselves opportunities and accomplishments.

If you are not happy with the story of who you are, try changing the way you tell it. See what possibilities you can write into the new you. See who you can be when you redesign the story of "who I am—really."

HISTORICAL PERCEPTIONS

Why is it that so many of us intensely relate to a particular period or periods in the past? How can our personal interests in history help us to better know ourselves? How does history play a role in who we are?

Each of us finds ways to incorporate history into our lives. Some of us by visiting historical sites, others by enjoying historical movies, books, or plays. There are those who take pleasure in collecting memorabilia from a particular era, event, or locale, while others will actually participate in reenactments or themed fairs. How do these interests define who we are?

When I began learning how to understand visions by using dream interpretation, I came across a book by Hugh Lynn Cayce (psychic reader and Edgar Cayce's son). The young Cayce wrote how through dreams we could discover our reincarnated path. However, he also explained how our personal interests and natural attraction to particular individuals and periods of time insinuated connections to reincarnation as well. He recommended that we pay attention to the types of books and movies we watched as well as those personalities from history we felt drawn to. He claimed these stories shed light on who we had been in the past, which ultimately offered us insight into who we are today.

I've found that these interests are not something we simply follow benignly, but rather we become passionate about them, allowing them to influence the clothes we

"All our knowledge has its origins in our perceptions."
Leonardo da Vinci

308

wear, the decorations we buy, and the way we live our lives. We might even pick up on this at a very young age.

Sometime during the fourth or fifth grade, I became fascinated by Native Americans, particularly with their hieroglyphics and their living off the land. I went so far as to make a native dress decorated with beads and fringe. I also made pages and pages of drawings using Native American symbol words that I had copied from library books. I found it fascinating that people might have an entire written language made up of glyphs rather than words.[2]

Several years ago, I had a session with a hypnotherapist who led me through a past-life regression. I'd never done anything like that before. During the session, I began to talk about the life of a famous Native American. Though I had heard this individual's name before, I knew nothing about him. Nevertheless, during the session I expressed many impressions about him, including personal feelings for his wife and family, religious beliefs, and some regrets on how he had lived out his life. I later researched this individual and discovered letters he'd written where I could verify many of my impressions. Not only did I seem to correctly know historic fact but I also knew the inner motivations of the man.

How did I know these things? Had I been reincarnated from him? I remained a skeptic. Yet I had tapped into enough of his thoughts, heart, and mind to be intrigued. Did this explain my childhood interest in Native Americans? Did this explain another part of who I am—really?

Is there such a thing as reincarnation? No one can definitively say. However, beginning in 1976, a series of events began that eventually led me to believe there is.

As a teen, I twirled baton and belonged to a group that wore Scottish kilts as their costume. As part of our routine, I'd been selected to be the feature, to do a bit of the Highland Fling, a traditional Scottish dance. Those who picked me from a group of girls said I seemed to do it the best, though I'd never done the dance before that day.

The director decided we should travel to Scotland and demonstrate our abilities abroad,[3] which we did. While there, we performed in many shows and also visited many historical sites. Edinburgh stands out in my mind more

"There are ways in which you can live on this plane and be aware of many other realities and, in doing so, enrich your existence here."

Iris Belhayes,
Spirit Guides

than any other city due to the many odd things that happened to me there.

The first occurred during a visit to historical Edinburgh Castle. On the grounds stands a small chapel dedicated to Saint Margaret who prayed there as her husband and son fought and died in a war during the 11th century. The tiny building houses nothing except a few plaques on the walls and a couple of display tables. Most of the kids in our group stuck their head in the door, took a quick glance in either direction, then went exploring else-where. I, on the other hand, didn't want to leave that place. I found myself mesmerized by the room. I walked in and lost all track of time or place. I had no idea I'd done this until my mother broke the spell by pointing out, "You seem to be very content in here." I had no explanation why. I can't even remember anything I saw while standing in there. I only knew she was right.

Had I been drawn by St. Margaret's energy—or something else? Later in the day, another odd event happened. We were staying at a college dorm within walking distance of Arthur's Seat, an old weather-beaten, craggy mountain that had been the home to many tales from lore.

I'd been infatuated with a boy in the group who would sometimes pay attention to me and other times not. Being young, I had my share of emotional ups and downs. I would get upset when he ignored me. We had a disagreement and I found myself running for safety. I felt as though I were running for my life and couldn't stop until I'd reached the saftey of the hill. There I remained until sometime later when the boy and a few other friends came to find me.

I never gave these incidents much thought until after reading Hugh Lynn Cayce's book.

I later read Margaret George's 880-page tale *Mary, Queen of Scotland and The Isles: A Novel,* where I learned of her daring escapes, one where she took refuge on Arthur's Seat. It also told of her being in the small chapel on the castle grounds. While I didn't want to think I might have been reincarnated from her (it seemed foolish to me) no matter what her final plight, I couldn't help but remember the panic that had run through me as I hid on Arthur's Seat. Had I reeinacted some prior flight?

Not long after reading the Cayce book, a friend invited me to her writer's group. One of the exercises began with

"What do we mean by the discovery of identity? We mean finding out what your real desires and characteristics are, and being able to live in a way that expresses them."

Abraham H. Maslow,
The Farther Reaches of Human Nature

the group's leader offering each person a verbal character sketch from whose perspective we were instructed to write the answer to a given question. The leader, who had quite a knack for doing this kind of thing, would stare into the eyes of each person for a moment before assigning the characters, who might be anyone from an ancient Egyptian slave to a 19th century Chinese monk, to a 20th-Century barmaid. Without having ever met me, and knowing almost nothing about me, she chose for me the position of handmaiden to Mary, Queen of Scots on the night of her beheading. Chills ran up my spine as she said it. Just having her tap into my interest in the queen seemed impossible and creepy.

I've had a variety of odd occurrences spanning many periods of time and places of historic reference, as I believe we all have in some form or another. What do they mean? What added dimension do they bring to our lives? They are another part of who we are. How should we use them? What can we do with this information?

For me, the most valuable aspect comes from looking at the people and places symbolically. By defining them in the same way I would interpret a mirror *(See: Chapter 19)*, I am able to see them in more concrete and usable terms.

For example, Mary, Queen of Scots was a woman thrust upon the throne, not by choice, but by the lineage of her birth. In her reign, she sought to bring together the English and Scottish peoples. She sought to uphold her Catholic faith. She sought to find balance between her royal duties and her personal loves and passions for life. In many of these things she did not succeed, partly because her true reign had been puppeted by her advisors, but also because of her incapacity to escape the boundaries set by her royal position and religious upbringing.

If I am to benefit from her memory and widespread historical presence, I must learn from her accomplishments and from her failures in much the same way I would learn from my parents. *(See: Section III)* I must look at what she stands for—to me—and see how those platforms apply to my life. Only by doing these things can her memory be of any good to me, regardless of any rhetorical connection I may or may not have had to her past. The same goes for any historical connections you may have.

"When we study our own consciousness, we find it has many different faces. These aspects occur both within and around us, comprising the fundamental basis of any reality we experience."

Anodea Judith,
Wheels of Life

311

ALIEN PERCEPTIONS

Around the same time I was fighting off severe depression and some time after seeing the angel materialize in my living room, I had a vivid vision, unlike any I had ever had before.

The vision was more like a lucid dream. Unlike a vision, this wasn't a series of disconnected, symbolic images. Although seen in the same way I would see a vision, in my mind, I could actively participate in the dream. Had it not been given to me in this form, I would not have given it a second thought. But because it came in the means that it did, I found myself dumbstruck and once again on a new search for who I am.

As I've already explained, during my period of severe depresion, I'd lost my will to live and had prayed to die. Even after having seen the angel and feeling much revived, I occasionally had bad days and suffered periods of doubt. On one of those days, I'd been wishing I could just "go home" when the following happened.

While standing in my living room, my mind's eye turned to seeing in the waking dream. I saw the roof of our home parted and opened, and from the clouds in the sky, an enormous spaceship appeared and hovered just above my head. From where I stood, I could make out beings at the helm through windows that circled the top half of the vehicle. These beings then began to have a telepathic conversation with me, the gist of which was that they assured me I could go home anytime I pleased. They reminded me, however, that I had not yet fulfilled my purpose.

As before, when Jesse appeared to me, I understood my purpose on a subconscious level, but in a place out of reach from my conscious comprehension. On one level, I could acknowledge my mission and its incompleteness, while on the other, I had no idea what they might mean. Something inside of me acknowledged the importance of my purpose and also my agreement made in some other place and time to fulfill it.

So I asked, "Will I fulfill my purpose?" and they answered, "Yes." Then they promised that if at any time in the future I changed my mind, I could return home.

There must have been other communications going on at some other level as well to bring me the inner assurance

"If I talk to you, if I tell you about the weird things which have been going on around me,' I heard myself saying aloud, 'you will surely think I'm nuts.'"
Rosemary Atlea,
Eagle and the Rose

"I still wonder. I wonder what effect this journal will have? No doubt, I won't be believed, and that's all right, because, in a sense, it leaves me free in ways that belief would not."
Whitley Strieber,
Whitley's Journal

that I felt. I don't recall any polite niceties such as "thanks," "good-bye," or "good luck." I only remember them turning the ship and leaving. The ceiling closed up, and once again I stood alone in my living room.

It occurred to me later that had the ship really been there, it would have been much larger than the house, and that due to its immense size, I wouldn't have been able to make out the inhabitants in the way that I did, let alone talk to them. But I didn't worry about any of those things since it had only been a dream of some sort—though it troubled me that I knew more about what had occurred than seemed logical. Then again, how logical could a space vehicle appearing in my living room be?

More importantly, the whole "spaceship thing" and it sbeing connected to God and purpose, threw my mind into a spin. I had never considered God and aliens as being connected, though I do remember a cousin and I discussing bible verses about angels and gods flying in clouds. She felt the references to clouds in the scripture referred to spaceships.

The consideration of God being alien sent me on a new search for answers and self-definition. I began reading, Whitley Strieber, Zachariah Sitchen, and other UFO authors. I particularly searched for information about blue-eyed blonds because Jesse was one. BEBs (blue-eyed blonds), as I came to refer to them, were often mentioned in books about aliens, but rarely elaborated on, so I still had no real understanding of what Jesse might really be.

I struggled to put a definition on who or what Jesse was because of the changes that had taken place in my life after his appearance. Something real had happened even if what I saw had been all in my mind.

Those few I told encouraged me to refer to him as an angel because their minds could accept his appearance if he were an angel—in other words, they weren't so inclined to send me away to a padded room for speaking of angels. Aliens were another thing.

As for me, I wasn't so sure. As I searched scripture, I found references that could be misleading. Definitions we unintentionally misinterpreted simply because our minds are closed to other avenues of thinking. I began writing a book that played on these definitions and their otherworld

"Do you want to know more about extraterrestrials? Do you want a definition of angels? We are you, yourself, in the distant past and distant future. We are you as you were, would have been and still are, had you not fallen from your original state of grace. We exist in a parallel universe of non-form, experiencing what you would have experienced had you not become associated with the materializing processes."
Kenneth X. Carey,
The Starseed Transmissions

"... that ETs are the new manifestations of angels or demons—
is a very popular one. It fits very
snugly with those who believe
that earth has been visited by
space travelers many times
before throughout our history. It
is equally acceptable to those
who feel that angels assume the
cultural or mythic form most
acceptable for any particular era
or milieu."

Malcolm Godwin,
Angels, an Endangered Species

possibilities. I started thinking of the biblical patriarchs in a different way once I realized that "foreign" in Hebrew could also mean "alien." "Angel," after all, simply meant "messenger," and some of the angels written about in the bible were more than just the typical harp-playing folk.

It made sense to me that angels were technically alien since, above all else, I knew for sure they weren't human. This, of course, did not change my feelings about God's angels, their calling, their ability to bring God's messages or to do His work. I just saw angels from a different perspective than most. It also occurred to me that there were countless people who believed in angels, something comforting and acceptable to most, while aliens were berated, scorned, and feared. Yet angels were definitely not the same breed as the "grays" credited with abductions and human experimentations.

I must not have been the only one thinking of such things because Scott Mandelker's book, *From Elsewhere: Being E. T. in America,* appeared on the bookshelves around the same time—and sold well. I remember taking the book on an airplane and reading it with the paper sleeve off because I didn't want anyone to know what I was reading. I figured I already had enough quirks for people to label me "crazy" and felt fortunate that I wasn't getting "communications from Neptune." Not because I couldn't believe in the possibility, but simply because I wasn't brave enough to tell others if I had. It was difficult enough telling people I saw visions and often said instead, "I had a dream," to ease their minds with something they would likely find more acceptable. Nowadays, it's more in vogue to speak of spiritual things and alien beings too, but at the time, it wasn't, so I kept quiet about all that I'd experienced.

In Chapter 17 *(Writing)*, I explained how writing fiction can allow us to write about what we might not be able to accept otherwise. After the experiences detailed above, I wrote two science fiction novels whose premises crossed alien boundaries, one discussing parallel universes, the other about a planet that had been destroyed. The premise of the second focused on the survivors who'd evacuated to another of the system's planets.

Through those stories I could allow myself to write

314

about alternative realities without feeling uncomfortable in dealing with issues that didn't fit in our day-to-day world. I could explain the unexplained without worrying about what anyone might think. After I wrote them, I put them away in a drawer and moved on to other things. However, many years later, I pulled them out again.

Sometime in the late 1990s, I made a new friend. Our first conversation lasted four hours. We immediately felt connected and have always known when the other was in some dire straits even though we live hundreds of miles apart. In one of our deep discussions, I mentioned my writings in passing. Coincidentally, she had also been writing a similar story about a destroyed planet, though her story focused on a different part of the solar system than mine. It was as if we both knew the same story, but from different perspectives.

Then, to make the story even more incredible, another friend pointed me to the channeled books of Patricia L. Pereira *(Songs of the Arcturians)*. Among her written transmissions from the Arcturians were descriptions of the destruction of a planet she referred to as "Cheuel." I found many parellels between her references and my novel.

There were hundreds of other oddities, too many to explain here. After a while, I just accepted the fact that I could add the label of "alien" in my ever-widening quest to discover "Who am I—really." I decided it didn't matter because this label was just another one of those things I kept in my imagination box, something I pondered from time to time, and didn't really affect whether or not I had to do laundry or go to the grocery store. In the long term, I decided we were all a little bit alien since we all had a soul—and that seemed alien to me.

BEYOND THE GALAXIES

Writing has a way of bringing out things that are hidden deeply in our minds and a way of connecting things we might not have connected under ordinary circumstances. This is not only true when searching for internal truths, but it works just as well for solving problems or creating new inventions. For me, writing became a catalyst for unearthing buried definitions of self. Not all of

"The horrors of that cataclysmic explosion continue to reverberate throughout the universe. The repercussions of the event resound through the corridors of your subconscious minds and filter into the depths of your sorrow-filled hearts. Cheuel's fiery demise is reflected in your dream images and meditative visions."

Patricia L. Pereira,
Songs of Malantor

315

"Unless you open yourself to something greater than yourself, you can never experience your complete self. And so you remain hemmed in by the conditions of what you think the self is."
Ken Eagle Feather,
A Toltec Path

these were discovered on my own. Some were the result of exercises which were part of Tom Bird's Intensive Writer's Program.

During the beginning of the program, I suffered terribly from writer's block and found myself unable to work on what would one day become this book. In an effort to help break me from the block's hold, Tom asked me to write about an imaginary character we began creating while on the phone. I called my character "Miranda," and quickly realized she was a remembrance of my sister. Whether reincarnation or simply a process of DNA, I wrote and experienced things about her death that were . . . well . . . disturbing. Disturbing because I relived her death. I relived the car hitting her. I relived her being unable to communicate in the hospital. I relived her being disconnected from the life support machines, even though all this happened before I was born.

All I can say is that it had to have been very difficult for a nine-year-old girl to understand what happened to her. How could she make amends for a split-second error like stepping off the curb into the path of an oncoming car? How exactly does one apologize for the immense amount of grief and pain a family endured due to having lost an integral part of themselves? How does one make up for the life of opportunity they had—and lost? How does a nine-year-old girl explain that she is still alive even though her body has been rendered useless?

What I came to understand through this particular piece of writing was that somehow, in some aspect, my sister lived inside of me. No one can explain this in scientific terms, but I know it's somehow true. I know this explains why I fear sudden death, and why, at nine years old, the same age she died, I began crossing my legs at the ankles when I slept so I wouldn't be mistaken for dead. No one told me to do these things. My sister and her death were rarely spoken of in our home.

My mother forbade me to take tap dancing because my sister had been a talented dancer. It pained my mother too much to have me be a dancer too. Yet no one could explain why, when I went behind my mother's back and put on my friend's tap shoes, I instinctively knew how to make them work.

No one could explain why for nearly the whole of my

life I carried with me an inner sorrow that would not leave or be released. While as adults we have many reasons to be sorrowful, a child has few unless in dire circumstances. Logically, I rationalized that it made sense to me that it might not be my sorrow but hers. Her sorrow for causing her family so much pain. Her sorrow for all that she lost.

It doesn't matter if anyone believes this because it is only something that lives inside me. It is just another aspect of who I am.

It does affect my choices. It does affect the decisions I make. I practically sweated blood when my husband had living wills written up and asked me to sign one. Did this mean I might have to relive my sister's death all over again when my turn to die neared?

It does affect my understanding of some things. All of my labels do. That is why they are important to me and why they are important to you. That is why you need to know what your labels are and where they come from. You don't have to share your labels with anyone; it was very hard for me to do, and I have only revealed these things for the sake of readers who may benefit from them. It also doesn't mean your labels have to rule or block your life. By uncovering them and defining them you have the power to set the boundaries they can keep. It gives you the power to put limitations on how your labels affect you. It gives you the power to heal the parts of your life you may not have understood before.

Knowing what I do about my sister, even if it is nothing more than one hundred percent pure imagination, allowed me to understand and heal the parts of my life she had touched. Knowing of her sorrow and remorse allowed me to understand my own. Discovering and defining your lables will do the same for you.

MORE WRITTEN REVELATIONS OF SELF

At another time during my work with Tom Bird and his Intensive Writer's Program, he asked me to create a character for each of my main attributes. I later learned that he expected me to write about only one or two, maybe three at the most, that really stood out. I came up with twelve. However, each one of them taught me something

"Discovering your specieshood, at a deep enough level, merges with discovering your selfhood. Becoming (learning how to be) fully human means both enterprises carried on simultaneously. You are learning (subjectively experiencing) what you peculiarly are, how you are you, what your potentialities are, what your style is, what your pace is, what your tastes are, what your values are, what direction your body is going, where your personal biology is taking you, i.e., how you are different from the others. and at the same time it means learning what it means to be a human animal like other human animals, i.e., how you are similar to others."

Abraham H. Maslow,
The Farther Reaches of Human Nature

about myself and were part of the "who am I—really" path. The twelve aspects were:

The Child (whom I called Little Miranda): There is a very large part of me that is a strong-willed child. She is awed by the forces of nature whether it be the tremendous blow of a hurricane or the wonders of a centipede's walk. She is full of love, understanding, and forgiveness, yet stubbornly independent.

Andrew, the scientist, is the logical one, the part of me that must have facts and evidence to prove a theory or to come out on top of an argument. He is the computer specialist and electronics wiz. He is quiet, reserved, the type that would sit at the back of the room and never open his mouth, but if he did, genius would pour out.

Edward is the analyst and statistician. He requires data. Lots of it. He must record everything—to a fault. He wants to know how much I weigh, how many times I biked around the block, what I did with draft number six after writing draft number seven. He can be a headache unless Andrew is in search of a fact. Edward labels or categorizes everything and if it's not done, he feels as if he's in chaos.

There are other aspects of me which I've defined, but which need little explanation. There is "Mrs. Cleaver" who represents the mother in me. The alien queen who was from the exploding planet explained earlier. There are also the healer, the teacher, the artist, the wife, the angel, and the writer/communicator. Last, but not least, is Sophia who culminates the overall wisdom of them all.

CORE ENERGIES

Way deep down inside, at the deepest point of who we are, is a core energy best described as an archetype known directly or indirectly to all. This core energy is that which directs the path and essence of our lives. Examples of these images might be Jesus, Mary, any of the patriarch saints, or any of the founding religious fathers, such as Buddha. Not all of the archetypes come from religion but many of them do because when these individuals walked the earth, their energies were such that those who came into contact with them were profoundly changed. This in turn caused

"When you see your likeness, you rejoice. But when you see your images which came into being before you, and which neither die nor become manifest, how much you will have to bear."
The Gospel of Thomas,
The Nag Hammadi Library

these individuals to be lifted up and worshipped as gods, even if they didn't mean to be.

As I've tried to show throughout this chapter, we are multifaceted beings. Thus we are always evolving, growing, learning, reaching up, metamorphosing, reaching for all that we are. When we reach into our higher mind, we eventually find the image of the core figurehead. This is not to say that this is the end point of who we are, for beyond the figurehead lies the interconnectivity to the all. Within that living component is another realm beyond the scope of this book.

For now, I will explain two energies so that you may better understand. The first is what I refer to as the seed energy. I like to use a sunflower as an example for the seed energy because it is beautiful, healthful, and produces many seeds.

For each thriving sunflower that grows, many seeds are formed. Of those that are later planted, a new plant just like its parent grows. This new plant is entirely new except for its DNA, which remembers its parent. The new plant may evolve in some way. It may adapt to new surroundings, but the important thing to remember is that it is an entirely new plant.

The seed energy comes to us through DNA, through ancestry, heritage, and reincarnation. These energies carry with them the innate challenges we must overcome, and the physical boundaries that we have set for ourselves. For example, a sunflower cannot become a rose, a beetle cannot become a grasshopper, a dog cannot become a horse. The seed energy dictates our boundaries.

The seed energy lives in annual cycles. It is born. It lives. It thrives. It produces flowers or fruits. It bears seed. Then it dies.

The second energy is the vine energy. When I think of the vine energy, I think of the ivy that grows thickly in my flower bed. If I want to grow it in another spot, I do not need seeds, rather I take a cutting from the growing plant. This means that when I place the cutting in the new flower bed, I am actually still only growing one plant. Though it has been separated from itself, it still is itself. No matter how many cuttings I take, no matter how many flower beds I start, I still have one plant separated from itself. Jesus said, "I am the vine." He said, "My father is in

"There are dimensions upon dimensions. There are as many viewpoints as can be imagined and almost as many worlds. And yet, we are all as much a part of one as the others. These dimensions interact with one another in a myriad of ways. There is no way that any part of All There Is can be cut off and exist separately."

Iris Belhayes,
Spirit Guides

319

me and I in him." They were the same "plant" just separated and planted elsewhere.

The vine energy produces our higher calling. It is the part of us that defines our highest purpose. Vine energy follows seasons but doesn't die annually rather, it constantly renews itself, provided the appropriate conditions exist.

In Section IV, I spoke of reaching the higher mind. Seed energy is the energy of the left and right hemispheres. Vine energy is the energy of the higher mind.

To live as the vine, we must tap into the higher mind. To reach the higher mind, we must seek out connection and the voice within. To find the voice, we must first find relief, heal our lives, seek our purpose, and come to know ourselves. When we know ourselves, we will know God. When we know God, we will know unconditional love and we will be one. We will be of the vine.

I AM THE RAINBOW

At the time I wrote this section, I saw a vision where I stood beneath a glimmering shaft of white light. The light felt loving, warm, comforting. Then the light turned into a rainbow, and I realized that each of the colors represented an aspect of me. We all have many aspects of self that we carry with us. We all have different labels that we can wear. Knowing how these can be used to benefit our lives ultimately helps us to heal our lives and live in total well-being. Be a rainbow and embrace all that you are, all that you can be.

"Behold the nature of light that is ours to command: the tools of our trade, the rainbow-hued optical wonders of purples, blues, oranges, yellows, pinks, violets, greens, and reds."
Patricia L. Pereira,
Eagles of the New Dawn

FLASHLIGHTS

When I first started sharing the concepts of this book, one of my friends, Pat, shared with me the following story.

Pat said that in our lives we are all trying to follow a dimly lit path. But every once in a while, we come across someone who has a flashlight. Pat said she thought I had a flashlight. She had met several people who she thought carried one.

However, what I explained to her was that we all can be flashlights. That is what the concepts in this book are intended to do—give to you the power so you can be a flashlight too.

IN CONCLUSION

I am not any one of the definitions listed in this chapter, I am all of them. All of these characters, all of these aspects, all of these labels which have been discussed in this chapter are in some way a part of who I am—really. They are all pieces I can pull when I tell the story of "who I am."

Many of us have forgotten about our other aspects or only focus on one part of ourselves, which limits what we can tell in our story and limits our ability to be who we were meant to be.

Take time to read through this chapter and its many sections carefully and search for all the many aspects of yourself by working through the different areas of thought.

Think of all the ways you can write the story of "Who I am," and start to use the power of those aspects to reach for and achieve your dreams. Go back, if necessary, and relook at the map you created under *Skills* and see if you have left off any important aspects of yourself. Go back, if necessary, and rewrite your goals and dreams to include any strengths you may have had forgotten. Go back to the sections on Heritage and think again of how history has been a part of creating who you are. Consider again how Writing may reveal those parts of yourself beyond your conscious acceptance of who you might be—really.

Most importantly, remember that connection is the tool you need to tap into your greatest potential.

"Your daily habits, including your thoughts about yourself and what you tell others about yourself, establish a specific continuity. Not only do these habits seal your identity in terms of what others expect of you, they also lock your focal point in place. . . . To break into the unknown, that continuity must be set aside; hence, erase it."

Ken Eagle Feather,
A Toltec Path

EPILOGUE 26

A few years ago, I joined an online Hodgkins disease support list. I thought I might be able to lend encouragement to those now plagued with the disease. What I discovered is that they could not focus on being well. They could only focus on their treatment.

When I signed on and wrote of my survival and of overcoming the disease, no one asked me how I did it. They could not think in those terms. They only wanted to know, "How many doses of radiation?" "What strength?" "What type of accelerator?" When I explained I'd forgotten all of that (I am not sure I ever knew it), they had no interest in talking to me.

What I suggest is that as long as you continue to put your focus on what it is to be ill, you will continue to be ill. The only way to turn that around is to change your focus to that of becoming well.

Change your focus. That is step one. Change of focus by talking to people who became well. Ask them what they did. Compare not treatments but actions and see where yours differ from theirs. Decide which of their well-being actions you can incorporate into your life. Do not allow yourself to become entrapped in the game Carolyn Myss calls "woundology." Avoid

"The only time you mustn't fail is the last time you try."
Charles F. Kettering

"When a woman focuses too much on healing a condition, she often does so to avoid facing the issues that led to the condition in the first place. Thus the healing process itself becomes addictive."

Christiane Northrup,
Women's Bodies,
Women's Wisdom

exchanging "war stories" and practice "well" stories instead. If you cannot speak of your own wellness, fill your mind with the stories of others who are. Allow their success to help germinate your own. If you don't personally know anyone who has made the journey to wellness, then search books, movies, and the Internet for others who have overcome whatever is challenging you.

If you've just been diagnosed with a major, life-threatening ailment, know that it might take some time before this book can help you because of the reasons described above. It is very difficult to change your focus when doctors are poking, cutting, x-raying, and examining you every thirteen seconds. It is even more difficult if the ailment also brings with it some type of pain. While all these things could be overcome with the exercises in this book, it will be much more difficult to do so during your diagnosis and treatment process, particularly if your disease is far advanced or your condition is severe.

At some point, however, whether during your initial medical treatment, or some time later, you'll come to a point where you take a somewhat selfish stance and decide no matter what the cost emotionally, you are going to do everything you can to heal your life. That can take many forms. It might be a subtle reaction where you pull back from the noise of life, or an extreme turnaround, where you make a dramatic U-turn from whatever you might have been doing previously. In either case, you'll have come to the point of commitment, as described in Section II, and are now ready to really use the principles described in this book. It's also at that point where your commitment causes you to take a new look at who you are and who you want to be.

I've given you the knowledge I've acquired in healing my own life and hope the five keys—*Relief, Commitment, Goals, Connection,* and *Synchronicity*—will be of help to you in finding healing for yours.

As you travel along your journey to total well-being, please drop me a note via the addresses provided in this book and share your journey with me. I love to hear how people have healed their lives, overcome their innate challenges, achieved their goals, and created a new life for themselves.

Remember the journey to well-being begins with you.

Each step you take, whether today, tomorrow, or next week, puts you one step closer to wellness. Choose to begin today.

I wish you the greatest success and send you my prayers for your full recovery, not only from any pain or physical ailment, but from whatever is blocking you from living your life and purpose to its fullest.

Jamie L. Saloff

"What the caterpillar calls the end of the world, the master calls a butterfly."
Richard Bach,
Illusions

To Contact Jamie:

Visit her website at:

www.ICanTransform.com
or
www.TransformationalHealing.net

or you may write to her at:

Jamie L. Saloff
C/O Sent Books
P.O. Box 339
Edinboro, PA 16412

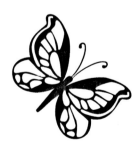

ACKNOWLEDGMENTS

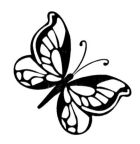

Writing a book is an adventure in itself with its own share of ups and downs, ins and outs, successes and failures. More than anything, it offered me an eclectic collection of supporters and friends who kept me going throughout the many years I worked on this and preliminary works. Without these people, I would have long ago given up on completing this extensive project, but probably at the cost of my health since it's so extensively tied to my innate challenges and purpose.

One of the greatest of those people is my husband, Tim, who from our first meeting, enjoyed reading whatever I had written and encouraged me to keep doing so, even when he didn't always agree with my way of going about it. Although his encouragement began years before I conceived this book, without his support I'd never have made it this far.

It was my husband who came home one evening after work and let me know he'd heard author Tom Bird on a local radio show. I'd heard he was offering a seminar on writing and wondered if it would be worth my while. My husband assured me that it would.

When I met Tom Bird, I began the most wonderful and difficult adventure of my life. The difficult part was due to my

"This means that in your body (and in your life) you have to be willing to go into and to be with what is happening in the moment. You then have to be willing to stay there long enough to tune into it and make the necessary adjustments. This is really the process of transformation."

Michael Lee,
Phoenix Rising Yoga Therapy

"*Sometimes being a friend means mastering the art of timing. There is a time for silence. A time to let go and allow people to hurl themselves into their own destiny. And a time to prepare to pick up the pieces when it's all over.*"

Gloria Naylor

own stubborness and refusal to listen to all Tom taught about the writing process. Because of my procrastination, on more than one occasion I put myself through hell while suffering through all the chaos that comes when sidestepping one's purpose. Nevertheless, Tom waited through all my whining and grumbling, offering whatever kick in the pants or firm guidance I needed at the time in order to keep redirecting me back toward my God-given path— Tom's specialty and calling. Above all else, Tom encouragaed me to be myself and he accepted me as me, no matter how many times my self-definition changed. I'll always be grateful for that.

God knows what we need and when we need it. There came a time when I needed something different from what Tom or my husband could offer. I remember from the first, my conversations with Dr. Nell M. Rodgers were different from those with anyone else. Like Tom, she accepted me for who I was, but more than that, took time out of an already overloaded schedule to offer me dedicated friendship and support. "Call me at 3 a.m. in the morning if you have to," she once said, and meant it. Fortunately, I never did, but always knew I could if necessary. Perhaps one of the best things about "Doc Nell", as she likes to be called, is that she isn't afraid to "call the kettle black." She taught me a lot about speaking and living my Truth, as every one of us likes to put a good spin on a situation. She wasn't afraid to stop me midsentence to point out an error in my thinking, and helped me stay on track so I could finish this project.

Without the many phone calls and emails I received from Mary McGovern, this book would not have been so nearly complete. Her confidence to reveal herself gave me the courage to do the same. I do not think I would have even considered writing all I did in the last two sections of this book without her support and inspiration, even more so when I decided to put my own name on the cover rather than a pseudonym.

I'd also like to thank Dr. Thomas Walker, Nancy Melinda Hunley, and Kenneth Fink, all who have offered heartfelt friendship and understanding about the writer's path. I also cannot forget my soul sister, Lisa Burt, who has more than once gone beyond the call of duty to be there for me over the years.

I am grateful to those who helped me with early read-throughs on this and prior drafts. Joey Korn and his wife Jill offered much needed feedback; Sunday Larson showered me with her always exuberant enthusiasm; Lois Hoover can turn a subject inside out and often led me to see an angle I might have missed; Marilyn Marszalek offered me encouragement, no matter how weird the material got.

Another dear group of friends lent me support throughout the years from the days we sat around one or the other's kitchen table reading, critiquing, and encouraging each other's writing efforts. An honored thanks to Thelma Kirsch, Cindi Palatos, Shirley Seineta, Gloria Mentch, and Peggy Wilson. Nor can I ever forget the efforts of (Saint) Charles Behrens, who was there for me during some of the darkest days I've ever known.

Thanks to Michael Seidman who, more than once, went out of his way for me and who taught me to hold on to my personal writing voice. His wisdom in the field of writing taught me a tremendous amount about crafting a manuscript, and I hope all of his teachings are reflected in this book, (though I'm sure his eagle eyes will spot every flaw).

Much appreciation is offered to Dr. Charlie Pados and his family. Although his chiropractic treatments helped me find relief when I no longer believed any could be found, I'm certain it was his smile and laughter that were the ultimate remedy.

When I began working on the concepts of this book, my good friends Pat Boyles and Liana Garwig, along with a few others who sometimes joined us, allowed me to practice my exercises on them, giving me insight into how to best describe them to others in my book. They never laughed at me and only offered constructive advice, even when I had them dancing in Pat's living room. Thanks to Victoria Peltz who occasionally joined us and with whom I exchanged countless emails and phone calls over the years in an attempt to understand the meaning of the universe.

Pennwriters members Sharon K. Garner and Catherine McLean offered me invaluable help on the final draft of this book, lending their editing skills which enhanced the book greatly and lifted it to a higher level than even I could have expected. Truly, God has given them both a tremendous gift.

"Live life fully while you're here. Experience everything. Take care of yourself and your friends. Have fun, be crazy, be weird. Go out and screw up! You're going to anyway, so you might as well enjoy the process. Take the opportunity to learn from your mistakes: find the cause of your problem and eliminate it. Don't try to be perfect; just be an excellent example of being human."
Anthony Robbins

"Friends are relatives you make for yourself."

Eustache Deschamps

Heartfelt thanks to Julie Mayer who never failed to ask, no matter when or where I saw her, "Is the book done?" Her prodding always succeeded in encouraging me onward. As did the crew at the Oakfield Recreational Club. Thanks to Ben and Terrie Berhalter, who led us to the ORC, and special thanks to Duane and Mickey, Wally and Sue, Fran and Shirley, Bruce and Sandy, Ron and Colleen, Ed and Barb, and Terry and Val, along with the rest of the ORC members who offered their support weekly without fail. (Fran, I am remembering all your wild tales and filing them for future reference!) To all the members of the ORC, thanks for allowing us into your extended family.

I am also sincerely grateful to Mary Fisher of Mary Fisher Design, whose expertise in graphic design was essential in taking this book to the next level. With her fabulous presentation ideas, it's to Mary I give credit for inspiring me to name the book *Transformational Healing*.

Thanks to numbers guru Daniel Hardt from Life Path Numerology whose daily, uplifting readings kept me believing I could accomplish this huge task.

I haven't forgotten our good friends, Dick and Pat Coscia, who listened to me talk about this book for years and never doubted I would finish it, as well as Beth Charles, who will be surprised to learn that her daily emails and occasional golf matches remind me to stay connected to family and home, an important value for anyone seeking healing. I am thankful too that I've been blessed with such a wonderful mother-in-law, Joann Saloff, who has been a second mom to me, and I miss my father-in-law, Bill Saloff tremendously.

I'd like to honor as well, several teachers who offered me the encouragement a budding writer needs. Our teachers are often forgotten when we travel farther down the road of life. Many of their beneficial influences are never again mentioned. I don't want that to be the case here. The teachers who offered me the most encouragement and guidance were Miss Bell, who taught me to read; Mrs. Lois Dunsmore, for the books she read to the class and who taught us tenth grade English grammar in fifth grade (much of which had been removed from the curriculum by the time I arrived in tenth grade); Mrs. Eva Joanou, who gave my fingers the joy of fingering the type-writer keys in precision (Oh, how my fingers throbbed after pounding that old manual typewriter!); Ms. Mary Libertin, who gave us the freedom to "just write" without rules; Mrs. Betty Rottenberg (now Horvath, I'm told), whose encouraging notes I still have and cherish; Ms. Judy Sullivan, who read my explicit horror story to the class while I was out ill (I wonder if she still has it as it was never returned); and Mrs. Kaye Varley, who gave me the most creative year of schooling I ever had.

I am grateful to those who helped me reinvent my physical self: Jason (the hair god) from Toni & Guy (yes, it is beyond a doubt, worth the drive to Pittsburgh); A.J. from AJ's Famous Labels, my absolute favorite dress shop in Erie; and photographer extraordinaire, E. J. Morris, who understands the difference between a snapshot and creating a lasting and memorable image.

I must not forget my parents, who never questioned my belief that I would one day be a writer and who always allowed me the freedom to make whatever decisions I felt necessary for my future. I miss them both every day but know they are watching over me.

Last, and never least, love and thanks to my sons Matthew and Mark. I've written this book in part on your behalf so that you might be able to bypass much of the hardships I faced in trying to discover the principles in this book. I also appreciate all the times you offered me quiet when I asked for it, helped around the house when I was desperate for it, and fun and laughs in between. I'm very proud to call you my sons and I'm always awed by the intellectual conversations we have.

Blessings to all of these angels in disguise.

"Friends are angels sent down to earth to make good days and help us find our way."
author unknown

APPENDIXES

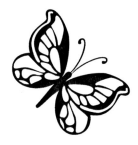

"If I'm afraid of something, that generally means I have to do it."
Madonna,
Elle magazine interview

APPENDIX A:
WORD ASSOCIATION:
HOW TO DO THE EXERCISES

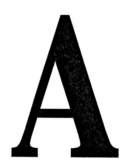

When working with the word-association exercises described herein, please remember the following:

STEP ONE

Writing forces the mind to clarify, define, and understand the thoughts written there. Words are no longer made up of symbols and code and ethereal essences, rather they become solidified and emphasize truth.

Do not discount the value of the written word. Do not presume you can obtain the same benefit by thought alone.

Use index cards, writing as quickly as possible on one, then another, and then another. Or use sticky notes and drop them in clusters onto a large sheet of poster board. During a lull in thought, rearrange the clusters to restimulate the mind into forward progress and deeper meaning.

STEP TWO

Always write whatever comes to mind, even if it appears to be off topic or irrelevant.

"Increasing your amount of information can help to manifest understanding you didn't even know you had. . . . grounding and activity, pulling energy down through the chakras, so the information can follow. . . . Like plugging in a lamp, if the information is there it will light up when connected to the proper context."

Anodea Judith,
Wheels of Life

Who can say why the mind connects the images and situations in the way that it does? And yet, today's seemingly irrelevant interactions and distractions may indeed be intertwined with those of your past.

Writing about a morning disagreement with your spouse may uncover a hidden message about an ailment from years before. A difficult situation at work may lend understanding to why you broke your wrist. It seems odd and impossible, but it's true. Try it and see.

STEP THREE

Always write ever so briefly using only one or two words or, at most, one short phrase or thought at a time. Then quickly move on to the next thought.

We are not asking ourselves to think or ponder or analyze each jot or note. Rather, we are attempting to travel deeper and deeper into our very core where the connection to our highest self resides, and with that connection we are given all the answers that we seek.

The answers we seek will do more than explain the underlying emotional connection between our ailment and our search for purpose. They will also offer us clarity and direction in terms we can understand to find and fulfill that purpose.

These answers have always been there for the asking, but we have blocked them in fear, having been programmed to do so by family, friends, education, religion, heritage, tradition, and society. Now we will break them free so they can guide us as they should.

STEP FOUR

In most cases, you will not need to save these stacks of cards or notes as it is not what the cards say that is most important, but rather the knowledge they uncover.

It is these previously unseen connections of the past to the present, the emotional underpinnings of our core, that we seek to record. Thus it is more important to write down your *conclusions*, as they are the signposts and maps you will later need.

". . . you will find that the act of carrying out the steps of the work and actually recording them in written form has the effect of stimulating a movement within you that draws forth awareness you would not have thought of in advance."

Ira Progoff,
At a Journal Workshop

APPENDIX B:
EXERCISE ONE
EXAMPLE:
SYMPTOMS, SYMBOLS, AND INSIGHTS

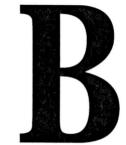

IMPORTANT INFORMATION
ABOUT THE FOLLOWING EXAMPLE

The example that follows is mentioned throughout the book and is based on Exercise One, Chapter 5.

My reasons for sharing this example with you are to:

- *Provide you with a detailed example of Exercise One, a core exercise for this book.*

- *Show you how an ailment or injury can provide you with a complex message containing multiple insights and direction for achieving wellness and purpose in your life.*

- *Demonstrate how leaps of thought are able to uncover previously undisclosed information, useful to the body-mind for healing.*

- *Explain how one ailment might merge with another for a similar message.*

"As difficult as it may be to consider, illness is also sometimes the answer to prayer, because it can be the means through which we discover our most valuable abilities and contribute the most to others. Such an illness can be thought of as a turning point at which you must exercise your power to choose."

Carolyn Myss,
Why People Don't Heal

Consultations:

Jamie offers personal coaching and a variety of online offerings.
Visit her website for more information.

www.ICanTransform.com

or

www.TransformationalHealing.net

The description that follows is innately personal to my own experience. If you are using this exercise as a companion to inner healing, you should work through the exercises yourself looking for your own connections and symbolic parallels because your insights will differ wildly from mine—which is exactly what makes the exercises in this book so uniquely personal and valuable to each of us.

Neither this or any other example in the book is intended to be a substitution for treatment or advice from your physician. All the exercises and insights in this book are provided solely for your deeper exploration and personal enlightenment. They are not intended to be exchanged for advice from your doctor. Please see your medical professional for any serious condition and treatment.

A SAMPLE EXERCISE IN FOUR PARTS

The sample exercise is presented in three parts as follows:

Part One is a flow chart showing words I wrote on index cards during my first assessment of the ailment. These were written one thought to a card in rapid succession and all the words were from one session. The flow chart appears on the next page.

Part Two details my initial thoughts and findings as I answered the questions to Exercise One *(See Chapter 5)*. My impressions flow from the associated words shown in Part One. You'll note they are not worked in any particular order.

Part Three includes later insights and strategies gained from subsequent sessions over a period of weeks. These writings are included directly after my initial findings in Part Two so that I could show them alongside the key words and impressions that led to their revelations .

Part Four is an Action List. The Action List, which is the last step of Exercise One, is a summary of beneficial action steps gleaned from the findings of the exercise.

"Sometimes our bodies will tell us a truth that our minds don't. We may say we're really not anxious—then notice that we're drenched with perspiration. No, no, nothing's wrong—so why is my stomach in knots? The body's responses cut through denial and rationalization, and the body won't lie to you."
Susan Forward,
Emotional Blackmail

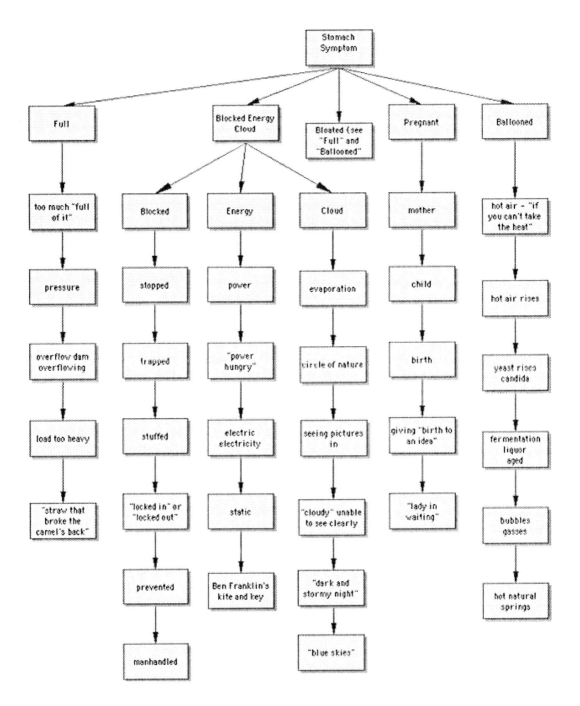

Exercise One Example Associated Words Flow Chart

Typically, these steps, when implemented, will help to resolve whatever emotional issues have been uncovered through the exercise process.

Because the writings that follow were taken directly from my journal, some of the passages are very frank and personal. I felt I needed to include these things in order for you to fully understand how your deeper issues are revealed and resolved through this process. The example shows what takes place during these sessions so you can fully understand what you are expected to do if you want the exercise to be effective. I did, however edit out all the irrelevant material which consisted of dead ends, personal unrelated qualms, and daily minutiae.

You'll note it takes a few tries before I reach any really valuable conclusions. This is because the ailment in particular emanated from a deeply buried ache that required several rounds to fully disclose and release all of its emotional connections. When attempting to interpret an ailment, the easy, more superficial meanings will surface first. The more severe the emotional wound and the more innate the connection, the more deeply embedded the meanings will be and the more rounds necessary to disclose them. Be diligent. The rewards are tremendous.

I've inserted additional explanations in parentheses, as needed, since the mind often connects groups of thoughts in a creative rather than in a logical fashion. Italicized words within the descriptions relate to key words relevent to the exercise.

"I was not interested in what I could bring to myself by being an actress, but in what I could bring out of myself."
Sophia Loren

HOW AN AILMENT HEALED MY LIFE
A COMPLETED EXAMPLE OF EXERCISE NUMBER ONE

During the course of working on this manuscript, I developed a chronic stomach problem. Being busy, I totally ignored it for a while. I do not analyze every hiccup or sneeze, nor do I expect others to. I don't believe it would be healthy to be that focused on one's physical health. Instead, I will usually wait until I recognize some aspect of my life is not moving forward as I'd like. I can usually find the answer as to why I've been stalled by interpreting an ailment.

In this particular case, I developed several other annoying symptoms that seemingly had no connection to my stomach. But, after all, I had ignored my stomach, so my body had to come up with some sidekicks to make sure its message got heard. That is usually the time when I also realize the problem isn't going to solve itself. I am going to have to uncover the underlying emotional connection in order for it to clear up.

It's always amazing to see what our *Body Songs* reveal. Initially, I thought I would discover the answer to my ailment in one sitting, as I often do. I figured it would take me an hour, maybe two. Instead, I ended up with fifty longhand pages spanning a period of many weeks. The emotional work was extensive; the rewards, immense.

"Words heal because they help us to raise our thoughts from fear to love."

Doreen Virtue,
The Lightworker's Way

KEY WORDS AND THEIR ASSOCIATIONS

(After relaxing as described in the beginning of the exercise on page 35, I began working through the remaining steps as follows:)

(Steps 1-2) Try to understand the ailment's malfunction and condition. Begin to put your thoughts into key words. Keep working with them until they feel defined. Let those thoughts take you wherever they will until the associations "ring true" or feel right to you.

(My key words[1] are listed in the flow chart on page 344. What follows are the key statements I felt most important after writing them.)

- *Feeling "ballooned," "full," "bloated"*

- *Feels like being four or five months "pregnant"*

- *Feels like energy in the solar plexus, visualized as a "cloud of energy" that doesn't know where to go or is blocked from being used*

(Step 3) The next step is to look at all the key words and to work through those that "ring true" or feel right to you. These words will feel like "button pushers" on your emotions. Save for later the words and statements without

344

an emotional charge in case you get stuck or need new directions to search.

Begin working with the words you chose, writing down your impressions and reactions to them. Continue using word associations, allowing whatever thoughts come to the surface to become a part of your description, even if they don't seem to fit at the moment. You may work through them in any order, come back to them at any time, or add new key words as they become apparent.

I HAVE BEEN POISONED

Stomach— "can't stomach this"
food—"food for thought"
digestion
gut—beer belly—pot belly
"stomachache"—pain

(None of the statements above led to any vital revelation at the time. In fact, my mind more or less went blank except for some statements about beer bellies and a memory of the Asian woman in the movie Pulp Fiction who said she wanted "a little pot belly." It was only later that I found the relevance in these statements. What follows is one of those revelations. More are included later where appropriate.)

For a long time, I thought I was eating something poisonous. Around the time I went to Arizona, it really started bothering me. I felt as though I wanted to cut open my abdomen and dig out whatever might be inside of me. Had I been able, I didn't think I'd find anything physical in there, nothing like a tumor or anything like that. Rather, I believed I'd find some inappropriate belief, or perhaps a buried trauma from childhood, since I'd experienced several frightening experiences in conjunction with my father's health, among other things.

I even went to a hypnotherapist in hopes she might be able to uncover the mysterious "poison" inside of me, but to no avail. I'd buried the answer so deep, my subconscious mind refused to release it at that time.

"Memories go underground because of conflict. Conflict is the key to repression."
Lenore Terr,
Unchained Memories

345

STOP PRESSURING ME!

"Blocked Energy Cloud"

What is a blocked energy cloud? How did I think up such a thing? How does a *"blocked energy cloud"* connect to my symptom?

> *. . . feels like energy in the solar plexus,*
> *visualized as a "cloud of energy" that*
> *doesn't know where to go or is blocked*
> *from being used.*

I've *blocked* some kind of *energy* and *trapped* it in my stomach. But what?

(I broke the phrase down into single words to get a better sense of the meaning of each word. Then I played around with them looking for the right meanings for me— now. I was waiting for one word or phrase to "ring true" or "click" inside of me.)

> Cloud— condensation
> evaporation
> circle of nature
> "blue skies"
> seeing pictures in
> "dark and stormy night"
> "cloudy"—unable to see clearly

> *". . . dark and stormy night. . . 'dark' is*
> *something hidden. . . What have I hidden from*
> *myself? 'Stormy'. . .is something tumultuous.*
> *Cloudy. . . unable to see clearly. What can't I see?*
> *What is it I don't want to see?"*

(Step 4) What in nature works like this? *(No ideas came to me. They should come quickly, if they don't, move on.)* What type of man-made objects function like this?[2] Isn't there something called a "cloud chamber" that scientists use? I wonder how it works?

(Then I saw a vision.) I see a vacuum tube that is closed on both ends. In the middle is a small black diaphragm. Something causes *pressure* in the tube and the *pressure* causes the diaphragm to pull down due to the

"Every single act of love releases blocked energy in your body. Unconditional love heals the body and the mind."

Wayne Dyer,
Manifest Your Destiny

346

vacuum in the tube. The pressure causes the pulling or expanded sensation I feel in my abdomen. Is there a diaphragm in my stomach? *(I don't know without looking it up, so I keep going.)*[3]

(Then the first of many conclusions emerges. Though minor and relatively insignificant, it's a start:)

Is there someone or something *pressuring* me to do something that I am *resisting*? Should I stop *resisting* or find the source of *pressure* and stop the source of *stress*?

Ultimately, *I* am the source of *pressure* as it is my free will to allow or disallow someone or something to *pressure* me. But what am I *resisting*? The *pressure* sensation feels like it is pulling down. Something is pulling me down, and I am *resisting*. What is pulling me down?

(To this statement, I drew a blank, so moved on to the next set of questions.)

WHEN DID THIS BEGIN?

(Step 5) When did this begin? When did I first begin to notice this condition?

The condition began within the past few months.

(I could not come up with a better answer, so I moved on. The key is to keep moving with the flow of thoughts. I discover the true beginning later on in my exploration.)

WHO ELSE IS DOING THIS?

(Step 6) What examples are occurring in my sphere of influence? What or who else is showing signs or symptoms of this type? Have I seen this in a recent movie, read it in a recent book? Have any of my coworkers, relatives, or friends been experiencing anything similar to this?

I have not seen the symptom in others as far as I can recall, though my sister-in-law did have some gall bladder trouble. I do have a friend who is *resisting* putting her house on the market. Perhaps I've been *resisting* change in my work and in my personal relationships. My boys have added *pressure* as they reach adulthood. I've been *resisting pressures* in regard to my work.

(Even if you don't gain anything valuable, keep moving forward. It takes time to draw out some of the deeper conclusions and often what is brought out in earlier

"We can create our own spiral of despair, or we can create a trampoline of happiness and attainment. Our thoughts have tremendous power."

Betty J. Eadie,
Embraced by the Light

347

rounds shows itself as more significant later when the true meanings begin to surface, as you will see. . .)

WHAT WOULD HAPPEN IF I WERE TO SAY OUT LOUD WHATEVER I WAS THINKING?

(Step 7) What can I do to change?

Am I *resisting* something I can stop? Or is it the *pressure?* How can I stop feeling the *pressure* from others?

Why do I feel *pressured* to do what others say—because I trust their judgment over mine?

What if I merely stated that as a fact—out loud—whenever I felt pressured? I could just stop and say, "I don't know what to do because I feel you are *pressuring* me." I wonder what would happen if I did?

Sometimes I don't trust my decisions. I used to find myself in a position where others were right and I was wrong. Now I worry about making the wrong decision, and more often than I should, I rely on others to make the right decision for me. The decision itself may not be as important as just stating the facts about how I feel. "I feel pressured because . . ." or "I'm not sure what the right decision is in this situation because . . ."

(I had not yet found any major revelations, so I kept working through the other associations, continuing to add to my revelations and action list—which appears at the end of this chapter.)

IF I STOP, I MIGHT DIE

(Notice how "pressure," which had arisen in the previous sections, had been one of the initial key words, indicating the significance of that word. So make note if a particular word, feeling, or symbol continues to pop up, it probably is attached to an important message for you)

Full—   too much—"full of it"
            pressure
            overflow—dam overflowing
            load too heavy—
            "straw that broke the camel's back"

Today, I did abs work with yoga. It's funny because I'd

> *"Don't make your interpretations too quickly. . . . Pay attention to colors, behavior, directions."*
>
> Ken Eagle Feather,
> *A Toltec Path*

348

been afraid to do the abs work even though I'd purchased the video over a month ago. I thought it would be too hard. But, this morning, I'd decided I'd do whatever I could, even if I had to stop partway through. I knew working my abs would help to release the pent up energy there, which is often connected to emotional garbage we've stored in our cells. Having explored the symbolism of a *blocked energy cloud* in my abdomen, I felt the yoga might help to release what my mind had been unable to.

To my amazement, the video wasn't very difficult. In fact, it felt really good to do the movements.

After I finished, I lay on the floor relaxing and allowing my mind to wander. I'd recently had a puzzling dream, so as I lay there, I pondered what it might mean.

In the dream, I kept saying over and over, "My head hurts." I didn't remember anything else about the dream.

Lying on the floor, I soon thought of my sister who had been hit by a car and died . . . she'd been hit in the head.

In a vision-like scene, I saw myself as my sister and could feel her pain and sense her fear. Soon, the pain and fear subsided, and I waited for the meaning of her feelings and of the dream to become clear.

The revelation for me was that I had feared my whole life that I would make some mistake or wrong move and die. This has caused me to always be on guard and to never really let go and fully enjoy life. This not only explained why I didn't want to make decisions for myself, as previously revealed to me, it also showed a deeper view of my life.

I don't even like to take time to sleep for fear I will suddenly die and miss out on some wonderful experience of life. This is because my sister and her premature death has been with me. It's as if I have this wide-eyed child alive and well inside me who wants to experience all there is to know about life. This inner child has become my drive. She wants to touch, see, and do everything. She doesn't want to miss a single moment.

This explains why I can't sit still and must constantly be working or doing something. I don't want to waste a single moment of my life. This is the message I have gleaned from the sister I never met.

What I'm seeing from this is that I have placed a lot

""Whatever you put your intention on increases. For the sake of the ecosystem and the new emerging civilization, remove your attention from the death process and place it on the process of birth instead."
Zoeu Jho,
E. T. 101

of pressure on myself to always do more. My body is trying to tell me to ease up a little.

Looking back at the key words I wrote for "full," *(too much, pressure, overflow)* I see how these words tie in to how hard I work and play. While I thought of my stomach as being full of air, the words brought forth from that connection show my life is full in other ways. Maybe too full.

Hidden Under the First Revelation I Discovered a Second

Bloated—

My search for well-being has turned into an interesting adventure. Over the past week I've been sorting through a collection of forgotten memories and past hurts I want to release, things like having to bid for family heirlooms on E-bay after my stepfather's death. His third wife sold them without a thought for us. It's very difficult to find forgiveness for someone who has reportedly flushed my mother's last remains down the toilet. (I do not know if this is true or not, but not knowing the truth is as devastating a thought as if it were true.)

This and other old scars have been troubling me for many years. I know it is time to release them before they become ailments and consume me. My gut seems to be helping out, showing me how *bloated* it has become with my unreleased thoughts.

I find it helps to write them down, to work through them, to let them go . . . when I can. Sometimes I can't. But I know why I can't. I feel bad for not having done more. At the time, finances, two small children, and miles between us prevented me from "being there" for my step-father. Perhaps that's why he remarried so soon after my mother's death.

Did that mean I did not even deserve a phone call when my stepfather died? Not even a letter? Is it right to have to read it two weeks later in the hometown paper? My mother-in-law called to tell me the news or I would never have known.

"Unlike other forms of life, though, people are easily led away from what's right for them, because people have Brain, and Brain can be fooled. Inner Nature, when relied on, cannot be fooled. But many people do not look at it or listen to it, and consequently do not understand themselves very much. Having little understanding of themselves, they have little respect for themselves, and are therefore easily influenced by others."

Benjamin Hoff,
The Tao of Pooh

These things make me angry because I was the "good" child, the "white sheep" of the family. I find it difficult to comprehend how anyone could be so cruel and for what reason? It's the shock of having no explanation that makes "forgive and forget" so hard.

Later in the day, I carried my feelings onto the golf course, where my husband and I played in league. Sometime during the first hole, I started having some stomach pain in the area of my bladder.

I didn't want to stop playing golf. I didn't feel bad, I just had this slight tenseness in my abdomen. I wondered if I could work through it while playing golf. I asked myself, what does this *feel* like?

I thought . . . pressure . . . it feels like pressure. (Oh, THAT again.) But we were in the middle of the golf game by now, and I couldn't focus enough to work through the word associations.

At home later that night, the pain turned into a burning irritation. I decided I had a bladder infection. I went and sat in the bathroom as sitting in there seemed to ease the pain. I took some over-the-counter bladder pills, drank a lot of water, and sat in the bathroom most of the night.

As the hours passed, I had a lot of time to think about the meaning of the malady. I felt the pain related to all the losses, fears, disappointments, and hurts I had been trying to release over the past few weeks. However, after treating the bladder infection for a couple of days, the burning had yet to subside. Despite the release and beneficial emotional healing I'd experienced from my interpretations so far, evidently something else still remained.

I spent some time in meditative thought, rethinking all of my associations and conclusions. What had I missed? Then it dawned on me. The "pain" I felt in my lower abdomen wasn't from my badder at all. In reality, I'd strained my stomach muscles from the yoga work I'd been doing all week. I had a good laugh about it, which in itself offered healing.

Nonetheless, the *burning* sensation had actually gotten worse. What did the burning relate to?

I sat contemplating the pain, having a hard time actually pinpointing what I felt. I kept waiting for the

"*Most psychiatrists and many psychologists and biologists now have come simply to assume that practically all diseases, and perhaps even ALL diseases without exception, can be called psychosomatic or organismic. That is, if one pursues any 'physical' illness far enough and deep enough, one will find inevitably intrapsychic, intrapersonal, and social variables that are also involved as determinants.*"

Abraham Maslow,
*The Farther Reaches of
Human Nature*

"Listening to our intuition, we will learn to be in the right place at the right time in order to provide our unique truth to others."

James Redfield,
The Celestine Prophecy

"click" inside my head indicating that I'd found the right connection, but none came.

Then I had it! I remembered a conversation I'd had with a woman just a few days before about yeast overgrowth in the body. I had a yeast infection! I immediately rushed out to the store, purchased a remedy, and within 24 hours my pain had gone. From my pain, I'd gained two more important insights.

At the time I'd spoken to the woman I'd thought it so odd, because for no reason, she had given me a detailed description of yeast overgrowth. She described yeast as a parasite. So I asked myself, "What is a parasite?"

I decided a parasite was, "an organism that lives off the energy of another." So I asked myself, "Are their any situations or persons who are drawing from my energy in that way?" I had named four before I'd even finished the thought!

However, the next day I wondered, "Is yeast a parasite?" I later looked it up (it isn't), but what mattered most at the moment was my *impression* of what it was. I'd read somewhere how yeast grew as quickly as weeds. Using the parallel of weeds overgrowing a garden *(from the exercise question 'what in nature works like this?')*, I surmised I must have been neglecting myself by working long hours over the past weeks. I also knew this interpretation coincided with the other key words and symptoms I'd been working with, which, in a sense, served as a secondary confirmation. I added a note not to let others drain me of my energy, as well, in keeping with the parasite image.

I DON'T REMEMBER HOW TO FEEL

> *Blocked—*   *stopped*
>   *trapped*
>   *stuffed*
>   *"locked in" or "locked out"*
>   *prevented*
>   *manhandled*

After a trying morning, I found myself wishing for some comfort. I allowed my mind to travel back, back,

back, to a time when my mother held me upon her shoulder and rocked me to sleep. She would sing "rock-a-bye-ba-bee, rock-a-bye, rock-a-bye, ba-bee," in rhythm to her rocking. As a toddler, I had my own little rocker and would mimic my mother's song singing, "bye, baby, bye."

Remembering my little chair, I thought of something I hadn't thought of for a long time—something important.

I'd always been a very curious child who longed to try and do many things. I couldn't have been more than two or three when I'd apparently seen my mother oil her sewing machine. *(I don't remember this part except from my mother's stories.)*

Now my father would allow me to help him in anything I could safely do, even if I could only be the "gopher" (go for this, and go for that). But my mother would only let me watch, so I would sometimes circle back and do things on my own when she wasn't looking.

As my mother used to tell the story, I went into her sewing closet and "helped" by putting glitter glue in all the oil holes of her sewing machine. I'm not sure if I just didn't know the difference between the tube of oil and the tube of glitter, or if I chose the glitter having seen her use it too. Maybe I liked how sparkly it looked. At any rate, my mother found my "help" a few hours later.

My mother's sewing machine was likely her most prized possession, and she told me it took her hours to dig all of the glitter out from the tiny oil holes with a darning needle. She said she wanted to find some way to impress upon me the wrong I'd done. *(This is the part I remember.)*

My mother said she looked down at me sitting happily in my little rocker, sucking my pacifier and holding my security blanket. In a flash, she plucked the pacifier out of my mouth and cut it up into the tiniest pieces she could, even the hard plastic back. She said I didn't say a word, but that my eyes were as large as dollars.

I think it must have been a terrible shock, particularly since the slicing and dicing of my pacifier occurred several hours after my glitter-glue adventure. I don't think I fully understood what I had done to cause my mother to become so angry.

Maybe this is when I first started *stuffing* my emotions. Even now, I am not quite sure what I might

"Visualize the challenge being over and being peaceful with everything around you."
Kryon (Spirit)
as channeled by Lee Carroll,
Kryon Cards

353

have done differently. I can't imagine any other appropriate reaction. Perhaps I could have cried or screamed, but neither would have erased from my mind the fear that even among those who loved me, I could not trust them. Their actions could be unpredictable. I learned I must *stuff* my emotions if I were to survive. In fact, we bragged about how all the Miller women on my mother's side of the family were able to tough their way through any difficult situation. The Miller matrons always found some way to survive, despite the Great Depression, despite a lack of funds, despite injury or ill health, all the while raising children and managing their day-to-day lives.

From that revelation—the reminder of the fearful incident and my reaction to it—within a few hours, I remembered other incidents where I'd *stuffed* my emotions.

In one situation, we rushed my father to the hospital late in the night. I might have been ten or eleven years old. My cousin and I sat in the waiting room while they assessed my father's condition. At last my mother came out from my father's room. She got very close to me and said, "The doctors do not think your father will make it through the night. You are not to tell him this under any circumstances. I want you to walk in there, paste a smile on your face, and kiss him good-night as if nothing is wrong."

I did as I was told and then we went home. Thus, once again, I'd been shown how it was not suitable to reveal one's feelings or fears. My father would come to be known as a survivor for pulling through all kinds of life-threatening situations, as he did this one . . . and following in his footsteps, so would I.

Other incidents like these surfaced like hot springs where the land seems to boil and bubble, releasing its pent-up heat, gases, and steam. I remembered each in turn and then let them go. I reminded myself that just because I'd been forced to not to express my true feelings then, didn't mean I couldn't now. I had the right to express my feelings appropriately and whenever I saw fit.

Energy blocked in my solar plexus could simply be my *holding back* my feelings and opinions. If I allowed myself to speak out those things I'd been holding in, if I stated them logically, calmly, but firmly, I would likely eliminate the pain associated with my symptom.

"When I hear somebody sigh, 'Life is hard,' I am always tempted to ask, 'Compared to what?'"

Sydney J. Harris

WHY I CHOSE TO SUFFER

I have continued to work diligently uncovering layers of hidden messages and have gradually been relieving myself from their emotional burden. Like an onion, underneath each layer I find yet another message and another belief, each more deeply seated than the previous, though all intricately entwined.

Here is an example of what I uncovered most recently. I had returned to bed after letting the dog out at sun-up. As is my custom, I used the time to ponder my many cluttered thoughts. Among them, I began thinking about the anger theme that had been hiding between the lines of my *Body Songs* exercise. I knew sooner or later I would need to deal with it.

Quite a few years ago I'd suffered from chronic body aches, which my doctors (depending on which one I asked) associated with my auto accident, thyroid, or misaligned spine. Each professional had his own opinion about what the pain might be, but none had succeeded in eradicating them permanently.

I'd known for a while how those burning aches were also an indication of a buried anger, yet I felt no anger on the surface. *(Of course not, that is precisely why they had resorted to Body Songs!)*

Obviously, I had not allowed this anger to surface nor to be released. In fact, I remembered one occasion, while working with Tom Bird in his Intensive Writer's Program, how he intentionally made me angry. We were on the phone and he said, "Let it out, get mad, yell at me." I felt my body tighten and contract. It took all my strength to say calmly through gritted teeth, "No. I'm not mad at you. I'm mad at myself."

He continued to take pokes at me for several more minutes, trying to get me to release whatever anger might be buried within me, but I refused. He hung up the phone knowing I wasn't going to let my hidden anger go.

So, while lying in bed and letting my mind contemplate those things., I picked up a stack of index cards and began listing all the situations which had perturbed me in one way or another. Most were common annoyances, like my sons constantly leaving messes and my husband not always understanding me.

Then I came to the problem of food, and how I'd eaten

"The very nature of God is to have goodness in so much abundance that it overflows into our unworthly lives. If you think about God in any other way than that, I'm asking you to change the way you think."

Bruce H. Wilkinson,
The Prayer of Jabez

an ice cream sundae while spending time with my mother-in-law the previous weekend. *(Remember "food" and "hunger" had appeared on my initial list of word associations.)*

I felt the anger welling up inside of me as I thought about how "everyone else" could eat whatever they wanted without a care. Why couldn't I? Why had I been chosen as the one who couldn't eat sweets without gaining weight, retaining water, or feeling awful side effects afterward? The more I thought about it, the more angry I became.

This angry feeling was still just a sensation, not the hot, broiled type, which appears during a shouting match. However, the more I thought about the things I wanted to eat, and the things I *should* eat, the angrier I became. This was the first I'd had any indication my body aches might be associated with the emotional pain hidden in my belly.

However, even that wasn't the million-dollar discovery. Something even bigger was about to come out. As I lay there thinking and ranting to myself about being *deprived* of these foods, a more significant connection revealed itself.

Just like the sugar and sweets I had often deprived myself of, I similarly felt deprived for having lost my mother, my father, my sister, my brother, and a total of more than thirteen significant relatives over the first half of my life. I felt angry for having been "singled out." Why had I been "chosen" to face these trying situations while others had their family gatherings, and even family issues. Yes, while they had to deal with their father's Alzheimer's, their mother's cancer, or Aunt Lila's senility, they also had their love, their companionship, their close-knit "forgive and forget because you are blood" connections. I didn't have that and not having it made me feel angry and deprived.

My feelings of anger and *deprivation* were echoed in my *Body Song* because deprivation is a feeling of "not having enough," so I ate more than I needed to fill the hole I felt in my belly. But the hole wasn't from a lack of food, so food couldn't correct or fill the need. The hole wasn't physical, it was emotional.

My mind had used food as a substitute for my perceived deprivation of love. And isn't that what love is— a kind of spiritual and emotional food? So I kept trying to

"So anything I view as lacking is because I see myself as removed from what I want rather than as connected to it."
Wayne Dyer,
Manifest Your Destiny

356

make myself feel "full" but had been filling it with the wrong kind of "food."

Therefore, I came to the realization that in order to resolve the constant tug of war resulting from this deprivation fear, I needed to come to terms with the loss of my family. I knew I could then easily separate the perceived missing love from its substitute—food. Then I'd be able to eat according to my physical need rather than from the emotional lack.

Coming to this deep realization helped me clearly see the situation and allowed me to ask for proper guidance. It allowed me to speak Truth to myself, to remind myself how all the losses and deprivation in my life were a part of my life's plan. They were a part of who I am and who I wanted to become. Without them, I wouldn't have had the understanding or knowledge I needed to write this book. The Truth is I *have* been singled out, I *have* been chosen to do the work I am doing, to live the life I am living.

"Thoughts have no power over us unless we give in to them. Thoughts are only words strung together. They have no meaning whatsoever. Only we give meaning to them. And we choose what sort of meaning we give to them. Let us choose to think thoughts that nourish and support us."
Louise L. Hay,
You Can Heal Your Life

WHEN THEY RESISTED GRIEF

Ballooned— hot air—"if you can't take the heat"
hot air rises
yeast rises—candida (tested negative)
fermentation—liquor—aged
bubbles—gases
hot natural springs
HOT—anger

My husband and I had a disagreement and, in anger, I shut myself in the bathroom. The first thing I did once in there was ask myself, "Why am I angry?"

My conversation with myself went something like this:

Why am I angry?

I am angry because he didn't make a decision about what to eat for dinner.

No, there is something deeper than that.

I am not angry for the reason I think. (A Course in Miracles lesson)

357

"When asked questions, the brain engages in a process called a transveridational search. That is a fancy way of saying that your unconscious mind will automatically search through your entire brain like a relentless, highly motivated research scientist might search through a complete library to come up with a correct answer. Your computer can search the entire hard drive for a specific file when asked to do so. Your brain automatically does the same thing."

Nell M. Rodgers,
Puppet or Puppeteer

What does my anger feel like?

I feel pressure or energy in the area of my heart and chest.

Why am I angry?

Because he didn't make a decision about what to eat for dinner.

No, that isn't right. I'm the one who didn't make a decision, but for a different reason. I'm afraid if I make the decision, it will be the wrong one because no matter what decision I make, he has a different opinion.

I suppose it wouldn't be so bad if I felt his opinions were wrong, but the fact is he often has better and more complete ideas than I—so much so that I have come to a place where I'm afraid to make a decision.

At the moment the last thought crossed my mind, I remembered something my friend Pat, who had passed away a few months before, once said about her husband. She said, "He can't ever make a decision and that drives me nuts. I don't know what difference it makes—if he makes a mistake or not, he should just decide and go from there. It doesn't matter if it's something as easy as choosing a shirt, he can't decide."

I felt like she might be standing right there in the bathroom with me, reminding me of our conversation.

Then the conversation with myself started again:

Why am I angry?

I am angry because I wanted to eat—I needed to eat—and he didn't make a decision. If I'd done it on my own, it would have been the wrong decision. If I'd made the wrong decision, he'd have been mad at me. Then I'd have been "punished" because he was mad.

But that is just my opinion. . .

Suddenly, the oddest thought came to me out of nowhere—(maybe Pat was still in the bathroom with me).

I needed to eat. I needed him to take care of me, and if he doesn't take care of me, there isn't anyone else who will.

Wow . . . what a loaded statement. I had shocked myself with my own words.

I started to cry because I realized my pain didn't come from my lack of food or from being hungry, my pain came from my feelings about my parents and family being gone.

There was more.

I thought about all these things for quite some time and I came to the following conclusion. When my sister died, my parents did not know how to release their grief. They only knew how to freeze it inside of themselves. But in order to freeze their pain, they had to also freeze the rest of their emotions as well. To freeze their emotions, they had to disconnect from each other, disconnect from themselves, disconnect from—*me.*

I'm sure in some psychological manual, it tells of the effects on a child when they are raised by parents who are disconnected in this way. But I don't think I need to look it up because I know what happens. That child becomes fiercely independent with a drive to prove how he or she doesn't need anyone to help them to succeed while, at the same time, deeply wanting with all of their heart to find someone who wants to care for them and love them unconditionally. This child may possibly fall into dysfunctional relationships with friends and family, playing a dual role of rescuer and rescuee. They might also harbor a deeply seated secret, believing, somehow, they are to blame for this lack of love from their parents because, no matter how hard he or she might have tried to win their love and to get them to show affection, they never wholly did. They couldn't. For in order for them to feel joy and love, they would have also had to feel their pain, and their pain was too large for them to bear.

So now it's mine to bear. I must acknowledge it and release it. But more importantly, I must be willing to feel the whole range of emotions, including pain, because it is only by doing so that I can overcome that burden which has been handed down to me.

"Don't drag the past around. Find the next thing that interests you."
Kazuya Tsurumaki, Director of the anime film *Evangelian*, EvaOtaku.com

Letting Go of Violent Energy

Energy—   *power*
           "power hungry"
           ("hungry," see stomach)
           electric—electricity
           Ben Franklin's kite and key
           static—chaos—anger

A few days ago, my husband innocently forwarded me one of those heavily passed around Internet jokes. The joke talked about the different viewpoints of a man and a woman on the issue of intimacy. Since my hysterectomy, I've been a lot more self-conscious about intimacy issues and the joke amplified my fears.

After I read the joke, I became very angry. I fired off a nasty email reply, really letting the spit fly. I don't even remember what I said. I just knew I wanted to express my anger. Then, feeling unsettled, I went into the kitchen where, like my mother used to do when she was angry, I started cleaning.

I could not believe how angry I felt. I had not felt such a rush of emotion in quite some time. I did not know how to respond to this feeling. Part of me wanted to repress it—as I often do—while another wanted me to release it on someone or something. Fortunately, my husband wasn't home, so I couldn't release it on him.

I remembered my mother once went into the basement and pounded a bunch of nails into a board to release her anger. I had a cake pan in my hand from the dishwasher and looked at it. I purposely banged it a few times on the dishwasher rack—hard. I liked the sound it made and the loud banging was a form of release, but I surprised myself by the strength of my anger. I had nearly poked a hole through the pan from the tines of the dishwasher rack.

Feeling guilty for damaging the pan, I put it away.

I still felt a need to release my anger. I found an old wooden spoon in the dishwasher. I picked it up and slammed it against the counter. It didn't leave a mark—which I deemed a good thing—so I hit the spoon against the counter a few more times before the force broke the spoon in half.

> *"Purification consists of getting rid of the toxins in your life: toxic emotions, toxic thoughts, toxic relationships."*
>
> Deepak Chopra,
> *The Way of the Wizard*

I still felt angry, but didn't want to break or damage anything. Right then, I remembered something I had read in a Stephen Wolinsky book. Wolinsky wrote about emotion as pent-up energy inside of us—nothing more, just energy. He taught his readers to allow themselves to feel that energy for what it was. So I assessed what sensations were occurring in my body and tried to visualize the energy inside of me.

I felt an area of energy in the region of my *solar plexus* and *womb*, particularly on the right side of my abdomen. I thought, "Oh, how appropriate, I am angry over a sex joke and my missing *womb* is involved in this *blocked energy*."

My mind then flashed through a series of split second thoughts:

- *This is where my stomach is distended*

- *Did needing a hysterectomy tie into sexual inhibitions and fears?*

- *Does this blocked energy tie into anything from my childhood?*

- *"I am not angry for the reason I think." (A lesson from A Course in Miracles)*

I continued to try to feel and visualize my anger, but I had a difficult time staying focused. My mind kept returning to my husband and the joke. I held on to the counter with my eyes closed and concentrated—hard—forcing my mind back again and again to the energy rather than the words and anger running through my mind.

I visualized the energy as a dark cloud or unrecognizable dark shape hovering inside of my body in the lower abdomen area. I thought again about the *Course in Miracles* lesson, "I am not angry for the reason I think."

A dear friend of mine had once told me, "Beneath anger you will find pain," so, while trying to focus on what my body physically felt—and not where my conscious mind had aimed its attack—I asked myself, "What (emotional) pain might I be feeling?"

As I thought about the blocked energy, my mind continued to flip back into "attack the husband" mode. In doing so, I noticed how my mind would flash through

"The most powerful unveiling of the hidden self comes when you acknowledge your feelings of the moment, that is to say at the time and during the situations in which feelings are first experienced."

Nell M. Rodgers,
Puppet or Puppeteer

361

memories, reminding me in quick succession of the many other times my husband's words or actions had hurt me. A few moments ago, these thoughts had provided fuel for my anger, but now I had a tremendous revelation.

The blocked energy in this area of my body stemmed from emotional pain I had stored away for years and years and years. Now, having revealed it, I saw these memories for what they really were—pain—all the hurtful things I'd packed away in my *gut* to keep myself from feeling them.

This brought me to the next stage where the energy now felt like pain—not a physical pain, but an emotional pain. That made me cry. Yet at the same time, I comforted myself by realizing I could now release all my pain, and how I wasn't really angry at my husband as much as I had been hurt inside.

The joke had triggered the memory of my buried pain. Although, had I not forced myself to feel and work through the physical pain, I would have remained in the "attack mode."

After a few minutes, the pain subsided and my tears stopped. I dried my eyes and even laughed about the broken spoon. I no longer had a need to break things or to yell at anyone, nor did I want to cause pain in vengeance. I understood now how my husband sending me the joke had given me the opportunity for healing.

But what about the nasty email I had sent? Luckily, I could rescind it by turning on his computer and deleting the email before he received it; thank goodness!

(This is not to say that we didn't later have a discussion about it because it wouldn't have been right to ignore something that had hurt me. Because we had the discussion several days later, after I had worked through all the anger, we were able to talk about it rationally and even laugh about it.)

I did not realize when I started out to do this exercise that I would be forced to face my feelings about intimacy, or that I would uncover long-buried hurts. But here they were in my face. Perhaps this is even an innate challenge asking to be conquered and overcome.

BENEATH ANGER YOU FIND PAIN

Pregnant— mother
child
birth
giving "birth to an idea"
"lady in waiting"

Why does this feeling in my abdomen remind me of being *pregnant?* I've had a hysterectomy, so I can't be pregnant. The swelling emanates from where my womb would be, and when the swelling occurs, I *look* pregnant.

I am remembering how I used to lie in bed with my hand on my pregnant belly. I had such a hard time becoming pregnant that I feared the baby would disappear in the middle of the night or that I would miscarry. I loved being pregnant! I'd wanted children so desperately, tried so hard, waited so long. The whole concept of birth and conception fascinated me.

What ideas have I recently conceived? Am I "pregnant with possibility"? Am I "pregnant with thought"? What ideas am I trying to "give birth to"? Am I *resisting* new ideas?

MY MOTHER'S HIDDEN ANGER

What else do bellies remind me of?

Once, while watching my mother dress, I asked her about the flab on her stomach. I mistakenly said I thought she "had let herself go."

Her blue eyes flashed with anger and she said, "This is from having YOU. This flab is from having children."

I felt bad for having said it. As I write this, I am wondering if she could have been *angry* about what pregnancies had done to her body. She'd always been conscious of her looks and weight.

I sometimes feel bad about my body. Perhaps I should have exercised more, tried harder than I did to maintain it. What can I do to change my feelings about my body?

After having children, I had a flabby stomach just like my mother's. I became very conscious of it. Something about it bothered me immensely. I didn't think about emotional connections at the time. I just knew I hated how

"It is what a man thinks of himself that really determines his fate."

Henry David Thoreau

363

I looked. I remember standing in the bathroom before my hysterectomy and feeling like I had something buried inside my belly I wanted to tear out. Even though I recognized something within me didn't feel right, I didn't yet know how to separate the physical from the emotional. I thought by losing the flab, I would stop feeling my emotional pain. But I hadn't removed the emotional pain, I had only removed the flesh.

I HAVE BEEN ABANDONED

What has been happening in my sphere of influence lately? I've been *angry* about my boys' lack of respect for the house. They leave the kitchen a mess and expect me to clean it up. Perhaps my children are mirroring the *anger* I am holding against myself.

Is there some way I have been disrespectful to myself? I have not been honoring self-made promises.

Does this in some way reflect on my own childhood or on feelings about my mother? Am I *angry* about something my mother did?

My mother didn't pay a lot of attention to me when I was growing up. I think I felt alone, abandoned, without support. She taught me a lot of things, but at times, I felt disconnected from her and my father. She spent hours and hours at her worktable, always at home, but never there.

All of my relatives have either died or abandoned me.

(I later realized that, like me, my living relatives were simply disconnected, having lived through the same traumas, they simply shut down their emotions.)

WHAT IS HIDDEN INSIDE ME?

What else could this feeling in my abdomen be compared to? I'm thinking of a clenched fist and how after menstruating the womb tightens. I have no womb now, there is just a hollow space where my womb used to be.

Wombs connect to *children* and *motherhood*. Am I *resisting* some *pressure* from my children? Or, in association with the feeling of the fist, am I *angry* for some reason with my children? With my mother?

(I wasn't quite sure what to do with this feeling at the time nor how it connected to my stomach problem. I did feel

"Resolve says, 'I will.' The man says, "I will climb this mountain. They told me it is too high, too far, too steep, too rocky, and too difficult. But it's my mountain. I will climb it. You will soon see me waving from the top or dead on the side from trying.'"
Jim Rohn,
The Treasury of Quotes

as though I had gone beyond the superficial layers and now had the opportunity to reach the deeper connections, provided I kept going.)

HOW A TOOTH RELATED TO MY STOMACH

Over these past weeks, I've done a tremendous amount of clearing work. So many issues from my past have surfaced for me to recognize and release. I have removed a huge burden from my life.

Today, I had a wisdom tooth extracted. I find this significant because this tooth in particular had been hidden in my mouth for years, and though it occasionally pained me, it had never been in a position before from which it could be removed. Over the past couple of months, it became visible, and then could easily be pulled.

To me, my tooth mirrors the other old pains I've "extracted" from my life. Now the tooth is out of my mouth forever. No more will it cause me trouble. I am free from its pain and from the issues that I've cleared.

THE HIDDEN TRUTH EMERGES

I am continuing to nurture the empty socket in my mouth having received lots of appreciated advice from family, friends, and medical providers on how to avoid a "dry socket." However, while pondering their advice, I caught myself thinking, "Caring for this blood clot reminds me of trying to hold on to a new fetus."

Whoa!

I had no idea how that thought had surfaced, but as soon as it had crossed my mind, I knew why. I had miscarried the first year of our marriage.

I don't suppose I ever cleared the experience, and while it's all but forgotten by the rest of the family, its unlikely I ever will forget. Although I could have only been a few weeks pregnant, it preceded years of concern and worry about my ability to conceive. Three years would pass before I would conceive again, years wrought with

"The body often tries to bring our attention back to 'the scene of the crime' to help us heal it."
Christiane Northrup,
Women's Bodies, Women's Wisdom

365

countless trips to gynecologists, hospitals for tests, and pharmacies for prescriptions and many pregnancy tests—all registering to the negative.

Did my having the miscarriage program my mind for those trials—trials that wouldn't come to an end until my hysterectomy some twenty years later? What can I learn today about this tragedy in my past? Should I analyze the loss? Or the psychological aspects set up because of it? Was I hurt more by the loss of a child or by the painful comments made by those who had no consideration for what I'd lost, what I'd felt, or what having a child would have meant to me? There wasn't just one incident, but many.

Pregnant or not pregnant, I knew something wasn't right. Early that morning, I'd started bleeding abnormally and passing a lot of clots. My cramps felt more like rhythmic contractions. I struggled between not wanting to get out of bed and having to rush to the bathroom. A call to the doctor's office instructed me to stay off my feet if at all possible.

Through all of this, I called off from work, swearing my friend and coworker to secrecy, as I hadn't told anyone of the in-home pregnancy test I'd taken just days before.

But she betrayed her promise and told everyone in the office. Within minutes, they were on the phone. In order to avoid being on my feet, I lay on the floor to talk to them. I felt myself bleeding, knew I was losing the baby, and heard them continuing to *congratulate* me. I kept saying, "No, I'm losing this baby," and they kept congratulating me anyway. It was all so surreal that I felt they were congrat-ulating me for my loss.

I didn't have a car, so my mother came and took me to the doctor's office. The gynecologist treated me as though I were an imposition on his day. His examination was rough, his words coarse. He sent me home to rest and to grieve alone. My mother understood. Perhaps she was the only one who did because she'd lost two children and had suffered a miscarriage besides. She took me to her house for the day so I wouldn't be alone.

I remember my father-in-law saying, "I didn't realize your condition was so serious. Had I known, I would have prayed for you more." At the time, his comments made me feel like I wasn't important enough. I knew it wasn't true, but in those early days, everything hurt.

My husband didn't—*couldn't*—understand. He wasn't ready for children. He had no way of knowing how such a thing affects a woman, affected me.

In my search for stomach-related connections, the word "womb" had surfaced, but I hadn't thought of the miscarriage then. Maybe I wasn't ready.

I don't know if I had ever been ready for womanhood. At fifteen, when menstruating, I hid under the bed. My mother didn't understand why. She had her crew of ladies working in the house that day and announced it to them. She sent me with my cousin—a male—to buy tampons. We stopped at a friend's house on the way and they had a large German shepherd who refused to remove his nose from between my legs. So, of course, my cousin had to tell our friends too.

I don't remember how I felt except I wanted it to be a private thing. Or maybe I felt like my older son, who cried when he lost his first tooth because "he didn't want to grow up." Or maybe I just felt embarrased, like when I shaved my excessively hairy legs for the first time in the sixth grade and didn't want anyone to know. That was the week my mother decided to show her friend just how hairy they were. They obviously knew I'd done something when, for over an hour, I adamantly refused to show them my legs.

I do know that from my hiding place under the bed I swore to those who would listen that I didn't care if my period ever came back—and it didn't for another whole year. Right up to the end, my periods were sporadic, unpredictable, and deadly. Even during my hysterectomy I'd nearly bled to death. I guess my body wanted to leave a lasting impression.

What can I learn from my miscarriage? Obviously, I'd been carrying around this *Body Song* for a long time.

From then on, I wanted children but couldn't seem to have any. I felt broken, believing something must be wrong with me. I spent countless hours in the gynecologist's office hoping with all hope that *this* time I would be pregnant. *This* time would be the one. But it never was. Not in those years. Instead, it was always an ovarian cyst or nerves or whatever made my hormones go awry.

"No one saves us but ourselves. No one can and no one may. We ourselves must walk the path."
Buddha

"Don't wish it were easier, wish you were better."
Jim Rohn,
The Treasury of Quotes

367

"Closing an old chapter of our lives is always easier than opening a new one."
Nell M. Rodgers

Is a miscarriage an ailment? Or just another horrible event? It's not a disease, an accident, or even a cut. It's just something that happens, often something that no one can explain. But what if it were an ailment? How would I interpret it? By the loss? By the cramps? By what means should I count it?

The one thing that remained prevalent through my miscarriage, both of my pregnancies, my hysterectomy, and many times in between, is the bleeding. Four times that I can remember, and there might have been more, I had to be given a blood transfusion to save my life, so perhaps the blood itself is the most important symbol to interpret.

What is blood to me? I know without even thinking, I know because it has always had the same meaning for me. Blood equals suffering and pain. I used to have a vision of standing in front of an altar, blood dripping from my wrists. I'd see this vision when I was suffering inside. I would stand before God and I would say, "Look how I'm suffering," and I would cry, and somehow I'd see the purpose in everything so I could go on.

Blood to me equals pain and hardship, like Jesus hanging on the cross. It's an emotional burden that must be borne.

But what is all this suffering I have borne so heavily that I had to physically bleed in order to express it?

I think it is not only the pain of my life, but pain from my ancestors. It's the pain of my grandmother with a six-month-old baby losing her husband during the Great Depression. It's my grandfather losing his wife to tuberculosis and his guilt for not doing enough to be with her, to help her more. It's the pain my aunt suffered when her only child committed suicide, leaving behind three children of her own under the age of ten. And it is my mother's and father's pain at the hardship of losing not just one child, but two.

I was born out of pain, brought to earth by God's hand, chosen to arise and learn so that I might come to understand the pain and be able to remove it.

Many, many years ago, I attended the service of a faith healer who offered her parishioners messages from God. She called me out of the crowd and compared me to

Moses. I didn't understand. I felt embarassed by the comparison. But I understand it now.

My path, my purpose, is to help relieve the burden of my ancestors' pain, and not just theirs, but that of anyone who will listen. Jesus said at his last supper, "This wine is the token of God's new covenant to save you—an agreement sealed with the blood I will pour out for you." *(Luke 22:20 New Living Translation)*

With his blood, Christ offered eternal life. With mine, I am offering the knowledge I have learned and the hope for relief from the emotional burdens we all carry. May we all live in love and peace.

PAST OR PRESENT—WE CAN CHOOSE TO HEAL OUR LIVES

(One afternoon I lay down to relax. I allowed my mind to rest and beome quiet. As I did, I saw the following visions:)

I came upon a time line and began to travel back through time, stopping at each point in my life which I believed to be the origin of my pain.

I remembered a trip to Sedona, Arizona, where I had met with my mentor, and my disappointment in the help he gave. But just as I thought this to be the origin, I remembered another time, back farther still, where I had stood in the bathroom looking down at my belly, loathing how it looked after two pregnancies and a laparotomy.

I remembered looking forward to my hysterectomy and thinking how, at last, my problems would be over. Yet, before I could claim this as the origin of my pain, my mind took me back farther still along the time line to where my appendix had been removed in the third grade. It had taken five nurses to administer the injection I'd received before surgery. Somehow, though but a child, I knew removing my appendix would not solve the mystery of the chronic stomachaches I frequently experienced, but not even this explained the origins of my pain.

Along the backwards tracking time line, I remembered an earlier time, a time when I was still very small and my mother held me down to administer suppositories

". . . if the goal in life is to discover our personal reasons for being here, to raise the vibration of the planet, and to move forward with self-realization, then we cannot spend all our time looking at what was."

Kryon (Spirit),
Channeled by Lee Carroll,
The Parables of Kryon

369

she believed would solve my intestinal troubles. It was here where I had my first inkling that the pain was not entirely my own, but also a reflection of the pain she carried and had never released.

On knowing this, I traveled backward farther still, before the time of my birth, and came to my sister who had complained of a stomachache on the day of her death. My mother would never forgive herself for sending my sister to school. Could she have prevented my sister's untimely death by keeping her home? But what had caused my sister's pain?

I once again drifted back, back, back, first through the lives of my parents, then their parent's lives. In my vision, I saw how it had pained my paternal grandmother to die before being able to see her son fully raised. She would never see him graduate from high school, meet his wife, hold her grandchildren. I saw how her pain had been passed on to my father by means of her impressions and interactions, both with her, and then through those with his grieving father.

Then, in my vision, I saw my maternal grandmother. I saw how her life had been scarred by the early loss of her husband, leaving her to raise her children alone through the Great Depression. Her grief would eventually turn into resentment, then anger, which she would wield over my mother until my mother left home at age fifteen.

In my vision, my paternal grandparents each took their pain and placed it into a glass tube, sealed it, then placed the tube in the belly of my father. My maternal grandparents each took their pain, placed it into a glass tube, sealed it, then placed their tube in the belly of my mother.

As my vision continued, I saw how my parents each removed the tubes from their bellies and poured them into a single tube which they placed into my belly, an exchange that took place both through the process of DNA at my creation, as well as through my impressions and interactions with them throughout their lives.

Thus I could see as I traveled back, back, back, how the pain I had carried in my life did not belong to me alone, but also to them. They had not learned how to remove it or dispel it, so they had each passed it on to the subsequent

"Aaron understood that all things learned during his lifetime would be passed on to his next incarnation, and he could hardly wait."

Kryon (Spirit),
Channeled by Lee Carroll,
The Parables of Kryon

generation in hopes of one day being free from what had grieved their hearts and minds.

At this point, the vision changed.

I saw myself standing in a field asking God, "How can I release and remove this pain I have carried for myself and for others? How can I heal my body from this pain that has plagued me for so many years?"

As I prayed, Jesus appeared and I said, "Jesus, please heal my pain and remove it from my body."

He replied, "We are one, you are in me and I am in you, therefore, be in me and be healed."

This puzzled me. I did not know how to "be in him," so I said, "Jesus, I do not know how to heal. I do not know how to 'be in you.'"

Jesus said, "Believe you are loved, for God is Love and since you are loved, then you are of God and you are healed."

"What is Love?" I asked.

"See yourself as made up of millions of molecules," Jesus said. "See all the molecules and then gradually focus down, down, down, until you only see one molecule. When you can see only one molecule, then see the space within the molecule. What you see and believe is you, is made from the solid-looking parts of the molecules. Love is the space in between the molecules. Instead of focusing on the solid-looking parts, focus instead on the space between the molecules. When you focus on the space between the molecules, then you will understand how God and Love are in everything that exists—everywhere—because the solid-looking parts you are focusing on exist only here and now, but when you focus on the space that is Love, you will see how this space is everywhere, running in and through all the other molecules, no matter where they are.

"It is by understanding how this space is Love and how you are one with this space, that you can see how you are connected to God," he continued. "This space is in you alongside the molecules you see as you, but also this space is intermingled with all the other molecules which exist throughout the universe. This is your connection to the all. Through knowing this vast space called Love, you can see how you are connected to a teacher in San Francisco, to a pizza baker in New York City, to a drug addict shooting heroine in a Chicago slum, and a cattle rancher in San

"All an atom is is the availability of potential."
Ramtha, (Spirit),
Channeled by J. Z. Knight,
A Beginner's Guide to Creating Reality

Antonio. By being one with this space called Love, you are also one with a nun in India, a starving child in Africa, a terrorist in Afghanistan, a coffee grower in Colombia, a scientist in Antarctica.

"But this love goes beyond your connection with other people as this space between molecules is also in the rocks of the mountains, the trunks of trees, the stems of grass. This space called Love exists within the drops of rain that fall to the ground, the rays of sun that warm it, and the air that rushes across the land. This space called Love exists even within the planets and the stars and all you see when you look into the heavens above. This space called Love is both within and around you. It is in your blood. It is in your bowels. It is in your brain. It is even in your breath."

I felt overwhelmed and awed by all I had just been told.

Then, as my vision continued, Jesus reminded me of an earlier vision where I had seen a long line of people dressed in white robes standing before the throne of God. At the time, I believed I was one of those individuals. Now he showed me a new meaning of my vision. He showed me how I was ALL of those individuals. He said, "Each of those individuals is a symbol of you. Each one of these 'yous' is making a different choice about the same situation. One of those 'yous' chooses to be angry about your pain. One chooses to ignore it. One chooses to cry about it. Another chooses to blame others for it. One of those symbols of you has chosen to be free from your pain. Choose to be that image of you."

"I do not know how to choose to be one of those others," I said.

Jesus said, "You choose when you react to any situation. Your actions are the evidence of your choice. Therefore, to change the you which you have chosen, change your actions, or change the thought that created the 'you.'"

"How do I do that?"

"To change your actions, simply begin to do things differently than you have in the past. As you make this change a habit, it will cause a different 'you' to step forward. To change the thought that creates the 'you,' you must find a contradiction in your beliefs. It is your thoughts and beliefs which create the individual 'yous' who

"I like to think of God as the ocean and myself as a glass. If I dip the glass into the ocean, I will have a glass full of God. No matter how I analyze this, it will still contain God. Now the glass of God is not as big as the ocean, nor is it omniscient or omnipotent, but it is still God. This metaphor allows me to trust both in myself and simultaneously in the wisdom that created me, and to see the oneness."
Wayne W. Dyer,
Manifest Your Destiny

stand in the line. When you find a contradiction in your beliefs, you then can replace that belief with a new one by finding evidence to support the new belief. By changing your beliefs, you are are creating a new thought which, in turn, creates another symbol of you. This adds more opportunity for your actions as you have more 'yous' to choose from."

Then the vision ended.

I pondered these things for a long time. It was a lot to take in. Later, the teacher voice showed me another way to see the molecules and the space in between. He showed me a bowl of ball-shaped cereal floating in milk. He said, the balls are the molecules and the milk represents the space called Love. He pointed out how the cereal was absorbing the milk. He said, "Even though the bowl seems to hold the milk in one place, know the space of Love that is God can not be held back or boundaried by anything."

Then I asked him, "Please explain about changing my beliefs."

He reminded me of the blue and white thermos. He said, "As long as you believed you were trying to remove the white lid from the blue thermos, you struggled as your choice matched your belief and fought to remove the lid. When you changed your belief, combined with the new evidence you had to prove the lid was not the lid at all, but actually the secured base, you then changed your actions. You no longer tried to remove the piece, now believing it to be secured. Your belief created a new symbol of you, a you that knew not to take off the base. When you believed the white strip to be a lid, the symbol of you that matched your belief stepped forward to take off the lid."

Thus I had gained a new perspective on Love, Belief, and Healing.

"Now is the time for the healing that you may have asked for earlier, for healing will come with action. Action is the result of knowledge."

Kryon (Spirit),
Channeled by Lee Carroll,
The Parables of Kryon

THE ACTION LIST

The Action List, as explained earlier, is the last step of Exercise One. It is a summary of beneficial action steps gleaned from the findings of the exercise. After creating the list, I put it in a prominent place in my office so I would see it often and remind myself to follow my own suggestions. The following list is based on the example exercise just detailed. Each time I interpret an ailment, I might need to add to my Action List. An item can be deleted from the Action List when it has become a habit and you no longer need reminded to "take action."

My Action List is as follows:

REACT:

1. Speak out my feelings. (This is disrespectful; I feel pressured, etc.)

2. I am allowed to relax, let go, and really enjoy life.

3. Wait, listen to the signs, and move with wisdom and guidance.

4. It is safe for me to feel and express all the available emotions.

5. I am an intelligent human being capable of making informed and prudent decisions for and about myself.

6. Remember no one item here is as vital as the others as unless the underlying emotional cause is addressed, the outer symptoms will not subside.

7. Food is not love. I have all the food I need. I will not starve, nor am I deprived. I am chosen, and I am loved.

8. Don't forget to take time off from work to rest, relax, and recharge.

RELEASE:

1. I have recognized innate challenges connected with these associations and have released them.

2. Feel my emotions as energy and allow them to flow for what they are. See their connections to my underlying state of being.

3. Allow myself to feel my feelings, and then acknowledge and honor those feelings; allow the body to release and heal.

This merely means assembling a list of that which no longer honors you in your life. This list may include characteristics which you would like to shed, or it may include persons, places, or conditions which no longer serve your sacred mission. It may mean moves, changes, and new plans."

Doreen Virtue,
Angel Therapy Newsletter

374

BIBLIOGRAPHY

"You are the only person on earth who can use your ability."
Zig Ziglar

BOOKS

Adrienne, Carol, Ph.D.: *The Purpose of Your Life: Finding Your Place in the World Using Synchronicity, Intuition, and Uncommon Sense.* Eagle Brook/William Morrow and Company, New York, 1998.

Adrienne, Carol, Ph.D.: *When Life Changes or You Wish It Would.* HarperCollins Publishers, New York, 2002.

Altea, Rosemary: *You Own the Power: Stories and Exercises to Inspire and Unleash the Force Within.* Eagle Brook/William Morrow and Company, New York, 2000.

Andersen, Hans Christian; Translated by Valdemar Paulsen: *The Ugly Duckling.* Checkerboard Press/Barnes & Nobel Books, New York, 1916, 1995.

Andrews, Lynn V.: *Love and Power.* HarperCollins Publishers/HarperPerennial, New York, 1997, 1998.

Armstrong, Lance; with Sally Jenkins: *It's Not About the Bike: My Journey Back to Life.* G. P. Putnam's Sons/Penguin Putnam, New York, 2000.

Bach, Richard: *Illusions: The Adventures of a Reluctant Messiah.* Creature Enterprises, Inc., Delacorte Press/Bantam Doubleday Dell Publishing Group, Inc., New York, 1977.

Bach, Richard: *Running From Safety: An Adventure of the Spirit.* Alternate Futures Inc., William Morrow and Company Inc./Bantam Doubleday Dell Publishing Group, Inc., New York, 1994.

Baker Eddy, Mary: *Miscellaneous Writings, 1883-1896.* The First Church of Christ, Scientist, Boston, MA, 1924.

Beattie, Melody: *Beyond Codependency.* Hazelden Foundation/Harper & Row, Publishers, Inc., New York, 1989.

Bickham, Jack M.: *Writing Novels That Sell.* Fireside, Simon & Schuster, New York, 1989.

Bird, Tom: *Releasing Your Artist Within.* Sojourn, Inc., Sedona, AZ, 2004.

Bird, Tom: ~~Write~~ *Right From God.* Sojourn, Inc., Sedona, AZ, 2001, 2003.

Bishop, Leonard: *Dare to be a Great Writer: 329 Keys to Powerful Fiction.* Writers Digest Books, Cincinnati, OH, 1988.

Blum, Deborah: *Love at Goon Park.* Persus Books Group, Cambridge, MA, 2002.

Boyd, T. A., quoting Kettering, Charles F.: *Professional Amateur.* Dutton, New York, 1957.

Brande, Dorothea: *Becoming a Writer.* Harcourt, Brace & Company/J. P. Tarcher, Inc., Los Angeles, CA, 1934, 1981.

Bro, Harmon: *Edgar Cayce on Dreams.* Castle Books, 1968.

Burley, Philip; Saint Germain (Spirit): *Saint Germain: To Master Self Is to Master Life.* AIM Publishers, Association for Internal Mastery, Inc., Scottsdale, AZ, 1997.

Buzan, Tony: *The Mind Map Book.* BBC Books, London, England/Plume/Penguin Group, New York, 1993, 1996.

Cameron, Julia: *The Artist's Way.* Tarcher/Putnam/Penguin Putnam, Inc., New York, 1992.

Cameron, Julia: *Supplies: A Pilot's Manual for Creative Flight.* Jeremy P. Tarcher/Putnam/Penguin Putnam, Inc., New York, 2000.

Carey, Kenneth X.: *The Starseed Transmissions.* HarperCollins Publishers, New York, 1982.

Carey, Kennneth X.: *The Third Millennium: Living in a Post-Historic World.* HarperSanFranscico, New York, 1996.

Carnegie, Dale; Carnegie, Dorothy: *The Dale Carnegie Scrapbook: A Treasury of the Wisdom of the Ages.* Dale Carnegie & Associates, Inc., Hauppauge, New York, 1959

Carnegie, Dale; Carnegie, Dorothy; Carnegie, Donna Dale: *How to Stop Worrying and Start Living.* Pocket Books/Simon & Schuster, New York, 1944, 1945, 1946, 1947, 1948, 1984.

Carroll, Lee; Tober, Jan: *The Indigo Children: The New Kids Have Arrived.* Hay House, Carlsbad, CA, 1999.

Carroll, Lee; Kryon (Spirit): *Kryon Cards: Inspirational Sayings From the Kryon Books.* Hay House, Inc., Carlsbad, CA, 2002.

Carroll, Lee; Kryon (Spirit): *The Parables of Kryon.* Hay House, Inc., Carlsbad, CA, 1996.

Chopra, Deepak, M.D.: *The Way of the Wizard.* Harmony Books/Crown Publishers, Inc., New York, 1995.

Christensen, Sue: *Making A Six-figure Income on Your Terms: Essential Life Balance for Today's Successful Real Estate Agents and Sales People in Any Field.* Destiny Publishing, Tucson, AZ, 2002.

Cott, Jonathan: *In Search of Omm Sety,* Doubleday & Co., New York, 1987.

Day, Laura: *Practical Intuition: How to Harness the Power of Your Instinct and Make it Work for You.* Villard Books/Random House, Inc., New York, 1996.

Dispenza, Joseph: *The Way of the Traveler: Making Every Trip a Journey of Self-Discovery.* Avalon Travel Publishing, Emeryville, CA, 2002

Dominguez, Joe; Robin, Vicki: *Your Money or Your Life: Transforming Your Relationship with Money and Achieving Financial Independence.* Penguin Books/Penguin Group, New York, 1992.

Dyer, Wayne W., Ph.D.: *Manifest Your Destiny: The Nine Spiritual Principles for Getting Everything You Want*. HarperCollins Publishers, New York, 1997.

Eadie, Betty J.: *Embraced by the Light*. Gold Leaf Press, Placerville, California/Bantam Doubleday Dell Publishing Group, New York, 1992, 1994.

Eagle Feather, Ken: *A Toltec Path*. Eagle Dynamics, Inc., Hampton Roads Publishing Company, Inc., Charlottesville, VA, 1995.

Edward, John: *One Last Time: A Psychic Medium Speaks to Those We Have Loved and Lost*. Berkley Books, N.Y., 1998, 1999.

Ehrmann, Max: *Desiderata*, from *The Poems of Max Ehrmann*. Bruce Humphries Publishing Company, Boston, MA., 1927.

Eldon, Kathy; Eldon, Amy: *Soul Catcher: A Journal to Help You Become Who You Really Are*. Chronicle Books LLC, San Francisco, CA, 1999.

Ford, Lacey: *The Men and the Machine*. Little, Brown, New York, 1986.

Forward, Susan, Ph.D.: *Emotional Blackmail: When the People in Your Life Use Fear, Obligation, and Guilt to Manipulate You*. HarperCollins Publishers, Inc., New York, 1997.

Fynn: *Mister God, This Is Anna*. Holt, Rinehart and Winston/Ballentine Books, New York, 1974, 1976.

Gendlin, Eugene T., Ph.D.: *Focusing*. Bantam New Age Books, Bantam, New York, 1978, 1981.

Gibran, Kahlil: *The Prophet*. Knopf, New York, 1923.

Gawain, Shakti; with King, Laurel: *Living in the Light: A Guide to Personal and Planetary Transformation*. New World Library, San Rafael, CA, 1986.

Gawain, Shakti: *Reflections in the Light: Daily Thoughts and Affirmations*. New World Library, San Rafael, CA, 1988.

Gibson, Lindsay, Psy.D.: *Who You Were Meant to Be*. New Horizon Press, Far Hills, NJ, 2000.

Grabhorn, Lynn: *Excuse Me, Your Life Is Waiting*. Beyond Books, Olympia, WA, 1999.

Godwin, Malcolm: *Angels—An Endangered Species*. Simon and Schuster, New York, 1990.

Hawking, Stephen: *A Brief History of Time*. Bantam, New York, 1998.

Hay, Louise L.: *Heal Your Body*. Hay House, Inc., Carlsbad, CA, 1982, 1984.

Hay, Louise L.: *You Can Heal Your Life*. Hay House, Inc., Santa Monica, CA, 1984.

Hoff, Benjamin: *The Tao of Pooh*. E. P. Dutton/Penguin Group, New York, 1982, 1983.

Jeffers, Susan, Ph.D.: *Feel the Fear and Do It Anyway*. Harcourt Brace Jovanovich, Publishers/Ballantine Books/Random House, New York, 1987, 1988.

Johnson, Spencer, M.D.: *Yes or No: The Guide to Better Decisions*. HarperCollins Publishers, New York, 1991.

Judith, Anodea: *Wheels of Life: A User's Guide to the Chakra System*. Llewellyn Publications, St. Paul, MN, 1992.

Knight, JZ; Ramtha (Spirit): *Ramtha: A Beginner's Guide to Creating Reality*. JZK Publishing, Yelm, WA, 1998, 2000, 2004.

Korn, Joey: *Dowsing: A Path to Enlightenment*. New Millennium Press, Augusta, GA, 1997, 2001.

Larsen, Sunday: *The Spinning Game, A Sedona Story*. DJ & Mumm, Salt Lake City, UT, 2003.

Lee, Michael: *Phoenix Rising Yoga Therapy: A Bridge From Body to Soul*. Health Communications, Inc., Deerfield Beach, FL, 1997.

Leeds, Joshua: *The Power of Sound: How to Manage Your Personal Soundscape for a Vital, Productive, and Healthy Life*. Healing Arts Press, Rochester, VT, 2001.

Lefko, Morty: *Re-create Your Life: Transforming Yourself and Your World With the Decision Maker Process*. Andrews and McMeel, Kansas City, MO, 1997.

Lindsay, Gordon: *The New John G. Lake Sermons*. Christ for the Nations, Inc., Dallas, TX, 1979 (Reprint).

Maltz, Maxwell, M.D.: *Psycho-Cybernetics*. Pocket Books/Simon & Schuster, Inc., New York, 1960.

Mandelker Scott, Ph.D.: *From Elsewhere: Being E.T. in America*, Birch Lane Press/Carol Publishing Group, New York, 1995.

Maslow, Abraham H.: *The Farther Reaches of Human Nature*. An Eslen Book/Viking Press/Arkana/the Penguin Group, New York, 1971, 1993.

McGovern, Mary: *The Reason We Are Here—The Truth*. VerAvail, Phoenix, AZ, 2004.

Myss, Carolyn, Ph.D.: *Why People Don't Heal and How They Can*. Harmony Books/Crown Publishers, Inc./ Random House, Inc., New York, 1997.

Robinson, James M., General Editor: *The Nag Hammadi Library in English: The Definitive New Translation of the Gnostic Scriptures, Complete in One Volume*. E. J. Brill, Leiden, The Netherlands/HarperSanFrancisco/HarperCollins Publishers, New York, 1978, 1988.

Northrup, Christiane, M.D.: *Women's Bodies, Women's Wisdom: Creating Physical and Emotional Health and Healing*. Bantam/ Bantam Doubleday Dell Publishing Group, Inc., New York, 1994, 1998.

Orloff, Judith, M.D.: *Dr. Judith Orloff's Guide to Intuitive Healing: Five Steps to Physical, Emotional, and Sexual Wellness.* Three Rivers Press, Crown Publishing Group, New York, 2000.

Pereira, Patricia L.: *Eagles of the New Dawn: Arcturian Star Chronicles, Volume Two.* Beyond Words Publishing, Inc., Hillsboro, OR, 1997.

Pereira, Patricia L.: *Songs of Malantor: Intergalatic Seed Messages for the People of Planet Earth: A Manual to Aid in Understanding Matters Pertaining to Personal and Planetary Evolution.* Beyond Words Publishing, Inc., Hillsboro, OR, 1998.

Progoff, Ira, Ph.D.: *At a Journal Workshop: Writing to Access the Power of the Unconscious and Evoke Creative Ability.* Jeremy P. Tarcher, Inc., Los Angeles, CA, 1975, 1992.

Prophet, Elizabeth Clare: *Forbidden Mysteries of Enoch: Fallen Angels and the Origins of Evil.* Summit University Press, Livingston, MT, 1983, 1992.

Purce, Jill: *The Mystic Spiral: Journey of the Soul.* Thames & Hudson, New York, 1974, 1980, 2000.

Renard, Gary R.: *The Disappearance of the Universe: Straight Talk About Illusions, Past Lives, Religion, Sex, Politics, and the Miracles of Forgiveness.* Fearless Books/Hay House, Inc., Carlsbad, CA, 2002, 2003, 2004.

Redfield, James: *The Celestine Prophecy.* Warner Books, Inc., New York, 1994.

Redfield, James; Adrienne, Carol, Ph.D.: *The Celestine Prophecy: An Experiential Guide.* Warner Books, Inc., New York, 1995.

Reilly, Harold J.: *Edgar Cayce Handbook for Health Through Drugless Therapy.* Macmillan Publishing, New York, 1975.

Rico, Gabriele Lusser, Ph.D.: *Writing the Natural Way: Using Right-Brain Techniques to Release Your Expressive Powers.* Jeremy P. Tarcher, Inc., Los Angeles, CA, 1983.

Rodgers, Nell M., D.C., M.N., R.N.: *Puppet or Puppeteer: You Hold the Key to the Life You Really Want.* Awesome Press, Decatur, GA, 2003.

Ruef, Kerry: *The Private Eye: A Guide to Developing the Interdisciplinary Mind Hands-on Thinking Skills, Creativity, Scientific Literacy.* The Private Eye Project, Seattle, WA, 1992, 1998.

Sarno, John E., M.D.: *Healing Back Pain: The Mind-Body Connection.* Warner Books/Time Warner Company, New York, 1991.

Schrader Gray, Lydia J.: *Children of the New Age.* The Edgar Cayce Publishing Company, Inc., Virginia Beach, VA, 1949.

Schulz, Mona Lisa, M.D., Ph.D.: *Awakening Intuition: Using Your Mind-Body Network for Insight and Healing.* Three Rivers Press, NY, 1998.

Self, Philip: *Yogi Bare: Naked Truth From America's Leading Yoga Teachers.* Cypress Moon Press, Nashville, TN, 1998

Strieber, Whitley: *Communion: A True Story.* William & Neff, Inc., Avon Books/The Hearst Corporation, New York, 1987.

Tanner, Wilda B: *The Mystical, Magical, Marvelous Would of Dreams.* Sparrow Hawk Press, Tehlequah, OK, 1988.

Terr, Lenore, M.D.: *Unchained Memories: True Stories of Traumatic Memories, Lost and Found.* Basic Books/HarperCollins Publishers, Inc., New York, 1994.

Thompson, Keith: *Angels and Aliens.* Ballantine Books/Random House, Inc., New York, 1991.

Thorpe-Clark, Susanna: *Changing the Thought: A Book of Insight.* Blue Star Productions, Sun Lakes, AZ, 2002.

Virtue, Doreen, Ph.D.: *Constant Craving.* Hay House, Inc., Carlsbad, CA, 1995.

Virtue, Doreen, Ph.D.: *Divine Prescriptions: Using Your Sixth Sense—Spiritual Solutions for You and Your Loved Ones.* Renaissance Books, Los Angeles, CA, 2000.

Waitley, Denis: *Timing Is Everything.* 1992.

Walker, Thomas, D.C.: *The Force Is With Us: The Conspiracy Against the Supernatural, Spiritual, and Paranormal.* 2004.

Wilkinson, Bruce: *The Prayer of Jabez: Breaking Through to the Blessed Life.* Multnomah Publishers, Inc., Sisters, OR, 2000.

Williams, Robert M.: *PSYCH-K . . . The Missing Piece Peace in Your Life.* Myrddin Publications, Memphis, TN, 2002.

Wolf, Fred Alan, Ph.D.: *The Yoga of Time Travel: How the Mind Can Defeat Time.* Quest Books, Theosophical Publishing House, Wheaten, IL, 2004.

Wolinsky, Stephen J., Ph.D.: *Quantum Consciousness: The Guide to Experiencing Quantum Psychology.* Bramble Books, Norfolk, CT, 1993.

Wolinsky, Stephen J., Ph.D.: *The Dark Side of the Inner Child: The Next Step.* Bramble Books, Norfolk, CT, 1993.

Wolinsky, Stephen J., Ph.D.; with Ryan, Margaret O.: *Trances People Live: Healing Approaches in Quantum Psychology.* The Bramble Company, Falls Village, CT, 1991.

BIBLES AND RELIGIOUS TEXTS

Amplified New Testament. The Lockman Foundation, 1954, 1958, 1962, 1964, 1965, 1987.

King James Bible. Zondervan.

New American Standard Bible (NASB). The Lockman Foundation, 1960, 1962, 1963, 1968, 1971, 1972, 1973, 1975, 1977, 1995.

New International Version. International Bible Society, Zondervan, 1973, 1978, 1984.

New Living Bible. Christian Literature International, 1969.

Holy Bible, New Living Translation. Tyndale Charitable Trust, 1996.

LYRICS

Cretu, Michael: "Cross of Changes," Enigma, *Cross of Changes*, Virgin, Schallplatten Gmbh, 1993.

Lynn, Jeff: "Eldorado," Electric Light Orchestra, *Eldorado*, 1974.

Mann, Manfred; Slade, Chris: "Questions," Manfred Mann Earth Band, *The Roaring Silence*, LP. Warner Brothers Music, 1976.

O'Day, Alan: "Angie Baby," 1974.

VIDEO

Yee, Rodney: AM PM Yoga, Gaiam, ©1997.

NEWSLETTERS, ARTICLES, POEMS, SHORT STORIES, WEBSITES, AND MISCELLANEOUS

Atkinson, Rita L.: *Introduction to Psychology*, Eleventh Edition, Harcourt Brace College Publishers, Orlando, FL, 1993. As recorded on: www.macalester.edu/~psych/whathap/UBNRP/Split_Brain/Split_Brain_Consciousness.html

Bird, Tom: *Riding the Wave*, The Bird's Word Newsletter, October 2000.

Bird, Tom: *Rollercoasters*, The Bird's Word Newsletter, February 2000.

Hay, Louise L.: *Present Moments* newsletter, April 2005.

Jolie, Angelina: During a televised interview with Barbara Walters in 2003.

Kravitz, Lenny: Yahoo online interview, 1988.

Madonna, *Elle Magazine,* February, 2001.

Quimby, Phineas Parkhurst: Is Disease a Belief?, 1859.

Saxe, John Godfre: *The Blind Men and The Elephant.*

Stevenson, Mary: *Footprints in the Sand.* 1936, 1984.

Strieber, Whitley: *Whitley's Journal,* "My Journey Til Now," July 29, 2005. www.unknowncountry.com
Vicente, Mark: *The Bleeping Herald, What the Bleep Do We Know Newsletter*, Vol. 4, Issue 1; August 2005. www.whatthebleep.com.

Virtue, Doreen,Ph.D.: *Angel Therapy Newsletter.*

ENDNOTES

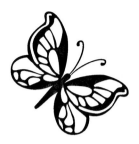

"The process of transformation requires that we trust sufficiently to enter this unknown domain."
Michael Lee,
Phoenix Rising Yoga Therapy

INTRO
Chapter 2
1. (Page 14) Mr. Toad is a copyrighted character from *Wind in the Willows* by Kenneth Grahame, ©1908

SECTION I
Chapter 4
1. (page 26) Not all chiropractors are created equal. Look for a qualified professional with satisfied customers.

2. (page 28) I later requested my medical records because I felt so high at the time I was sure I'd received some hallucinogenic drug, but the records showed it had been many hours since I'd had even a Tylenol.

3. (page 32) As posted on the St. Charles Science Fiction-Fantasy Society website; www.scsffs.org.

SECTION II
Chapter 8
1. (page 79) Ironically, in not going to my mother's funeral, I was retracing my mother's own steps and challenge. I did not think of it at the time, only later, when I was writing this book. My mother had missed her mother's funeral due to being on full bed rest with a difficult pregnancy. She carried the baby to term, but three days later Marshall Bruce died. My mother later said that if she had it to do over again, she would have gotten out of bed. (She didn't say whether she would have gone to the funeral; there was no love lost between the two.) She felt that the troubled pregnancy was God's sign that something was wrong. Of course, with today's medical technology, Marshall's congenital heart problem might have been repairable.

2. (page 94) Muscle Testing is a process introduced by George Goodheart, D.C., founder of Applied Kinesiology. Most commonly, the person being tested will stretch out an arm at a right angle to their body. A second individual will ask the first person a question. The validity of the answer given is judged based on the strength in which they can keep the arm outstretched while the questioner applies firm pressure to the individual's arm and wrist immediately after asking the question. If the first individual is offering a response that his or her body/mind perceives as true, he or she will be able to hold the arm outstretched and strong. If he or she is offering a response that his or her body/mind perceives as false, the individual will not be able to withstand the firm pressure from the second person and the arm will easily be pushed down. Think of it as a built-in lie detector test.

Section III
Chapter 9
1. (page 99) Mind Map is a registered trademark of the Buzan Organization, ©1990.

2. (page 102) Inspiration software is a registered trademark of Inspiration Software, Inc. The software is available by visiting their website at www.inspiration.com or by calling 800-877-4292 or 503-297-3004.

Section IV
Chapter 14
1. (page 145) Robert Kraft's reply during a CNBC interview when asked how he knew how to choose personnel for his team.

Chapter 15
1. (page 149) My paternal grandmother died young of tuberculosis. She left little behind, a few photos, some news clippings, and a couple of postcards. To the average person, not playing music would mean little. However, in my family, Bessie's disinterest meant a sure sign of her health's decline, one I saw in my father's latter days as well.

2. (page 149) I will never forget the occasion when I had been outside playing and I heard hilarious laughter coming from inside. My father had the kind of laugh that filled the whole house and made everyone who heard him laugh too, so I went to see what might be so funny. I found my mother sitting at our small, play-by-numbers chord organ and my father standing beside her, sax in hand, both still laughing. My mother said, "Your father was playing the sax and blew so hard he shot his false teeth out of his mouth and across the room." I don't think any of us ever forgot that day.

3. (page 150) My father always used the LP *Provocative Percussion*, "I'm in the Mood for Love," for this purpose.

4. (page 153) Always protect your hearing. Never turn up the volume enough to damage your ears. Joshua Leeds (*The Power of Sound*), recommends not wearing headphones for workouts or exercising.

5. (page 154) If you do not have this particular song available for your first experiment, choose an instrumental track that is approximately ten to twenty minutes long. Techno and movie soundtracks are best, usually something slightly repetitive but not too monotonous. I like the Oakenfold track because it offers a variety of sounds and transitions, but if you do not have that CD, you might try something by Danny Elfman, Juno Reactor, Chris Spheris, Enigma, or Mike Oldfield. Other alternatives would include Infinity, Inferno, and Biosphere. If you don't mind a little heavy metal, try Linkin Park, particularly their song, "Somewhere I Belong." (Note: Most New Age tracks are not effective. Check my website for more titles.)

According to Joshua Leeds (*The Power of Sound*), certain beats per minute (bpm) are conducive to different desired brain states. For concentration use 50-70 bpm, kick up the tempo to 90 bpm for energizing, and lower them for relaxation and calming. Leeds refers to rap music as sonic Valium, heavy metal as music that "hits right in the gonads." He recommends classical for babies and for enhanced learning.

Chapter 16

1. (page 160) Rollerblading *can* be passive. With good quality blades and a flat-surfaced road, skating takes relatively little effort. The trick is in the blades and the quality of the bearings. With a quality pair of blades, one push returns triple the momentum given.

2. (page 161) Always protect your hearing. Never turn up the volume enough to damage your ears. Joshua Leeds (*The Power of Sound*), recommends not wearing headphones for workouts or exercising.

Chapter 17

1. (page 174) The core of Julia Cameron's *Artist's Way* program hinges upon the use of 'morning pages,' something she refers to as 'three pages of handwritten text jotted as soon as possible after

rising.' Both Bird and Cameron fully explain their connective writing methods in their mentioned books. If writing is the strongest means of connection for you, I recommend you read their books.

Chapter 19

1. (page 193) You don't need to press on your eyes to see visions (clairvoyance). Actually, seeing visions has nothing to do with the physical eyes at all. Visions occur in the mind.

2. (page 200) The structure of reverse engineering is based loosely on the paper "A Pattern Language for Reverse Engineering" written by Serge Demeyer, Stephane Ducasse, and Sander Tichelaar, Software Composition Group, Institut fur Informatick (IAM), Universitat Bern, Berne, Switzerland. For more information, visit http://www.iam.unibe.ch/~scg/.

3. (page 215) The *Romper Room* show apparently appeared in two different forms. One where the show was syndicated and shown in a variety of areas. In some venues, however, the show was franchised and had a unique host for that area, such as New York City. Thus, not everyone grew up with host "Miss Sally." In addition, the show ran from the late 40s until the early 1990s and, as you can imagine, retired more than one host.

4. (page 226) From the book, *Introduction to Psychology*, by Rita L. Atkinson, see reference under websites in the Bibliography.

Chapter 20

1. (page 255) Words of Saint Teresa of Avila as quoted by Malcolm Godwin in *Angels: An Endangered Species (See: Bibliography)*.

Chapter 21:

1. (page 263) My father-in-law also said that angels sometimes appeared on swings that appeared to lower from and rise to heaven.

SECTION V:

Chapter 24

1. (page 287) Life Balance software is available for PC and Mac from Llamagraphics at 1-800-505-6198, or visit www.LlamaGraphics.com.

2. (page 289) You can learn a lot about how you spend your money through reading Joe Dominguez and Vicki Robin's book, *Your Money*

or Your Life: Transforming Your Relationship With Money and Achieving Financial Independence. How-ever, if you want to take that knowledge to the next level, in keeping with today's financial times, I highly recommend reading the *Rich Dad, Poor Dad* series of books by Robert Kiyosaki. You might also enjoy reading books by Suze Orman.

Chapter 25

1. (page 305) Do not make the mistake of confusing identities with impersonations. An impersonation could be illegal, dangerous, or even deadly.

2. (page 309) This also relates back to my interest in interpreting our lives through images. Though at the time, I thought I was learning about Native Americans and their writing, I was also learning how to communicate through pictures and glyphs.

3. (page 309) The leader of our baton corps, Veronica (Roni) Caruso, hoped to one day see baton twirling as a part of the Olympics. She'd learned that the main reason it twirling wasn't included was due to it not being a world sport, so she had taken us abroad to help spread interest in the skill. Roni has a unique personality that motivates people, particularly kids, toward higher achievement. She has always been a children's and animal advocate and is still going strong as of this writing even though she is in her 70s. I'll always be grateful for her inspiration.

APPENDIXEX
APPENDIX B

1. (page 344) In regard to the key words and the flow chart, feasibly all the text words shown in the diagram could be further flushed out, as could those subsequent words, and so forth. However, after the initial idea stage has been completed, it's best to move on to writing and answering the questions. The latter will not only pull from a deeper part of you, but will also connect the chosen words with hidden associations—and this is what you want. By revealing any hidden emotional pains or past transgressions, you will be more able to heal and clear them from your life.

2. (page 346) I remember once asking my husband about how a carburetor worked. He immediately thought I had detected something wrong with the car and didn't undersand how a carburetor might relate to food allergies I wanted to interpret. In this particular case, I learned how a carburetor regulated air and gasoline or the flow of fuel to the engine of the automobile. His descriptions helped me to understand how my body needed enough air along with the food I was eating. I found I often held my breath and needed to relax and breathe while eating, which helped solve a mysterious malady.

3. (page 347) I later looked up diaphragms on the Internet. We have a diaphragm above our stomach. I also f ound an experiment for school children about how lungs work. They cut off the bottom of a pop bottle and covered it with a cut open balloon. Then they taped a second balloon around the mouth of the bottle with the balloon hanging down into the bottle. When the first balloon is pressed or pulled, it affects the second balloon. In the case of the experiment, it acted like a lung. For the sake of my vision, it explained how pressure could cause my stomach to bloat.

INDEX

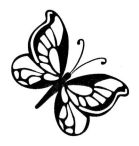

"Apparently there is nothing that cannot happen today."
Mark Twain

Quotations Index

"To solve any problem, here are three questions to ask yourself: First, what could I do? Second, what could I read? And third, who could I ask?"

Jim Rohn,
The Treasury of Quotes

WE'D LOVE TO HEAR FROM YOU

write Jamie at:

jamielinn@saloff.com

or visit Jamie's website at:

www.ICanTransform.com
or
www.TransformationalHealing.net

Printed in the United States
37238LVS00003B/6